Optimizing Medical Education With Instructional Technology

Erdem Demiroz
Trakya University, Turkey

Steven D. Waldman
University of Missouri - Kansas City School of Medicine, USA

A volume in the Advances in Medical Education, Research, and Ethics (AMERE) Book Series

IGI Global
DISSEMINATOR OF KNOWLEDGE

Published in the United States of America by
IGI Global
Medical Information Science Reference (an imprint of IGI Global)
701 E. Chocolate Avenue
Hershey PA, USA 17033
Tel: 717-533-8845
Fax: 717-533-8661
E-mail: cust@igi-global.com
Web site: http://www.igi-global.com

Library of Congress Cataloging-in-Publication Data

Names: Demiroz, Erdem, 1981- editor. | Waldman, Steven D., editor.
Title: Optimizing medical education with instructional technology / Erdem Demiroz, Steven D. Waldman, editors.
Description: Hershey, PA : Medical Information Science Reference, [2019] | Includes bibliographical references.
Identifiers: LCCN 2018007452| ISBN 9781522562894 (hardcover) | ISBN 9781522562900 (ebook)
Subjects: | MESH: Education, Medical | Educational Technology
Classification: LCC R737 | NLM W 18 | DDC 610.71/1--dc23 LC record available at https://lccn.loc.gov/2018007452

This book is published in the IGI Global book series Advances in Medical Education, Research, and Ethics (AMERE) (ISSN: 2475-6601; eISSN: 2475-661X)

British Cataloguing in Publication Data
A Cataloguing in Publication record for this book is available from the British Library.

For electronic access to this publication, please contact: eresources@igi-global.com.

Advances in Medical Education, Research, and Ethics (AMERE) Book Series

ISSN:2475-6601
EISSN:2475-661X

MISSION

Humans are living longer now than ever as a result of advances in the medical field. Having the tools available to train knowledgeable and ethical future generations of doctors and medical researchers is essential to continuing to advance our understanding of the human body and develop new ways of treating and curing sickness and disease.

The **Advances in Medical Education, Research, and Ethics (AMERE)** book series highlights publications pertaining to advancements in pedagogical practice for developing future healthcare professionals, research methods, and advancements in the medical field, as well as moral behavior and practice of healthcare professionals, students, and researchers. Featuring research-based book publications that are highly relevant to the healthcare community, this series is ideally designed for library inclusion at medical universities and research institutions as well as personal use by medical professionals, researchers, and upper-level students entering the field.

COVERAGE

- Clinical Research
- Conflicts of Interest
- Ethics in Medicine
- Healthcare Pedagogy
- Medical Curricula
- Medical Simulation
- Patient Data
- Professional Development
- Research Methods
- Scientific Misconduct

The Advances in Medical Education, Research, and Ethics (AMERE) Book Series (ISSN 2475-6601) is published by IGI Global, 701 E. Chocolate Avenue, Hershey, PA 17033-1240, USA, www.igi-global.com. This series is composed of titles available for purchase individually; each title is edited to be contextually exclusive from any other title within the series. For pricing and ordering information please visit http://www.igi-global.com/book-series/advances-medical-education-research-ethics/132365. Postmaster: Send all address changes to above address.

Titles in this Series

For a list of additional titles in this series, please visit:
https://www.igi-global.com/book-series/advances-medical-education-research-ethics/132365

Exploring the Pressures of Medical Education From a Mental Health and Wellness Perspective
Christina Ramirez Smith (University of the Bahamas, Bahamas)
Medical Information Science Reference • ©2018 • 349pp • H/C (ISBN: 9781522528111) • US $225.00

Impact of Medical Errors and Malpractice on Health Economics, Quality, and Patient Safety
Marina Riga (Health Economist-Researcher, Greece)
Medical Information Science Reference • ©2017 • 334pp • H/C (ISBN: 9781522523376) • US $200.00

Advancing Medical Education Through Strategic Instructional Design
Jill Stefaniak (Old Dominion University, USA)
Medical Information Science Reference • ©2017 • 349pp • H/C (ISBN: 9781522520986) • US $205.00

Organizational Culture and Ethics in Modern Medicine
Anna Rosiek (Nicolaus Copernicus University in Toruń, Collegium Medicum in Bydgoszcz, Poland) and Krzysztof Leksowski (Nicolaus Copernicus University in Toruń, Collegium Medicum in Bydgoszcz, Poland)
Medical Information Science Reference • ©2016 • 448pp • H/C (ISBN: 9781466696587) • US $225.00

Handbook of Research on Advancing Health Education through Technology
Victor X. Wang (Florida Atlantic University, USA)
Medical Information Science Reference • ©2016 • 588pp • H/C (ISBN: 9781466694941) • US $335.00

Optimizing Medicine Residency Training Programs
Jayita Poduval (Pondicherry Institute of Medical Sciences, India)
Medical Information Science Reference • ©2016 • 300pp • H/C (ISBN: 9781466695276) • US $220.00

For an entire list of titles in this series, please visit:
https://www.igi-global.com/book-series/advances-medical-education-research-ethics/132365

IGI Global
DISSEMINATOR OF KNOWLEDGE

701 East Chocolate Avenue, Hershey, PA 17033, USA
Tel: 717-533-8845 x100 • Fax: 717-533-8661
E-Mail: cust@igi-global.com • www.igi-global.com

This book is dedicated to Agostino Molteni, M.D., Ph.D., educator extraordinaire.

Table of Contents

Detailed Table of Contents

Health disparities and social determinants of health are directly linked to access, quality of healthcare, and increase in morbidity and mortality in minority and diverse communities. It is accepted that physicians lead healthcare teams; therefore, academic medical centers must assume the responsibility to provide training to reduce health disparities. The nation's academic medical centers and teaching hospitals have a responsibility to provide education on how healthcare disparities impacts diverse patient populations. This chapter provides a detailed overview of the curriculum development process and design of two asynchronous learning modules on health disparities and social determinants of health for graduate medical learners enrolled in multiple clinical specialty areas throughout one academic medical center's three geographic regional campuses. Formative and summative evaluation processes allowed the curriculum design team to revise the module design process, in situ and throughout the creation of the modules as well as evaluate learner growth and satisfaction.

Technological advancements and imaging evolution in contemporary medicine continue to change the ways medical education and clinical care are delivered. Historical methods of learning anatomy through human cadaveric dissection may be supplanted by three-dimensional renderings, injection models, and virtual reality simulations. The cost effectiveness of new imaging and study modalities may demonstrate major advantages in the logistics of information delivery, cost containment, and skills development in the current healthcare environment.

Technological advancement is steadily reshaping the field of medical education. In histopathology and especially dermatopathology training, the transition from glass slide microscopy (GSM) to virtual microscopy (VM) is serving as an instructional tool for medical students, residents, fellows, and experienced physicians. Online slide atlases and digitalized content are being utilized by educators and trainees to enhance and assess both individual and collaborative learning. With the expansion of mobile technology, new avenues are emerging for image attainment, in addition to remote instruction and consultation in resource-limited areas. Various computer-based applications ("apps") and social media sites also serve as digital assets in education and training and allow for rapid dissemination and sharing of information around the world.

This chapter serves to provide medical educators with an overview of competency-based education (CBME) and the clinical skills necessary for medical school graduate. Technology that supports the teaching, learning, and assessment of CBME and clinical

and the benefits for both clinicians and patients. For clinicians, mobile devices and apps may serve as diagnostic aids, med calculators, and clinical references. They can also be used for medical education purposes and access of electronic medical records. For patients, mobile devices and apps are often utilized to find resources and information about diseases, to help with disease management, and to promote lifestyle modification and fitness. Nevertheless, despite the numerous benefits of mobile devices in practice, potential risks and drawbacks must also be considered.

The authors have developed a pedagogical approach to the teaching of histology and histopathology using a team-based, collaborative learning model. To accomplish this, students are assigned to small groups of "microdissection" teams, mirroring the approach used in gross anatomy dissection. These collaborative groups present the case, including history, relative labs, imaging, gross pathology, and microanatomy, to their classmates. Each clinical case contains normal and abnormal virtual microscopy slides with links to key areas of interest, as well as hyperlinked references to the medical literature (the electronic pathology text or an article from a general medical journal, e.g., The New England Journal of Medicine®). In order to facilitate this collaborative process, they use Microsoft Office 365® and the included OneNote® program. The approach has facilitated integration of histopathology into the curriculum with more interactive laboratories stimulating active learning to build improved diagnostic skills for the learners.

The impact of technology can be felt throughout the medical education continuum. From online learning environments in blended learning approaches to exclusively providing the preclinical curriculum online, there is a growing need to optimize the way that technology supports self-directed learning in the next generation of medical professionals. In this chapter, the authors address issues of best practice surrounding the development of virtual content for medical education. The information presented will be integral for medical education professionals, basic science/clinical faculty, and educational assessment specialists with an interest in the use of technology for

Foreword

The resource book *Optimizing Medical Education With Instructional Technology* provides a broad perspective of changes in the medical field as the growth of integration in new technologies in education.

The chapters develop core themes relevant to understanding the changing nature of medical education. There are chapters that provide research-based discussions of specific transformative technologies including the integration of mobile devices in medical education and clinical settings. Mobile devices offer opportunities to provide access to medical data such as monitoring atrial fibrillation that change the level and quality of interaction among patients and medical personnel.

Several chapters are devoted to developing comprehensive research-based responses to the changing nature of medical classrooms and the interactions among learners and educators as a result of the integration of instructional technologies. There are chapters about simulations to teach anesthesia, flipping classrooms to blended forums and the development of collaborative mentoring learning forums instead of the traditional lecture-based classroom.

Additionally, there are chapters written from the perspective of the learners as new technologies are integrated into a more constructivist learning program such as a competency-based learning program.

Finally, there are chapters that deal with overarching social issues that are discussed in chapters on the integration of instructional technologies to reduce health disparities. The issue of the ethical integration of new technologies into medical education is discussed including both the potential and the problems inherent in the integration of instructional technologies into medical education.

In summary, this resource book develops a broad and comprehensive research-based review of the current state of integration of instructional technologies in medical education that provides the reader with a coherent perspective on the state of change in medical education resulting from the integration of transformative new technologies.

Donna Russell
Walden University, USA

Preface

Nihil sub sole novum

I bet your first thought was, "Let's just skip the Preface," or perhaps, "What does that mean?" or "I wonder if that is how you say the bottom of my feet hurt in pig Latin?" or "Seriously?" For the one or two of you that just had to know what *nihil sub sole novum* actually means, I suspect that you already looked it up on Google! (You can bet that your students certainly did.) If you didn't bother, you really should read this Preface because you clearly are not currently of an instructional technology mindset!

The fact that there is a generational gap between those who educate and those who learn is nothing new. For each generation, new technology has been a major factor in how that generation was ultimately defined. One can only imagine the impact of radio and television on the Baby Boomers, the impact of the personal computer and cable television on Generation X'ers, and the impact of the internet, cell phones, and smart devices on the Millennials. While wanting to avoid overgeneralization, there is no doubt that the technology that helped define each generation also helped define each generation's preferred culture of learning. So, insofar as medical education is concerned, there really is nothing new under the sun.

Much has been written about the unique learning styles of our current generation of learners, the Millennials. Current pedagogical thinking states that Millennials are extremely adept and discerning curators of information and that they approach learning in a manner that is different than the students of previous generations. This is not surprising in that millennials grew up with the ability to access almost all of the information that the world had to offer with the simple click of a mouse. They didn't need a classroom, they didn't need a teacher, they didn't need mom and dad. If they didn't understand something the read on the internet, they simply texted a fellow classmate. Is it any wonder that web-based self-directed learning is the gold standard by which the Millennial learner will judge all other educational techniques?

If we assume this fact to be correct, then those who are serious about using instructional technology to enhance medical education have an important first step to guide them when attempting to create a culture of learning for today's learners. A culture of learning that not only quickly gains the learner's attention, but is then able to keep it. This means that regardless of the teaching format or instructional technology chosen, the information to be taught must be easy to access, easy to share, easy to edit, easy to annotate, and whenever possible, personalized, visually appealing, technology-enhanced, gamified, mobile device friendly...... and if that were no enough.....it should preferably be free and without those annoying pop ups, satisfaction surveys, and pesky advertisements. If you are a really gifted educator, the educational content you are attempting to convey must also be as up-to date as "CNN breaking news" and must be totally socially conscious. Here's a value-added tip: if your goal is to win the teacher of the year award, you must find a way to link all content you plan to teach to:

- Katy Perry. @katyperry. Bio: Love. . . .
- Justin Bieber. @justinbieber. Bio: Let's make the world better. . . .
- Barack Obama. @BarackObama. Bio: Dad, husband, President, citizen. . . .
- Rihanna. @rihanna. ... Bio: ProFilter Foundation back in stock.
- Taylor Swift. @taylorswift13. Bio: The old Taylor can't come to the phone right now.
- Lady Gaga. @ladygaga. Bio: Needs no bio.
- Ellen DeGeneres. @TheEllenShow. Bio: Comedian, talk show host and ice road trucker.
- Or when in doubt, to any one of the Kardashians.

A second step to designing a culture of learning that works for today's learners is to match the instructional technology and teaching format that you are going to use to the type of information you are trying to teach. Just using technology will not get you where you need to be. For example, to improve clinical skills, small group active learning, high fidelity simulation, and hands-on simulation labs are the way to go. To help learners acquire basic knowledge required to pass certifying examinations, computer- aided instruction, small group competition, and gamification of the information to be presented will improve both learning and retention. To train learners in best practices of how to deal with difficult patients, manage critical events, and improve decision making in ambiguous situations, the use of virtual patients, role playing, human patient simulation, and creative projects such as student production of training videos to share with other learners will yield great results.

The third step in successfully using instructional technology to tailor your educational approach to work for today's learners is to understand that the skill sets that may have made you a great teacher at the bedside or at the lectern may not translate well to contemporary technology-driven pedagogy. In order to excel, you not only need to master the technology, but you need to understand the theoretical underpinnings that make the use of these instructional technologies in medical education effective.

Erdem Demiroz, our chapter authors, and I hope that *Optimizing Medical Education With Instructional Technology* will make the implementation of these steps a little easier.

Steven D. Waldman
University of Missouri – Kansas City School of Medicine, USA
September 2018

Acknowledgment

We would like to thank our invaluable authors who drafted their expertise, knowledge and experiences for this book, Reid Waldman, Emine Demiroz, Ali Yılmaz, Çağlar Ozan Tekinalp, Umitcan Cengel, Ogun Kaya, and IGI Global team who contributed to this project, and spent hours to make it ready for publication.

Chapter 1
Asynchronous Education for Graduate Medical Trainees to Reduce Health Disparities and Address Social Determinants of Health:
Online Education for Graduate Medical Trainees

Joyce E. Balls-Berry
Mayo Clinic, USA

Cheryll Albold
Mayo Clinic, USA

ABSTRACT

Health disparities and social determinants of health are directly linked to access, quality of healthcare, and increase in morbidity and mortality in minority and diverse communities. It is accepted that physicians lead healthcare teams; therefore, academic medical centers must assume the responsibility to provide training to reduce health disparities. The nation's academic medical centers and teaching hospitals have a responsibility to provide education on how healthcare disparities impacts diverse patient populations. This chapter provides a detailed overview of the curriculum development process and design of two asynchronous learning modules on health

DOI: 10.4018/978-1-5225-6289-4.ch001

INTRODUCTION

The many chronicled associations between health disparities, social determinants of health, rising healthcare cost and minority status illustrates the need for the healthcare workforce to be trained in culturally appropriate evidence based medicine (Braveman, Egerter, Woolf, & Marks, 2011; LaVeist & Pierre, 2014). Initiatives such as the Healthy People 2020, the National Partnership for Action to End Health Disparities, the National Prevention Strategy, and the Sullivan Commission on Diversity in the Healthcare Workforce implore health care profession to consider not only the patient, but also the overall community and how the built environment impacts the diversity of the healthcare workforce (Jackson & Gracia, 2014; LaVeist & Pierre, 2014). For instance, LaVeist and Pierre (2014) posed a 3 Ds (determinants, disparities, and diversity) conceptual framework that incorporates social determinants, health disparities and equity, and workforce diversity. The authors suggest that using this framework would lead to six public health benefits; improved quality of care, increased cultural competency, expanded access to care to under-resourced communities, improved research, and benefit society and minority providers in private practice (2014).

Additionally, policy changes under the Affordable Care Act of 2010 (ACA) (Office of the Legislative Counsel, 2010) support health disparities education and training. A key feature of ACA relates to the elimination of health disparities by creating new approaches to reduce social determinants of health (LaVeist & Pierre, 2014; Office of the Legislative Counsel, 2010). A provision of ACA is to create new training opportunities for healthcare teams, which are most often led by physicians. Thus, there is a societal imperative for the next generation of physicians to be competent in recognizing and meeting the needs of diverse patient populations.

Arguably, the responsibility to increase understanding and provide education on how health care disparities impacts diverse patient populations, largely falls on academic medical centers and teaching hospitals. However, few Graduate Medical Education (GME) programs have formal training in the complexity of sociocultural risk factors and other health care inequities, which customarily result in poor health outcomes, often for the most vulnerable patient populations, especially racial/ethnic minorities, immigrants, and those with issues of functional literacy.

Fortunately, public accountability through accreditation and other forces are driving curricular transformations in medical education. Several stakeholder organizations such as the Institute of Medicine (IOM), American Board of Medical Specialties, Association of American Medical Colleges, the taskforce that developed the "Kelly Report: Health Disparities in America (Kelly, 2015)" and other proponents have issued a call to action and advocate for cultural competency as an important aspect of the training and clinical practice skills development of the nation's physicians. Most relevant to this article, the Accreditation Council for Graduate Medical Education (ACGME), the largest accreditor of graduate medical training programs in the United States, designated health care quality, with an emphasis on educating medical residents and faculty on reducing healthcare disparities, as one of the six focus areas (patient safety, healthcare quality, care transitions, supervision, duty hours/fatigue, and professionalism) of the Clinical Learning Environment Review (CLER) program. Implicit in this learning environment mandate is the need for ACGME sponsoring institutions to implement curriculum that will provide residents/ fellows education and patient care experiences in recognizing and reducing health care disparities for the nation's increasingly diverse patient population (Maldonado, Fried, DuBose, Nelson, & Breida, 2014). In order to achieve this as an objective, curriculum development in this area must utilize inter-professional curricula design teams that consist of not only subject matter experts, but also include the expertise of institutional quality and GME leaders who have working knowledge of program accreditation and professional medical society standards. In particular, Bass and Chen (Thomas, Kern, Hughes, & Chen, 2016) chapter authors in *Curriculum Development for Medical Education: A six step approach*, argue a key component of medical education curriculum design is the understanding and incorporation of the competency development expectations of accrediting agencies and professional organizations. Thus, a critical initial step to developing the two asynchronous learning modules was to engage key educational stakeholders in the design and development of health disparities curricular content that meets institutional goals, learner's needs and the specific practice based learning and systems-based physician competency requirements of ACGME.

Residents and fellows are diverse learners in various stages of training and based across multiple specialties and disciplines. Concomitantly, the increasing demands of the medical profession severely constrict the amount of time teachers and learners have available for traditional classroom and seminar based learning. To keep pace, medical education curriculum must leverage technology and other innovative content delivery platforms. It was within this context that the institutional charge came to the authors to create an effective, efficient, cost effective, and contemporary training, suited to graduate medical physician learners, in two key areas; addressing social determinants of health and institutional response to health disparities. This chapter describes the approach used, by the curriculum design team at a large national academic medical center, for the development of asynchronous education related to social determinants of health and health disparities for use by graduate medical education.

LEARNING THEORY AND ASYNCHRONOUS CURRICULUM DESIGN

In graduate medical education the learners are adults. Commonly regarded as the father of adult learning, Malcolm Knowles' (Knowles, 1990) andragogy theory, differentiates, in contrast to children, both the motivations and processes by which adults learn. Andragogy is based on the framework of self-directed learning generally characterized by an intrinsic motivation, which in turn stems from the relevance of the subject matter to the learner's life – most often their career aspirations. Therefore, the activity of learning is towards a goal or resolution of a problem using strategies that incorporate the learner's experiences and builds upon already acquired knowledge. Knowles posited six key cultivating factors of adult learning (Knowles, Holton, & Swanson, 2012):

1. Need to know (content is relevant to life or work of learner)
2. Self-concept (learner as responsible for actions and decisions)
3. Learner's experiences (learner's experiences are valuable)
4. Readiness to learn (learner acknowledgement of changing environment)
5. Orientation to learning (learner belief that the learning will prepare them for the task)
6. Motivation to learn (learner personally wants to know the information)

This theory, emphasizing learner independence, self-motivation and self-guidance, is complementary with the principles of instructional design and online learning, especially because the delivery of content is asynchronous in e-learning settings (Demiroz, 2016). The incorporation of these six adult learning principles undergirded the approach utilized to create asynchronous curriculum suitable for the institution's numerous graduate medical education training programs. The principles provided the scaffold for structuring the curriculum in that; twenty first century physicians in training, as medical professionals (self-concept), need education on health disparities to meet the outcomes required by their ACGME program accreditation standards (need to know) and to provide the best care to all patients. Moreover, the curriculum was designed to help them develop sufficient knowledge, awareness and cultural competency to effectively treat patients of all backgrounds. As future independent clinicians (motivation and readiness to learn), they are responsible for making decisions that impact the lives of their patients and their families (orientation to learning). Another curricular goal is increased knowledge and self-awareness in order to recognize how their own socio-cultural perceptions (learner's experience) can influence their clinical decision making. As a result, they are uniquely positioned during training for their medical specialty – when learning has the most relevance for self and patient, to learn culturally based material that could ultimately improve the care they will provide in their clinical practice (motivation).

INSTITUTIONAL DESCRIPTION, SCOPE AND PURPOSE OF EDUCATIONAL INITIATIVES

Mayo Clinic is a nonprofit academic medical center based in Minnesota with two major campuses in Arizona and Florida. The institution's logo features three shields representing patient care, research and education. Biomedical education programs are provided through the five schools of the Mayo Clinic College of Medicine and Science. As the largest school in the College, the Mayo Clinic School of Graduate Medical Education (MCSGME) offers training in over 280 medical specialty and subspecialty fields on campuses located in three regions (Midwest, Southeast, and Southwest) of the United States. The scope of this project was to create an asynchronous curriculum that provided a basic overview of healthcare disparities for the MCSGME's post-graduate medical learners. This task meant selecting a design team with knowledge of the learner mix and health disparities subject matter expertise. Ultimately, the team was comprised of curriculum design experts, GME leadership and instructional designers. To achieve these goals, the MCSGME collaborated with the Center for Clinical and Translational Science (CCaTS) Education Resource and Community Engagement Programs. CCaTS offers graduate training to Mayo Clinic learners on healthcare disparities as part of the Master's and doctoral degrees in Biomedical Sciences. For over the last decade, CCaTS sponsors a traditional class on health disparities taught to graduate students and other fellows to increase knowledge of healthcare disparities with an emphasis on biomedical research and health care. In the last six years, the course has evolved from a traditional lecture based course to a blended learning course. The course directors created the curriculum specifically to increase knowledge in the overall definitions of health disparities and the impact of social determinants of health on patients and the greater community (Balls-Berry, et al., 2012).

Figure 1 depicts the composition of collaborative curriculum design team and illustrates the process used by the team for the creation of the modules. The design team met several times to determine the process for module development. During the first meetings, the first author developed a list of internal resources for health disparities curriculum and served as the course director. The second author identified ACGME CLER requirements for education on health disparities as well as developed strategies for deployment of the curriculum to residents and fellows

Figure 1. Collaborative curriculum design team module development process

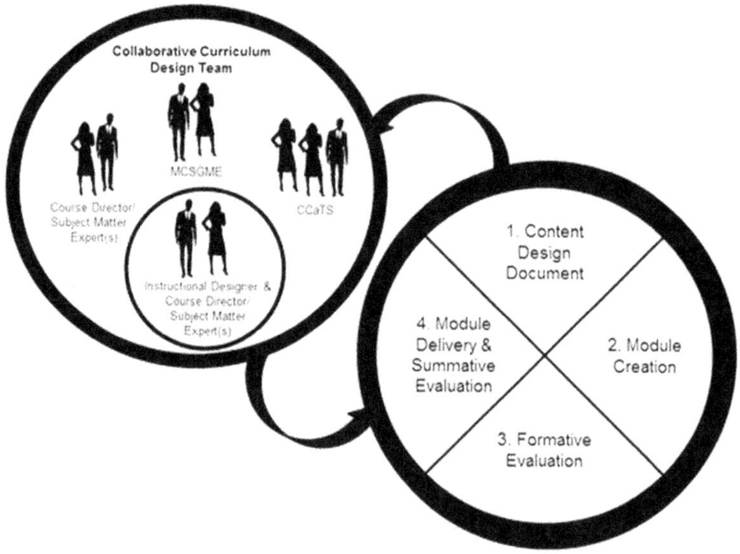

enrolled in the MCSGME graduate medical education training programs. CCaTS provided instructional and curriculum design support for the module development and determine the platform for module delivery.

Once assembled, members of the design team developed the scope and purpose of the educational initiatives for learners. The project scope was to create a basic understanding and definition of health disparities, social determinants of health, and highlight available institutional resources for physicians to address health disparities for their patients. The design team began the process by revisiting the andragogical process used for the development of other similar asynchronous courses such as a previous course developed to increase knowledge of community-engagement in research (Balls-Berry et al., 2017).The application of adult learning theory proved relevant and using a Mayo Clinic "3 shield approach" allowed the design process to focus directly on graduate medical learners. The "3 shield approach" relates directly to the institution's tripartite missions of patient care, research, and education that guide the structure of all activities conducted by the institution. Figure 2 shows the juxtaposition between these areas with the extant internal resources aimed at reducing health disparities in each shield. Under patient care, it was crucial to identify internal educational stakeholders that had expertise and working knowledge of the types of healthcare disparities that were the most prevalent across the institutions three regional campuses. This meant identifying efforts by Employee and Community

Figure 2. Mayo Clinic 3 shield approach to health disparities education

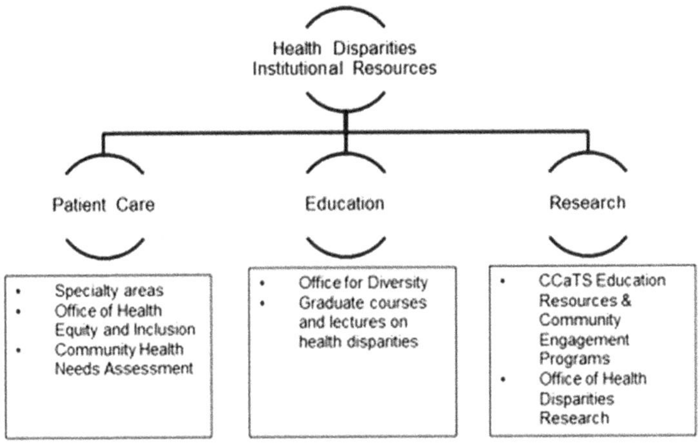

Health programs, at each location, and examining data collected from the local Community Health Needs Assessments (CHNA). Mayo also has an Office of Health Equity and Inclusion that seeks to increase equitable care provided to Mayo Clinic patients. The office conducts research, provides access, and develops processes to implement and support efforts for greater inclusion of diverse patients.

The education shield houses the College of Medicine's Office for Diversity. This office focuses on increasing the diversity in the educational programs thereby the diversity of the healthcare workforce. The Office works closely with the GME programs to recruit and retain diverse trainees. The third shield, research, has several opportunities to engage in efforts to reduce health disparities. The research infrastructure has CCaTS and the Office of Health Disparities Research. CCaTS Education Resources has experts in health disparities curriculum development. The CCaTS Community Engagement Program also has expertise in community-engaged research design focused on increasing health equity and reducing health disparities. The Office of Health Disparities Research supports all health disparities research efforts conducted at Mayo Clinic.

The combination of these multiple institutional resources allowed for the design team to have access to a wealth of information when determining content for the basic overview of the healthcare disparities module.

After identifying available internal resources, the team conducted a literature review with the objective to identify current practices related to curriculum design for health disparities for medical learners. The final deliverables, determined by the team, was the development of two self-directed on-line modules with each module containing a maximum of one hour of content.

TECHNOLOGICAL LEARNING PARADIGMS

Over the last ten years, there has been a monumental shift in education content delivery from use of traditional static proprietary materials (e.g. books and journals) to globally accessible and open asynchronous platforms. Free Open Access Medical education (FOAM) is one of the most widely known progenitors of the open-sharing, collaborative and non-traditional approach to medical educational content delivery. It has been described as "a dynamic collection of resources and tools for lifelong learning in medicine, as well as a community and an ethos". FOAM is continually "evolving and growing rapidly, and from anarchic beginnings is increasingly attracting interest from practicing clinicians, trainees, educators, researchers and publishers alike" (Nickson & Cadogan, 2014).

Dabbagh and Bannan-Ritland (2005) characterize a meaningful online learning environment to be accessible, based on pedagogy, and one, which utilizes internet technologies to promote learning and knowledge sharing through impactful activity and interface. FOAM achieves this through multiple asynchronous learning options via various platforms, including but not limited to: blogs, podcasts, websites, tweets, web-based application, videos, digital photographs, graphics and more (Nickson & Cadogan, 2014).

The Successive Approximation Model (SAM) is a non-linear approach to the instructional design of e-learning content. Its developers (Allen Interactions) describes SAM as an "an agile e-learning development process built specifically for the creation of performance-driven learning" (Allen Interactions, 2017). In its most simple form it consists of preparation, iterative design, and iterative development phases. Accordingly, SAM provides a greater "emphasis on learner experiences, engagement, and motivation over content organization, presentation of information and post-tests" (2017).This approach takes into account the complexity of learning style and helps educational curriculum designers to consider new approaches for content delivery while staying true to the core concepts of the subject. The SAM approach is a useful tool for subject matter experts to organize content delivery, knowledge checks, and evaluation of the information taught to the learners.

CONTENT DESIGN DOCUMENT

Using the SAM approach, the collaborative curriculum design team created a *content design document* that outlined the curriculum design process for both modules. Again it was critical to engage key stakeholders as project personnel such as the subject matter expert/course director, instructional designer, graduate medical school administration, and other stakeholders with an interest training physician leaders, and educational curriculum consultants.

Table 1 shows the multi-faceted components of the design document which served as the operational structure for the modules' development and organization. The design document was comprehensive and contained a brief introduction that describe the history and background of the project as well as stated the business need. The business need describes the main purpose for the curriculum design and in this case it was creating health disparities curriculum for graduate medical education. The next component in the design document was the tool utilized for articulating and tracking project milestones. This section contained the project management dashboard. The dashboard listed each task related to the curriculum design process including each meeting and the length of the meetings. The point of contact for each task were listed by their initials and a suggested due date was added to each task. A status column was included that provided information on the progress of each task. The tasks were marked "not started", "in progress", "overdue", or "complete". The last column gave detailed notes for each task. The content background section described in detail the learning management system that would be used for the module delivery. In this case, the modules were delivered on a system called MyLearning that is managed by CCaTS Education Resources. The duration section describe the suggested length for each module being 15 minutes for the active engagement component with 45 minutes of additional resources like readings, web resources, and detailed guides

Table 1. Content design document components

Component
Introduction • Project History/Background • Business Need/Application • Project Information • Personnel
Milestones Tracking
Content Background
• Access • Duration • Learners • Environment • Objectives • Materials, Tools and Equipment
Outline/Treatment
Learner Activities and Assessment
Program Evaluation

on available resources at Mayo Clinic to help residents and fellows address health disparities identified by patients.

The learners for the modules were described as all residents and fellows enrolled in one of the 280 graduate medical education-training programs. The geographic and multi-specialty dispersion of these learners necessitated an electronic and open access delivery platform. In this case, the training was self-directed online and available for learners to complete at their leisure by defined dates from MCSGME. Each module had a list of learning objectives related to addressing the social determinants of health, health disparities, and recognizing the physician's role in addressing health disparities in during a one-on-one patient encounter. The materials, tools, and equipment needs for the creation of these modules were the lecture materials, readings, of resources for physicians to address health disparities of patients the learning management system, and access to design equipment (Articulate Storyline, audio equipment to record voiceovers for the module, and Videoscribe for the creation of interactive videos). Modules were limited in scope and contained a basic overview of health disparities and social determinants of health. Moreover, the modules allowed the graduate medical learners to consider how to apply the course content in their specialty areas.

The outline component served as a treatment for the development of the modules including the script and video delivery of the health disparities content. The outline detailed each scene or slide in Articulate Storyline. This including giving details on the special effects, voiceover, sources of media and resources.

The learning activities component provided information on how learners knowledge would be evaluated using the learning management system. The system would deliver a few short quiz questions and provide direct feedback to learners. The program evaluation section of the design document provided details on the review process by the design team.

A TALE OF TWO MODULES

Again with SAM as a methodology, the curriculum design team met to outline each module. The foundation of the modules began with a historical overview of health disparities. The course director/subject matter expert provided the curriculum design team with detailed information about the content of the curriculum and the basic details that the learners needed to show basic knowledge of health disparities. To ensure the training would be relevant to physician learners and incorporate adult learning principles, the design team employed the six domains of quality healthcare (Agency for Healthcare Research and Quality, 2016):

1. **Safe:** Avoid injuring or harming patients from care meant for their treatment
2. **Effective:** Use scientific knowledge to avoid the misuse, underuse, or overuse of treatments/services to those who may benefit or not benefit;
3. **Patient-Centered:** Care based on patients cultural needs of the patients which includes not only their needs but values, norms, and preferences;
4. **Timely:** Decrease patient waiting which may increase their risk for health disparities and cause more harm;
5. **Efficient:** Avoid wasting resources like materials, equipment, supplies, energy, and ideas; and
6. **Equitable:** Delivering the most appropriate care to all patients regardless to patient's demographic or affinity group.

Physicians are the leaders of healthcare teams and provide care to increase patient's wellness; therefore, in addition to the quality healthcare domains used by the curriculum design team, the first author created a set of core competencies related to increasing the cultural awareness of physicians in order to reduce healthcare disparities. The competencies centered on the historical landmarks such as the Heckler Report. Over 30 years ago Margaret M. Heckler, United States Department of Health and Human Service Secretary, created a taskforce on Black and minority health (1985). The taskforce categorized minority health concerns and developed a comprehensive list of recommendations that would address health disparities and social determinants of health. This report preceded the current healthcare reform efforts like the Affordable Care Act. During the design process, the curriculum team decided to utilize the Heckler Report and the "Kelly Report: Health Disparities in America (Kelly, 2015) ." The Kelly Report led by Congresswomen Dr. Robin Kelly and presented at the Congressional Black Caucus Conference in September 2015 emphasized the health disparities and the impact on minority and under-resourced communities. The report describes the current healthcare arena in the United States and centers around some of the early success of the Affordable Care Act (i.e., more individuals with health insurance and the creation of the Patient Centered Outcomes Research Institute) (2015).The report also underscores the high prevalence of social determinants of health that plague minority and under-resourced communities. Moreover, it is a charge to change how care is provided by members of the healthcare team to the most vulnerable patient populations. This also represents an opportunity for medical education to incorporate these findings into the contemporary curriculum. In aggregate, the curriculum design team used the Heckler and Kelly Reports, the Triple Aim, recommendations from the American Board of Medical Specialties and the Association of American Medical Colleges to develop competencies that elucidate the skills needed by physicians to provide quality and equitable healthcare.

The competencies have five overarching responsibilities to increase patient action (i.e., adherence and compliance) to physician recommendations. The responsibilities and competencies are:

1. Assess the health disparities that impact patient population
   a. Identify factors that affect health disparities and health equity
   b. Ability to apply the health disparities theories
   c. Use practice-based learning to demonstrate an understanding of health disparities
2. Measure the impact of health disparities on healthcare outcomes
   a. Demonstrate mastery in the overall impact on health disparities on health outcomes
   b. Knowledge of the federal changes to increase health equity
3. Evaluate patient's risk for health disparities
   a. Demonstrate mastery of the levels of prevention
   b. Ability to identify complex patient characteristics that increase health disparities
   c. Determine available resources and assets to reduce health disparities
4. Master communication skills to increase patient action to reduce health disparities
   a. Implement cross-cultural communication best practices to increase patient action
   b. Recognize and create strategies tailored to the patient's needs
5. Identify tools and resources to reduce health disparities for the creation of reasonable patient action plans
   a. Identify factors that enhance or impeded patient actions
   b. Determine resource needs to create patient action plans

The subject matter expert and the instructional designer collaborated on the creation of the modules. Figure 3 depicts the modules created for the learners. The first module, "Overview of Health Disparities", had learning objectives Define health disparities and health care disparities 1) Define health disparities and health care disparities; 2) Describe factors that impact health disparities and health care disparities; 3) Determine physician actions to avoid health care disparities; and 4) Identify Mayo Clinic resources available to address health care disparities. The content provided a basic overview of health disparities, information internal and external resources to address health disparities, and tools that learners may use to gain insights on health disparities experienced by their patients.

Several multimedia interactive platforms were considered to imbue multicultural competencies for the module. The main platform selected was Articulate Storyline.

Figure 3. Health disparities modules for the graduate medical learners

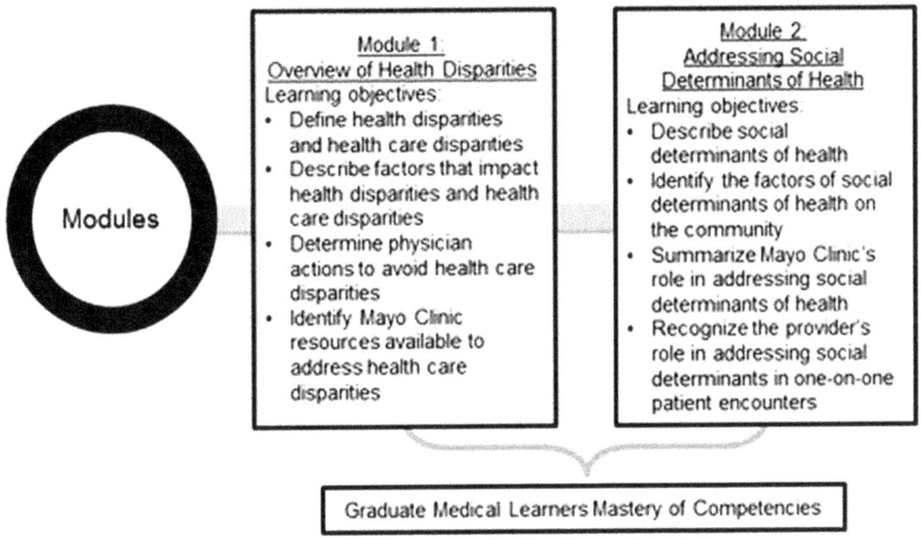

This platform is used for the creation and delivery of educational content that moves beyond the traditional PowerPoint slides. To make the module more engaging, interactive tools like Videoscribe were added for the learner to switch and click on different content. Videoscribe allows for the creation of animations and cartoons to describe various processes and creation of other graphics. Additionally, the module includes videos and links to external sites.

The second module, Addressing Social Determinants of Health, had learning objectives: 1) Describe social determinants of health; 2) Identify the factors of social determinants of health on the community; 3) Summarize Mayo Clinic's role in addressing social determinants of health; and 4) Recognize the provider's role in addressing social determinants in one-on-one patient encounters. The content provided learners with details on social determinants of health and the negative influences it has on health. The module included information on the generational factors and health while also providing details on Mayo Clinic's response to social determinants to health. The learners received recommendations on how to address social determinants of health during the patient visit.

FORMATIVE EVALUATION

Prior to launching the modules, alpha and beta testing was conducted with the collaborative design team and other stakeholders. Design team members reviewed the alpha version of the modules and provided feedback on the organization of the content and interface. The instructional designer used this feedback to revise and refine the modules. The beta test involved reviewing the next version of the modules. This evaluation allowed for feedback on the interface and accessibility of the module via the learning management system. The final version of the module was delta tested for timing, engagement, and ease of navigation for learners. This part of the evaluation involved making sure active links worked and that resources on health disparities were up-to-date.

The formative evaluation process also provided the collaborative curriculum design team a systematic process to analyze the curriculum design and implementation process. For instance, the team was able to make changes to the project timeline and applied knowledge gained more efficiently in the creation of the second module such as reducing in-person meetings and electronic document review by email saved time. An additional benefit was this method provided a log of changes for the instructional designer. There were also quality changes made to the design document that CCaTS Education Resource based on this process which are now utilized with other similar projects.

MODULE DELIVERY AND SUMMATIVE EVALUATION

There were several digital platform options to deliver the content to the graduate medical learners. One option was Blackboard as the learning management system. The institution uses Blackboard for management of online and traditional courses. However, there was a major concern with using Blackboard related to its challenging enrollment and management of such a large group of learners. Therefore, CCaTS Education Resources had to determine an alternative option for delivering the modules. During the design process, the collaborative design team settled on using MyLearning. This learning management system was already available and used successfully by Human Resources to provide asynchronous required trainings to Mayo Clinic employees. Moreover, MyLearning does not limit the number of learners and the completion of the module is documented on an institutional transcript. Another interesting feature of the MyLearning was the ability to collect pre and post module evaluation data. This was useful for demonstrating each learner's growth and development as a result of the content and satisfaction with the modules as an effective and efficient learning tool.

The modules were made available to the current residents following the institution's first ACGME CLER site visit. . Annually, the incoming residents and fellows are required to complete both modules in succession during the first weeks of beginning training. Each learner completes the modules during the time-period as directed by MCSGME. However, the electronic platform allows them to complete the modules during their own time and is accessible within their clinical work areas or off campus. To date, the modules have over a 99% completion rate. The modules utilize an integrated, real-time, assessment process to test knowledge change for learners who completed both modules. Each module contains a knowledge check point and asked questions that relate to use of the content in their clinical practices.

Because the SAM e-learning design philosophy emphasizes the learner experience over content, a final step was to evaluate the trainees' level of satisfaction with the modules. Table 2 summarizes the post module evaluation results. A Likert scale asked learners to rate their level of agreement from 1 to strongly disagree to 4 strongly agree on areas of module quality, length, content, and utility.

The Health Disparities curriculum (module #1) was completed by 1896 residents and fellows. A total of 420 learners completed the module post evaluation. The response rate for the module evaluation was 22%. A majority of the respondents agreed the quality of the module was excellent (77%). They also agreed that the length was appropriate (74%). A majority agreed that the content was relevant to their work (73%), they would share the knowledge with others (72%), and it was a good use of their time (66%).

Table 2. Post module evaluations

Module 1 Post Evaluation n=420	Strongly Disagree n (%)	Disagree n (%)	Agree n (%)	Strongly Agree n (%)
The quality of the module was excellent	7 (2%)	26 (6%)	324 (77%)	63 (15%)
The length of the module was appropriate	7 (2%)	22 (5%)	309 (74%)	82 (20%)
The content is relevant to my work	11 (3%)	33 (8%)	304 (73%)	72 (17%)
I will share this knowledge with others	12 (3%)	44 (10%)	302 (72%)	62 (15%)
This was a good use of my time	18 (4%)	59 (14%)	278 (66%)	65 (15%)
Module 2 Post Evaluation n=776	**Strongly Disagree n (%)**	**Disagree n (%)**	**Agree n (%)**	**Strongly Agree n (%)**
The quality of the module was excellent	12 (2%)	39 (5%)	592 (76%)	133 (17%)
The length of the module was appropriate	12 (2%)	38 (5%)	556 (72%)	170 (22%)
The content is relevant to my work	17 (2%)	63 (8%)	559 (72%)	137 (18%)
I will share this knowledge with others	19 (2%)	91 (12%)	532 (69%)	134 (17%)
This was a good use of my time	29 (4%)	100 (13%)	529 (68%)	118 (15%)

The Social Determinants of Health curriculum (module #2) had 1919 completers. 776 respondents completed the module post evaluation; the response rate for the module evaluation was 40%. A majority agreed that the module was excellent (76%), the length was appropriate (72%), the content of the module information was relevant to their clinical work (72%), they would share the knowledge with others (69%), and completing the module was a good use of their time (68%).

DISCUSSION AND CONCLUSION

The struggle to reduce healthcare disparities in the United States continues. In the last 30 years reports like the Heckler Report and more recently the "Kelly Report: Health Disparities in America" ascertain that little success has halted the decline in health disparities (Heckler, 1985; Kelly, 2015). Although these reports underscore many policy changes that have resulted in gains, a disproportionate number of minorities and under-resourced citizens still do not have access to the preventative care that promotes well-being. Fortunately, these reports also provide recommendations on necessary steps to improve the quality of care and increase cultural awareness of the healthcare needs of minority and under-resourced communities. Chief among them is increasing the awareness of health disparities and cultural competence of the nation's healthcare workforce. Overall, contemporary healthcare providers may lack of awareness of social determinants of health, health disparities or even cultural norms of the patients they serve. As physicians are implicitly future leaders in transforming and improving the nation's healthcare system, it is pivotal to focus their attention on these issues while they are still in training. As a result, the incorporation of health disparities in the graduate medical education curriculum is increasingly becoming a proactive strategy to reduce health disparities and increase health equity.

The responsibility to increase the cultural awareness and knowledge of health disparities of the next generation of physicians traditionally falls on academic medical centers which in turn have delegated this task to the nation's GME programs (Drobac & Morse, 2016; Maldonado et al., 2014). National stakeholder health organizations, policy makers, medical societies, and accrediting organizations are setting expectations for physician learners at all stages to develop or improve the socio-cultural knowledge, attitudes, and competencies needed to reduce health disparities in the patients they serve.

However, a barrier to delivering non-clinical curriculum during graduate medical training relates to the competing demands placed on physician learners and preceptors who also have concurrent patient care responsibilities. To overcome these challenges, modern medical education must consider alternative formats for how non-clinical education content is delivered to graduate medical learners.

In this chapter, the authors described the development and use of asynchronous curriculum to increase graduate medical learners' knowledge of health disparities and social determinants of health as well as raise awareness of institutional based cultural resources to enhance their clinical practice. The process of developing the web-based modules embraced electronic learning technologies paradigms and open access platforms such as that lauded by FOAM proponents and utilized SAM, a systematic approach to electronic curriculum design. For example, Articulate Storyline was selected because it provides a usable platform for curriculum design that compliments other platforms like Videoscribe, websites, and other forms of multimedia. Unlike PowerPoint, Articulate Storyline is more interactive and has additional features that allow for a more streamlined design process. Another feature of the design process was the addition of real-time assessments and engagement in the modules. Finally, the team decided to keep the entire module to one hour of content with only 15 to 20 minutes dedicated to Articulate Storyline.

The module design process used a team-based approach engaging multiple stakeholders. The collaborative curriculum design team used a multifaceted approach to determine available resources, prioritize content area, and determine the most appropriate institutional supported learning management system for the delivering the modules to learners in multiple clinical specialty areas across the institution's three national campuses. From a content perspective, one of the key deliverables was to not only increase functional awareness of the social determinants of health and health disparities, but also to bring attention to the available resources for physicians within the institution to address these issues.

Each module had measurable learning objectives designed to meet the ACGME's CLER standards and the educational needs of MCSGME. A formative evaluation process allowed the curriculum design team to revise the module design process throughout the module creation. Not discussed in the article were the learner pre-assessments to determine applicability of the content, which was another valuable outcome. In fact, most of the learners reported that the content was useful in their clinical work area and maintained that they would share the information learned with others. Although, the 99% completion rate can be attributed to the mandatory nature of the modules, through analysis of the optional module post evaluation data, we were able to establish that the learners found the modules a good use of their time. Administering the pre/post module evaluation provided useful information to the design team which will be used to improve the quality of the module and applicability of the content. Throughout the design process, the team had to overcome a variety of barriers. First, and most important, was determining the appropriate team to engage in the project. Second, there was a short timeframe to create the modules in order to respond to the CLER accreditation requirements. Of course, this was done in the midst of the collaborative curriculum design team members each having other priorities related to their other job duties. Third, the platform to deliver the content had to be easily accessible to diverse learners in multiple clinical and specialty areas and documentable to the ACGME.

The collaborative curriculum design team used best practices for designing the modules but took it a step further by developing next practices that are measurable for creating asynchronous curriculum for adult learners. Our next steps are to create more curricula that is specific to the disparate populations of each regional Mayo Clinic campus.

REFERENCES

Agency for Healthcare Research and Quality. (2016). *The Six Domains of Health Care Quality*. Retrieved from https://www.ahrq.gov/professionals/quality-patient-safety/talkingquality/create/sixdomains.html

Allen Interactions. (2017). *Agile eLearning Development with SAM*. Retrieved from http://www.alleninteractions.com/sam-process

Balls-Berry, J. E. (2012). *Mayo Clinic Learners' Perceptions of Health Disparities*. Paper presented at the 13th RCMI International Symposium on Health Disparities, San Juan, Puerto Rico.

Balls-Berry, J. E., Billings, H., Ernste, L., Valdez Soto, M., Frimannsdottir, K., Weavers, K., ... Patten, C. A. (2017). Development of a self-directed, online-learning curriculum to increase community-engaged research in clinical and translational science. *J Clin Transl Sci*, *1*(2), 135–139. doi:10.1017/cts.2016.19 PMID:28649456

Braveman, P. A., Egerter, S. A., Woolf, S. H., & Marks, J. S. (2011). When Do We Know Enough to Recommend Action on the Social Determinants of Health? *Strong Medicine for a Healthier America*, *40*(1Supplement 1), S58–S66. doi:10.1016/j.amepre.2010.09.026 PMID:21146780

Dabbagh, N., & Bannan-Ritland, R. (2005). *Online Learning: Concepts, Strategies, and Application*. Upper Saddle River, NJ: Pearson/Merrill/Prentice Hall.

Demiroz, E. (2016). Principles of Instructional Design for E-Learning and Online Learning Practices: Implications for Medical Education. In V. Wang (Ed.), *Handbook of Research on Advancing Health Education through Technology* (pp. 419–451). Hershey, PA: IGI Global; doi:10.4018/978-1-4666-9494-1.ch018

Drobac, P., & Morse, M. (2016). Medical Education and Global Health Equity. *AMA Journal of Ethics, 18*(7), 702–709. doi:10.1001/journalofethics.2016.18.7.medu1-1607 PMID:27437820

Heckler, M. (1985). *Report of the Secretary's Task Force on Black & Minority Health*. Retrieved from https://minorityhealth.hhs.gov/assets/pdf/checked/1/ANDERSON.pdf

Jackson, C. S., & Gracia, J. N. (2014). Addressing Health and Health-Care Disparities: The Role of a Diverse Workforce and the Social Determinants of Health. *Public Health Reports (Washington, D.C.), 129*(Suppl 2), 57–61. doi:10.1177/00333549141291S211 PMID:24385666

Kelly, R. (2015). *Kelly Report: Health Disparities in America*. Washington, DC: United States Congress. Retrieved from https://robinkelly.house.gov/sites/robinkelly.house.gov/files/2015%20Kelly%20Report.pdf

Knowles, M. S. (1990). *The Adult Learner: A Neglected Species*. Houston, TX: Gulf.

Knowles, M. S., Holton, E. F., & Swanson, R. A. (2012). The Adult Learner: the Definitive Classics in Adult Education and Human Resource Development (7th ed.). New York, NY: Taylor & Francis.

LaVeist, T. A., & Pierre, G. (2014). Integrating the 3Ds--social determinants, health disparities, and health-care workforce diversity. *Public Health Reports (Washington, D.C.), 129* (Suppl 2), 9–14. doi:10.1177/00333549141291S204 PMID:24385659

Maldonado, M. E., Fried, E. D., DuBose, T. D., Nelson, C., & Breida, M. (2014). The role that graduate medical education must play in ensuring health equity and eliminating health care disparities. *Annals of the American Thoracic Society, 11*(4), 603–607. doi:10.1513/AnnalsATS.201402-068PS PMID:24708150

Nickson, C. P., & Cadogan, M. D. (2014). Free Open Access Medical education (FOAM) for the emergency physician. *Emergency Medicine Australasia, 26*(1), 76–83. doi:10.1111/1742-6723.12191 PMID:24495067

Office of the Legislative Counsel. (2010). *Compilation of Patient Protection and Affordable Care Act*. Retrieved from http://housedocs.house.gov/energycommerce/ppacacon.pdf

Thomas, P. A., Kern, D. E., Hughes, M. T., & Chen, B. Y. (Eds.). (2016). *Curriculum Development for Medical Education: A Six-Step Approach*. Baltimore, MD: John Hopkins University Press.

KEY TERMS AND DEFINITIONS

Asynchronous Education: Self-directed online training provided to learners.

Cultural Awareness: It is the understanding and gaining knowledge about the differences and similarities between diverse groups of people regarding their demographic characteristics.

Curriculum Development: Creation of educational material for learners using pedagogical principles.

Graduate Medical Education: Training provided to physicians after completing undergraduate medical education. Residency and fellowships are in specific clinical areas.

Health Disparities: The differences in preventable disease burden to attain overall wellness faced by under-resourced or vulnerable communities.

Health Equity: Refers to people achieving the highest quality of health.

Social Determinants of Health: The circumstance of where a person lives, works, interacts, plays, and learns affect overall wellness.

Chapter 2 Technologic Advances in Neurologic Practice and Education: The Cell Phone Replaces the Direct Ophthalmoscope

Charles Donohoe
University of Missouri – Kansas City School of Medicine, USA

Sean M. Gratton
University of Missouri – Kansas City School of Medicine, USA

Vivek M. Vallurupalli
University of Missouri – Kansas City School of Medicine, USA

Steven D. Waldman
University of Missouri – Kansas City School of Medicine, USA

ABSTRACT

Although the visualization of the ocular fundus yields important clinical information regarding the optic nerve and retinal vasculature, proficiency in using the traditional handheld direct ophthalmoscope by both practicing physicians and medical students continues to deteriorate. A replacement for the direct ophthalmoscope is long overdue. The authors suggest a role for non-mydriatic fundus photography as having potential to resurrect the dying art of visualizing the fundus in both clinical practice and medical education. This chapter reviews the substantial barriers in both patient care as well as graduate and undergraduate medical education created by technical difficulties encountered using the direct ophthalmoscope to visualize the ocular fundus. The authors propose that a smartphone-compatible adaptor to view the ocular fundus will replace the direct ophthalmoscope.

DOI: 10.4018/978-1-5225-6289-4.ch002

INTRODUCTION

Although the visualization of the ocular fundus yields important clinical information regarding the optic nerve and retinal vasculature, proficiency in using the traditional handheld direct ophthalmoscope by both practicing physicians and medical students continues to deteriorate. A replacement for the direct ophthalmoscope is long overdue. The authors suggest a role for non-mydriatic fundus photography as having potential to resurrect the dying art of visualizing the fundus in both clinical practice and medical education. This chapter reviews the substantial barriers in both patient care as well as graduate and undergraduate medical education created by technical difficulties encountered using the direct ophthalmoscope to visualize the ocular fundus. The authors propose that a smartphone compatible adaptor to view the ocular fundus will replace the direct ophthalmoscope. This device is a technological 'work in progress' and is just becoming commercially available but will ultimately fill the current unacceptable void in patient care and in educating students on the importance of fundoscopy.

A CHANGING LANDSCAPE

Advances in technology have been a primary driving force in medical progress. The direct ophthalmoscope introduced by Herman von Helmholtz in 1851 dramatically changed the practice of ophthalmology and provided the first view of the human fundus and the first in vivo views of central retinal artery occlusion in 1855 and papilledema in 1860 (Swanson, Ku, & Chou, 2011)

The handheld version of this device was introduced in 1915 and traditionally medical students have been expected to own and carry this instrument with the goal of becoming proficient in its use in examining patients. Over time technical difficulties using the direct ophthalmoscope have frustrated medical students and non-ophthalmologists to a point where funduscopy is now routinely omitted from the physical exam. The magnitude of these technical difficulties has created avoidance behavior in clinicians allowing crucial clinical findings such as papilledema, optic disc swelling due to increased intracranial pressure, to escape detection with tragic consequences including blindness.

The authors, practicing neurologists, routinely encounter pseudotumor cerebri syndrome (PCS). This condition frequently seen in obese females is characterized by increased intracranial pressure not associated with a tumor or mass. Over time, this pressure can damage the optic nerve. Brain imaging findings are often negative or non-specific and the only diagnostic marker is a swollen optic nerve visualized on funduscopy. These patients present with headaches associated with visual complaints who often have been evaluated in multiple emergency rooms, undergone normal computed tomography (CT) scanning and magnetic resonance (MR) brain imaging without their medical providers even attempting to visualize the fundus.

Rarely this can end tragically in permanent visual loss. Equally disturbing is that review of these patient's medical records documents a templated notation in the physical exam as 'normal eye exam'. The patient when questioned is firm in their contention that 'no one ever looked in my eyes '. This practice ultimately can form the core evidence for an unpleasant medical malpractice action and provides a glimpse into the dismal state of clinical funduscopy outside of ophthalmology.

A solution to this problem, the digital non-mydriatic fundus camera, has been available for 20 years. The first photographs of the human fundus were captured in the late 1800s. Fundus photography became available for clinical use in the 1950s and eventually became digital and diagnostic even through an undilated pupil (Mottow-Lippa, Boker, & Stephens, 2009). Until recently these nonmydriatic fundus cameras were available only in the offices of ophthalmologists and optometrists despite the fact that high-quality images can be obtained within minutes even by non-physicians with minimal training (Lippa, Boker, Duke, & Amin, 2006).

his chapter reviews the technical difficulties with the direct ophthalmoscope, the advantages of available non-mydriatic fundus cameras and the recent experience with their use beyond ophthalmology in the emergency room and neurology clinic. A portable and affordable modification of the standard fundus camera reduced to the size of a cellphone attachment is now positioned to replace the handheld direct ophthalmoscope.

THE CURRENT STATE OF OPHTHALMOSCOPY

Examination of the ocular fundus with a direct ophthalmoscope has been part of the physical examination since the middle of the 19th century (Sherman, 1989). Visualizing the retina, optic nerve, and retinal vessels is a valuable endeavor that can divulge diagnostic and prognostic information about many neurological and systemic diseases. Mackay, Garza, Bruce, Newman, and Biousse delineate some of the advantages of direct, including its wide availability, portability, relatively low cost, and ability to provide a magnified view of the posterior pole (Mackay, Garza, Bruce, Newman, & Biousse, 2015). Despite these factors, each clinician weighs the value of direct against its challenges, and many seem to be concluding that the commitment required to achieve proficiency is not worth the potential benefit, leading to an erosion of the overall ability of non-ophthalmologists to view the fundus (Mottow-Lippa, 2009).

The future of direct can best be predicted by examining trends in medical education. A decline in medical student ability to view the ocular fundus can potentially lead to widespread deterioration of the skill. Despite vigorous efforts to reinforce ophthalmology education in medical school curricula, studies suggest that the trend has not been reversed (Mottow-Lippa, 2009). Numerous studies have examined the patterns of medical student use of the direct ophthalmoscope. The Teaching to Medical Students (TOTeMS) study compared the accuracy and preferences of medical students learning to examine the ocular fundus using a human volunteer, a simulator, and fundus photographs. 77% preferred fundus photography to direct (Kelly et al., 2013). Additionally, students were more accurate in their interpretations using fundus photography compared to direct ophthalmoscopy. A follow-up study, TOTeMS II, examined the same group of students one year later, and found that accuracy was once again better in the fundus photographs group compared to direct ophthalmoscopy, but that there was a decline in performance in both groups over time. These students reported performing direct ophthalmoscopy on clinical rotations less than 10% of the time, and, alarmingly, 20% reported the primary reason for not examining the ocular fundus was discouragement by a preceptor (Mackay et al., 2014). Students have also been shown to prefer the panoptic ophthalmoscope to the classic direct ophthalmoscope; however improved accuracy did not accompany this preference (McComiskie, Greer, & Gole, 2004). Not surprisingly, medical student ophthalmoscopy skills can be improved with training (Milani et. al, 2013), but decay when not practiced regularly (Mottow-Lippa, 2009; Lippa, 2006).

Data support similar trends in the use of direct ophthalmoscopy in physicians after medical school. In the Emergency Department setting, only 14-48% of patients presenting with headache and other neurological emergencies had ophthalmoscopy documented (Bruce, et al., 2011). Another study with a mix of Family Medicine, Internal Medicine, and Emergency Medicine residents and staff physicians found that only 26% routinely performed direct ophthalmoscopy, and even fewer, 13%, felt confident in their skill level (Donohoe C, Gratton S, & Vallurupalli VR, 2018). Lack of confidence in the ability to perform and interpret direct ophthalmoscopy combined with the ever-increasing time pressures on physicians of all specialties is leading to the virtual abandonment of this essential aspect of the physical examination.

Examining the ocular fundus of patients with headache and visual loss is particularly important as fundus findings can help to identify debilitating and even life-threatening pathology. In the Fundus Photography vs Ophthalmoscopy Trial Outcomes in the Emergency Department (FOTO-ED) study, of 354 adult patients visiting the Emergency Department with headache, acute neurological deficit, or acute visual change, 10% had relevant findings on non-mydriatic fundus photography, including papilledema, severe hypertensive retinopathy, optic atrophy, and retinal vascular occlusions (Bruce et al., 2011). This alarmingly high rate of pathology identified by fundus photography combined with the decline of the use of direct funduscopy creates circumstances that will invariably lead to missed diagnoses, morbidity including permanent visual loss, and medicolegal repercussions.

AN EMERGING TECHNOLOGY FOR VIEWING THE OCULAR FUNDUS

Given the difficulty of direct ophthalmoscopy in the clinical setting, some developers have sought an entity that is more familiar to clinicians as a possible solution: the smartphone. In fact, it has been estimated that up to 98.9% of physicians currently own smartphones with 92.6% of them finding their device useful in the clinical setting (Mobasheri et. al, 2015). The torrid pace of technological advancement has resulted in smartphones being used to transform medicine through various applications and features. In the realm of ophthalmology, smartphone capabilities have already begun to be implemented to view, diagnose and document pathologies of the eye. Given their ease of use and portability, this form of "smartphone ophthalmoscopy" has served to obtain high-quality pictures of the eye in settings such as emergency rooms, for inpatient consultations, and examinations under anesthesia, etc (Haddock et. al, 2013).

Typically, the mechanism of smartphone fundus photography involves use of the camera and flash light capabilities of a smartphone with an external apparatus to direct the light and magnify the viewing angle, in order to view the fundus of the eye. One such apparatus, the D-Eye device (Figure 1), is a magnetic fundus lens that attaches to the iPhone and utilizes an application and the iPhone camera to take both photographs and videos of the fundus (D-EYE Srl, Padova, Italy). This recently developed Food and Drug Administration-approved device (Figure 2) and corresponding HIPPA-compliant smartphone application has shown promising utility.

In one study comparing the D-Eye device with conventional indirect ophthalmoscopy, 172 eyes from 87 pediatric patients aged 3 – 18 years were examined with both methods. The mean cup-to-disc ratio quantified using the D-Eye apparatus and smartphone photo capabilities was 0.239 (±0.091), while the same ratio measured with the conventional indirect ophthalmoscopy method was 0.238 (±0.095) (Dickson et al.). Notably, this particular smartphone ophthalmoscopy technology showed a vast improvement in accuracy of measuring cup-to-disc ratios in comparison to the standard, cumbersome direct ophthalmoscope. Direct ophthalmoscopy has been reported to accurately measure the cup-to-disc ratios only 10% of the time versus retinal tomography. D-Eye smartphone technology, on the other hand, had an exact cup-to-disc ratio agreement of 73.2% to indirect ophthalmoscopy (Dickson et al., 2017).

Figure 1. Commercially available D-Eye ophthalmoscopy device
Source: With kind permission from Spencer Lee of D-EYE Srl, Padova, Italy

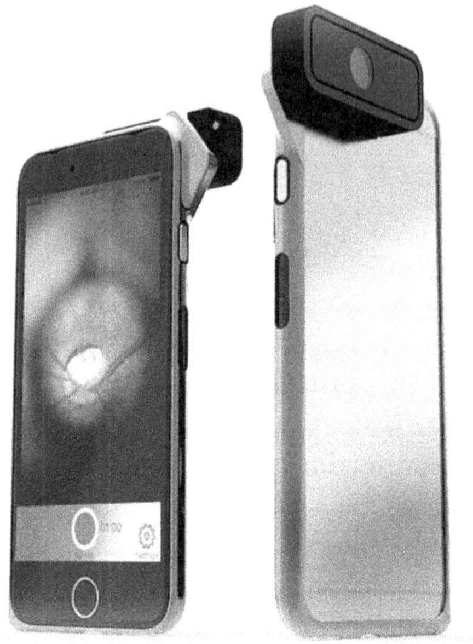

Figure 2. Demonstration of smartphone ophthalmoscopy device
Source: With kind permission from Spencer Lee of D-EYE Srl, Padova, Italy

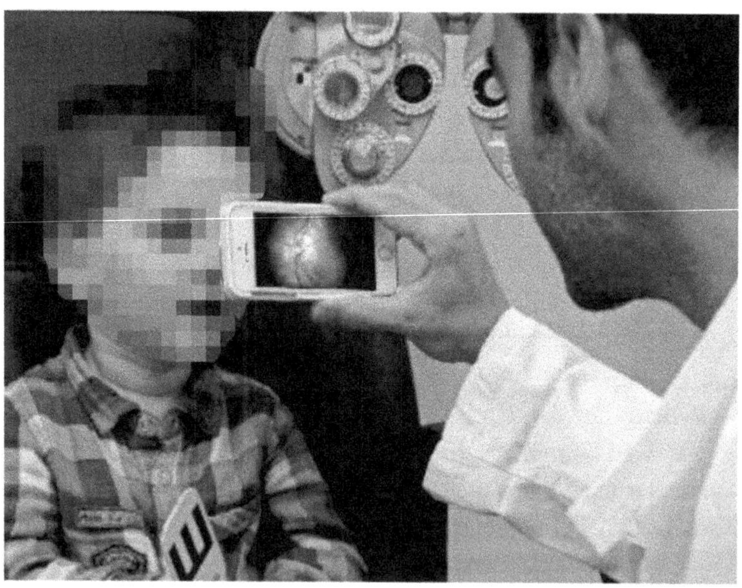

Another study compared the ability of the smartphone ophthalmoscope to grade diabetic retinopathy with the proven retinal slit lamp biomicroscope. In 120 patients (240 eyes) with type I or type II diabetes mellitus, the smartphone with D-Eye apparatus showed agreement within 1 step on a 5-step grading scale of 96.7%, and a specificity of 98% at detecting clinically significant macular edema in these same patients (Russo et al., n.d.). This substantial agreement with slit lamp biomicroscopy for diabetic retinopathy shows intriguing clinical value for smartphone ophthalmoscopy that is further strengthened by the affordability, accessibility and portability of the latter technology.

Along with the noteworthy accuracy at quantifying cup-to-disc ratios and grading diabetic retinopathy, the D-Eye apparatus along with a smartphone proved very capable at detecting fundus abnormalities. In comparison to indirect ophthalmoscopy, the D-Eye method yielded specificities of 0.97 and 0.98 at detecting fundus abnormalities and measuring optic nerve size, respectively. In addition, many distinct pathologies can be detected using the D-Eye method, including: optic nerve hypoplasia, peripapillary atrophy, optic disc drusen, optic disc coloboma and Wyburn-Mason syndrome (Dickson et al., 2017; Figure 3). Smartphone ophthalmoscopy technology is still considered to be a "work in progress" that is only recently becoming commercially available in clinical settings. Regardless, these studies highlight the great utility and reliability of smartphone technology in a clinical setting. Further development will increase the breadth of such capability.

The immense technological development of smartphones has resulted in devices that are now more portable, efficient, and powerful than ever before. From a global perspective, the smartphone and its capabilities offer unique benefits. Certain regions, especially in developing nations, have limited access to the conventional forms of ophthalmoscopy along with a paucity of eye specialists to diagnose and treat these common eye pathologies. In these areas, smartphones possess an immense advantage: their portability, affordability and cost-effectiveness (Lord, Shah, San-Filippo, & Krishna, 2010; Pasquel et al., 2016). Their ease of use allows for local personnel to be trained to obtain picture or video of retinas which could be saved and interpreted remotely by eye specialists. In fact, retinal images acquired from smartphones have already been used to successfully diagnose retinopathy of prematurity in certain resource limited areas in Sub-Saharan Africa (Oluleye, Rotimi-Samuel, & Adenekan, 2016). In a similar light, further development and availability of the smartphone ophthalmoscopy capabilities could establish them as a major facilitator of retinal examinations for various pathologies in areas with limited resources.

Figure 3 Representative retinal images of various pathologies taken with D-Eye device: (a) normal optic disc; (b) optic nerve coloboma; (c) image of a 0.5 cup/ disk ratio; (d) congenital cataract and nystagmus; (e) optic nerve hypoplasia and peripapillary atrophy; (f) Wyburn-Mason syndrome; (g) image of the optic nerve pit; (h) optic disc pallor; (i) congenital cataract

Source: Image reproduced with kind permission from Donny Suh M.D., University of Nebraska Medical Center, Omaha, Nebraska; Dickson et al.

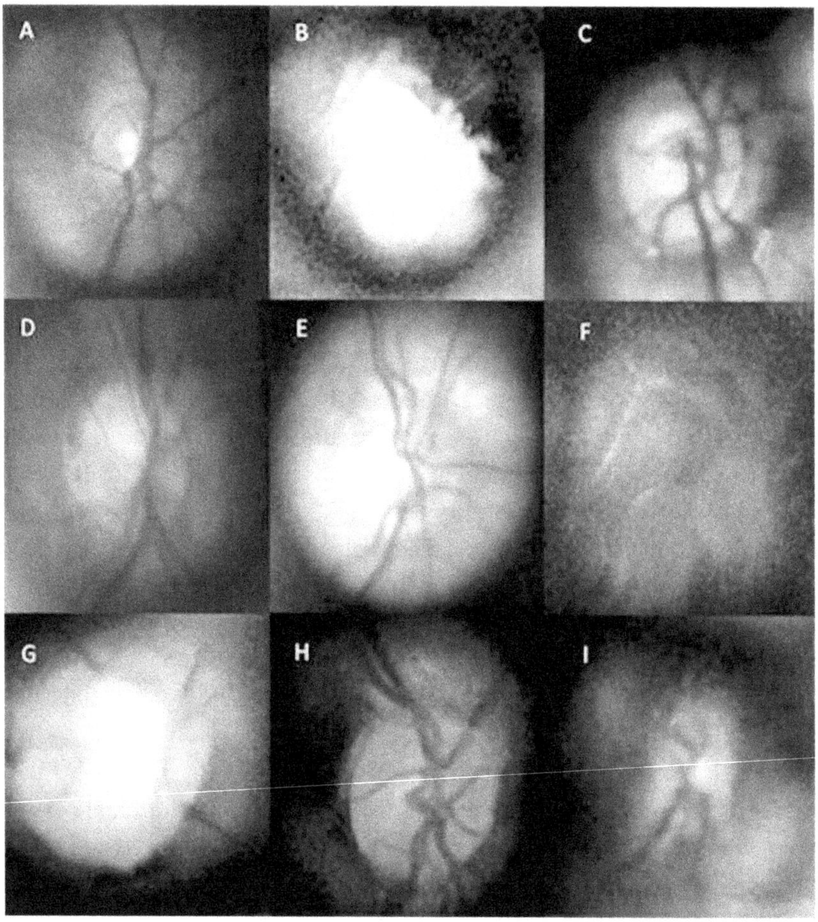

CONCLUDING REMARKS

The venerable handheld direct ophthalmoscope is an outdated, cumbersome technology that is no longer suitable for clinical practice or medical education. New or preowned standard non-mydriatic fundus cameras are both recommended as short-term replacements. Portable cellphone based retinal cameras are being refined and becoming commercially available. It will still be challenging changing the engrained tradition of purchasing and even carrying a handheld direct ophthalmoscope but rarely actually examining the retina or optic nerve.

The authors support the rapid transition to cellphone based fundus cameras. Exposing medical students and residents in training to improved high quality images of the retinal vasculature and optic nerve will help expedite this technological advancement. This should reinvigorate interest in clinical funduscopy beyond the specialty of ophthalmology. These goals coincide with a powerful movement in medicine fueled by technology that makes accurate information easily accessible to non-specialist medical providers. The application of evolving technologies ultimately foreshadows patients monitoring their own medical care and providing a potential solution to the unsustainable costs of our healthcare system.

REFERENCES

Breen, D. P., Duncan, C. W., Pope, A. E., Gray, A. J., & Al-Shahi Salman, R. (2008). Emergency department evaluation of sudden, severe headache. *QJM: An International Journal of Medicine*, *101*(6), 435–443. doi:10.1093/qjmed/hcn036 PMID:18443002

Bruce, B. B., Lamirel, C., Wright, D. W., Ward, A., Heilpern, K., Biousse, V., & Newman, N. J. (2011). Nonmydriatic ocular fundus photography in the emergency department. *The New England Journal of Medicine*, *364*(4), 387–289. doi:10.1056/NEJMc1009733 PMID:21268749

Dickson, D., Fouzdar-Jain, S., MacDonald, C., Song, H., Agraz, D., Morgan, L., & Suh, D. (2017). Comparison study of funduscopic exam of pediatric patients using the D-EYE method and conventional indirect ophthalmoscopic methods. *Open Journal of Ophthalmology*, *145*(03), 145–152. doi:10.4236/ojoph.2017.73020

Donohoe, C., Gratton, S., & Vallurupalli, V. R. (2018, April). *Implementation of Smartphone-Compatible Non-Mydriatic Ocular Fundoscopy in the Evaluation of Headaches in Clinical Settings.* Poster session presented at the 2018 UMKC Health Sciences Research Summit, Kansas City, MO.

Haddock, L. J., Kim, D. Y., & Mukai, S. (2013). Simple, inexpensive technique for high-quality smartphone fundus photography in human and animal eyes. *Journal of Ophthalmology*, 518479. PMID:24171108

Kelly, L. P., Garza, P. S., Bruce, B. B., Graubart, E. B., Newman, N. J., & Biousse, V. (2013). Teaching ophthalmoscopy to medical students (the TOTeMS study). *American Journal of Ophthalmology*, *156*(5), 1056–1061. doi:10.1016/j.ajo.2013.06.022 PMID:24041982

Lippa, L. M., Boker, J., Duke, A., & Amin, A. (2006). A novel 3-year longitudinal pilot study of medical students' acquisition and retention of screening eye examination skills. *Ophthalmology*, *113*(1), 133–139. doi:10.1016/j.ophtha.2005.09.003 PMID:16310854

Lord, R. K., Shah, V. A., San-Filippo, A. N., & Krishna, R. (2010). Novel uses of smartphones in ophthalmology. *Ophthalmology*, *117*(6), 1274–1274. doi:10.1016/j.ophtha.2010.01.001 PMID:20522335

Mackay, D. D., Garza, P. S., Bruce, B. B., Bidot, S., Graubart, E. B., Newman, N. J., ... Kelly, L. P. (2014). Teaching ophthalmology to medical students (TOTeMS) II: A one-year retention study. *American Journal of Ophthalmology*, *157*(3), 747–748. doi:10.1016/j.ajo.2013.12.013 PMID:24528937

Mackay, D. D., Garza, P. S., Bruce, B. B., Newman, N. J., & Biousse, V. (2015). The demise of direct ophthalmoscopy: A modern clinical challenge. *Neurology. Clinical Practice*, *5*(2), 150–157. doi:10.1212/CPJ.0000000000000115 PMID:26137422

Maizels, M. (2001). Headache evaluation and treatment by primary care physicians in an emergency department in the era of triptans. *Archives of Internal Medicine*, *161*(16), 1969–1973. doi:10.1001/archinte.161.16.1969 PMID:11525699

McComiskie, J. E., Greer, R. M., & Gole, G. A. (2004). Panoptic vs conventional ophthalmoscope. *Clinical & Experimental Ophthalmology*, *32*(3), 238–242. doi:10.1111/j.1442-9071.2004.00810.x PMID:15180833

Milani, B. Y., Majdi, M., Green, W., Mehralian, A., Moarefi, M., Oh, F. S., ... Djalilian, A. R. (2013). The use of peer optic nerve photographs for teaching direct ophthalmoscopy. *Ophthalmology*, *120*(4), 761–765. doi:10.1016/j.ophtha.2012.09.020 PMID:23246117

Mobasheri, M. H., King, D., Johnston, M., Gautama, S., Purkayastha, S., & Darzi, A. (2015). The ownership and clinical use of smartphones by doctors and nurses in the UK: A multicentre survey study. *BMJ Innovations*, *1*(4), 174–181. doi:10.1136/bmjinnov-2015-000062

Mottow-Lippa, L. (2009). Ophthalmology in the medical school curriculum: Reestablishing our value and effecting change. *Ophthalmology*, *116*(7), 1235–1236. doi:10.1016/j.ophtha.2009.01.012 PMID:19576494

Oluleye, T. S., Rotimi-Samuel, A., & Adenekan, A. (2016). Mobile phones for retinopathy of prematurity screening in Lagos, Nigeria, Sub-Saharan Africa. *European Journal of Ophthalmology*, *26*, 1–102. PMID:26044377

Pasquel, F. J., Hendrick, A. M., Ryan, M., Cason, E., Ali, M. K., & Narayan, K. M. (2016). Cost-effectiveness of different diabetic retinopathy screening modalities. *Journal of Diabetes Science and Technology*, *10*(2), 301–307. doi:10.1177/1932296815624109 PMID:26719134

Russo, A., Morescalchi, F., Costagliola, C., Delcassi, L., & Semeraro, F. (n.d.). Comparison of smartphone ophthalmoscopy with slit-lamp biomicroscopy for grading diabetic retinopathy. *American Journal of Ophtalmology, 159*(2), 360-364.

Sherman, S. E. (1989). The history of the ophthalmoscope. *Documenta Ophtalmologica*, *71*(2), 221–228. doi:10.1007/BF00163473 PMID:2663401

Swanson, S., Ku, T., & Chou, C. (2011). Assessment of direct ophthalmoscopy using plastic canisters. *Medical Education*, *45*(5), 520–521. doi:10.1111/j.1365-2923.2011.03987.x PMID:21486343

Chapter 3
Simulation Technology in Anesthesia Education

Morgan E. Gonder
University of Missouri – Kansas City School of Medicine, USA

Maxwell Holtmann
University of Missouri – Kansas City School of Medicine, USA

Steven D. Waldman
University of Missouri – Kansas City School of Medicine, USA

ABSTRACT

This chapter provides an overview of increasing role of simulation technology in anesthesia education. A brief history of the role of simulation is discussed, spanning across the introduction of the first medical simulators of the 18th century to the role of modern simulation technology in education today. The capacity in which anesthesia education is conducted has dramatically improved with the advancement in simulation technology and use of part-task and full-body simulation trainers. In this chapter, focus is placed on the indications and utility of simulation for airway management, bronchoscopy, and central line placement education, as well as whole-body simulation models and their role in practicing complex scenarios. Key elements that ensure a successful simulation scenario are outlined, and the advantages and barriers to the use of simulation technology in anesthesia education are discussed.

DOI: 10.4018/978-1-5225-6289-4.ch003

INTRODUCTION

Since the late 20th century, anesthesia has served as a leader in the advancement of medical education by integrating technology and simulation into educational practices. Simulation can be defined as being the imitation of real processes or situations for the practice of skills, problem solving, and judgment; and it is often combined with software-based simulation, mannequins, and virtual reality to facilitate learning (Rosen, 2008). The incorporation of simulation technology for educational purposes advances not only students' acquisition of procedural skills but also improves patient care and safety (Jones, Passos-Neto, & Braghiroli, 2015). The importance of improving patient safety was brought to light in 2000 when the National Institute of Medicine report *To Err is Human* revealed that the number of deaths due to medical errors in the US exceeded the numbers deaths caused by breast cancer, motor vehicle accidents, and AIDS (Kohn, Corrigan, & Donaldson, 1999). Still more contemporary estimates suggest that each year, as many as 400,000 American patients die due to medical errors, making medical errors the third leading cause of death in the United States (James, 2013). These alarming statistics and the increased demand to improve patient safety have influenced educational institutions to contemplate new methods of instruction in order to curve these numbers. Simulation technology is one method being used to improve medical education.

Before the advent of simulation-based education, the old paradigm of medical education largely consisted of an apprenticeship model in which trainees work with attending physicians to care for their patients and in which clinical decisions are shared among the attending physicians, residents, and medical students. While this "hands-on" model was sufficient for more commonplace medical problems, it did not adequately provide students and residents with experience in handling risky procedures (Jones et al., 2015). Alternatively, simulation provides a safe and controlled environment in which inexperienced trainees can rehearse high-risk procedures without posing a risk to actual patients (James, 2013). Simulation also permits for customization; allowing students to gain valuable experiences in technical training, communication, or even leadership skills—with unlimited repetition (Jones et al., 2015). This repetition enables students to learn from their mistakes so to master the correct response or technical skill. Richard Satava summarizes, "The greatest power of virtual reality is the ability to try and fail without consequence to animal or patient. It is only through failure – and learning the cause of failure – that the true pathway to success lies" (Satava, 2001). Simulation affords students the ability to make mistakes in a stress-free environment, discuss poor decisions, explore better options, and retain memories that improve patient care. Thus, simulation provides an innovative approach to medical education—one in which trainees can practice medical skills to be better prepared for clinical encounters, thereby potentially reducing patient risk (Jones et al., 2015). Furthermore, medicine is not alone in its endeavors to incorporate simulation into educational pursuits—as simulation has been an accepted part of training, assessment, and research in aviation, nuclear power, and the military (Chang, 2013). In fact, aviation saw a 50% reduction in aircraft accidents after incorporation of simulation-based learning models into their educational curriculum for pilots (Tegtmeyer, Ibsen, & Goldstein, 2001).

Although traditional anesthesia residency training consists of didactic lectures and observation with procedure practice occurring on patients with supervision, simulation has been found to be a more effective training tool to teach the skills necessary to perform invasive procedures (Good, 2003). In anesthesia, these procedures include endotracheal intubation, bronchoscopy, and central venous catheter insertion, among many others. In the following chapter, we will introduce the history of simulation technology and review the use of part-task trainers and high-fidelity mannequins. Particular attention will be given to the use of simulation to facilitate learning airway management, bronchoscopy, central venous catheterization, and complex-scenario educational experiences. The advantages and potential barriers to widespread use of simulation technology will also be explored.

A BRIEF HISTORY OF SIMULATION TECHNOLOGY IN ANESTHESIA

Medical education has greatly evolved over the last 200 years from requiring a simple apprenticeship to a graduate level education—necessitating competency in knowledge, technical skill, and professional behavior (Rosen, 2008). This transition in curriculum has largely been a reflection of improved medical knowledge, research, and advances in technology. Although the introduction of human patient simulation toward the end of the 20th century was a major step in the evolution of health sciences education, simulation has been present in medicine for centuries. During Antiquity, models were built of clay in order to demonstrate clinical features of disease processes (Jones et al., 2015). As history progressed, so did the quality of simulation. In 18th century Paris, an obstetrical mannequin named the Phantom was created from a human pelvis and a dead baby in order to aid in instruction on delivery techniques for decreased adverse events associated with delivery (Rosen, 2008). Although Italy was the primary source of medical simulators in the early 18th century, dominance in clinical simulation moved north to France, Britain, and Germany in the 19th century (Owen, 2012). Examples of simulation education are present throughout history and can be found in many different cultures and countries; however, the roots of modern day medical simulation are largely based on advances in aviation simulation technology used for training (Cooper & Taqueti, 2008; Loftin, 2002; Rosen, 2008).

In 1929, Edwin Link created the first patented prototype flight trainer called the "blue box" with the hope of creating a comparatively safer and less expensive way to learn the skill of flying (L3 Link, 2017; Rosen, 2008). Although the "blue box" was initially utilized as an amusement park ride, by the mid 1930's the blue box's teaching capabilities were being recognized and utilized by the military (Rosen, 2008). Use of this trainer flourished during WWII due to military needs, which also led to the creation of the first bomber crew trainer and airplane specific simulation model (ibid.). During the 1950's, the use of the trainers again increased due to military expenditure caused by the Korean War and the Federal Aviation Administration requirement for simulation recertification to maintain commercial pilots' licenses (Dorey, 2010; ibid). The 1950's also brought the first computers, leading to the creation of more realistic flight simulation technology (Strachan, 2000).

In 1954, Link Aviation was sold to General Precision Equipment Corporation (GPE) (L3 Link, 2017). Under this new leadership, GPE collaborated with the National Aeronautics and Space Administration (NASA) to incorporate the first analog and digital computers into new advanced simulators in the 1960's (Myers, 1998). From this point, simulation technology continued to thrive in military, which prior to the 1990's was responsible for 80% of all the modeling and simulation used for education. After the 1990's the world of gaming took over the role of leader for the production and use of simulation technology (Drake, 1998).

Building on the success of simulation technology used for aviation education, the modern medical world saw its first simulation model in 1960 (Laerdal Medical, 2006). This model was referred to as Resusci-Anne and was used to teach mouth-to-mouth cardiopulmonary resuscitation (Jones et al., 2015). Resusci-Anne was created by Ausmund Laerdal, a toy manufacturer, inspired by the work of Peter Safar, who described the efficacy of mouth-to-mouth cardiopulmonary resuscitation (ibid.). When looking for what form his medical model should take, Laederal decided to take his inspiration from the death mask of a famous young French drowning victim from the 1890's, the Girl from the River Seine (ibid.; Laerdal Medical, 2006). It can only be assumed that this young girl might have benefited from the life-saving techniques of mouth-to-mouth resuscitation—a fact that Laederal hoped would inspire students to learn the proper technique of cardiopulmonary resuscitation with the model (Jones et al., 2015; Laerdal Medical, 2006). Although Resusci-Anne was initially designed only for mouth-to-mouth breathing, with the continued help of Safar she quickly evolved, and a spring was added in her chest for the practice of cardiopulmonary resuscitation (CPR) with cardiac compression simulation (Jones et al., 2015). Resusci-Anne also enabled physicians to practice hyperextension of the neck and chin lift for improved airway obstruction management (ibid.). Due to the undeniable benefit of cardiopulmonary resuscitation, Rescusci-Anne became the most widely used CPR mannequin of the 20th century; however, a new model named Harvey came into existence in 1968 (Jones et al., 2015; Michael S. Gordon Center for Research in Medical Education [GCRME], 2007). Harvey was developed at the University of Miami to mimic any cardiac disease by simulating blood pressure, breathing, pulses, heart sounds, and heart murmurs as well as lung disease (GCRME, 2007). The ability for learners to auscultate both heart murmurs and lung sounds using Harvey creates a realistic experience that easily translated to real patients. The 1960's also brought the development of a patient simulator referred to as Sim One created by Abrahamson, Denson, and their fellow colleagues at the University of Southern California (Good, 2003). This simulator featured a heartbeat which was synchronized with the temporal and carotid artery pulsations with a measurable blood pressure and spontaneous breathing. The eyes and mouth of the Sim One stimulator also opened and closed through a computer program control that allowed the simulator more lifelike qualities and responses to treatment. Sim One was one of the first models that could respond to several intravenous anesthetic medications, as well as to inhaled oxygen and nitrous oxide. These capabilities (built on those initially seen in Harvey) allowed first-year anesthesia residents to learn not only endotracheal intubation but also the basic skills of intravenously inducing general anesthesia (Good, 2003; Abrahamson, Denson, & Wolf, 1969)

As technology continued to improve during the 1980s and 1990s, software and computerized simulation systems were developed with the capability to mimic physiologic responses—allowing for immediate action feedback for learners (Jones et al., 2015). These systems relied on new technology such as the Macintosh computer and waveform generators in order to simulate physiologic responses to the use of anesthesia (Good, 2003). In the mid-1980s, teams of anesthesiologists at the University of Florida and at Stanford University each used this new technology in order to develop simulators with real-time physiologic feedback. At the University of Florida, anesthesiologists developed the Gainesville Anesthesia Simulator (GAS) with the objective to increase first-year anesthesia residents' skill acquisition and improve senior anesthesia residents' ability to detect and correct rare and complex failures related to the anesthesia gas delivery equipment (Good, 2003). While at Stanford University, a group led by David Gaba developed the Comprehensive Anesthesia Simulation Environment (CASE) and used the system to create and apply an educational curriculum known as Anesthesia Crisis Resource Management (ACRM) (Good, 2003). Both the GAS and CASE simulation systems underwent refinements throughout the 1980s and early 1990's before being manufactured on a larger scale and made commercially available for the use of other educational institutions (Good, 2003). The 1980's also brought the development of skill trainers for procedures such as fiberoptic bronchoscopy, epidural catheter insertion, and central venous catheter insertion (Chang, 2013).

The application of simulation technology for anesthesia education took another turn in the early 21st century as virtual reality simulation came into existence (Jones et al., 2015). In 2007, an internet-based forum called "Second Life" was created, providing medical students with the capability of practicing taking a patient history and clinical examination in a virtual world (Jones et al., 2015). The early 2000s also saw the development of The Society for Simulation in Healthcare, a group dedicated to the advancement of simulation as a tool for healthcare learning. This group also spearheaded the creation of an annual international meeting in 2004 and began publishing an official journal in 2006 entitled, "Simulation in Healthcare" (Chang, 2013). Due to the commitment of the Society for Simulation in Healthcare and those dedicated to the pursuit of simulation learning, today there are numerous simulator systems being professionally manufactured. These simulation systems feature ever-enhancing technology, physiological sophistication, and realism in order to continually improve the simulation learning experience (Cooper & Taqueti, 2008; Good, 2003; Rosen, 2008). In 2011, a survey conducted by the Association of American Medical Colleges found that simulation technology was used by up to 94% of 90 United States medical schools responding to the questionnaire (Passiment, Sacks, & Huang, 2011). In the same survey, approximately 86% of the 64 teaching hospitals questioned were using simulation for educational purposes at some point during a five-year span of residency education. These percentages represent a growing trend towards the use of simulation education in anesthesia training as well as in other medical specialties in both the United States and around the world (Good, 2003; Passiment et al., 2011).

CURRENT USE AND EFFICACY OF SIMULATION TECHNOLOGY IN ANESTHESIA LEARNING

Due to the procedural competency and crisis management skills necessary to advance in the field of anesthesiology, educational experiences in a low-stakes virtual environment enhance learning and increase patient safety (Yang, Wei, Xue, Deng, & Zhi, 2016). This section will review the use and efficacy of part-task trainers and full body mannequins for anesthesiology education. Anesthesia has long been at the forefront of simulation technology integration for education, as reflected by the large variety of task trainer models and full-scale mannequin simulators available for use.

Part Task Trainers

Part task trainers are simplified models designed and used to teach the introduction to specific skills. These trainers allow learners to gain knowledge of the basic set-up for procedures, positioning, and steps for a successful procedure on models with normal anatomy. By first becoming familiar with a procedure using part task trainers, learners can subsequently be better prepared when managing actual patient undergoing procedures. The use of simulation allows for a low-stakes, safe environment for improved learning where instructors can openly give feedback.

Airway Trainers

Proper airway management represents a fundamental skill for any anesthesiologist. In clinical practice, the failure to secure or manage a patient's airway – especially when presented with a difficult airway – can be a challenging task. Furthermore, the associated morbidity and mortality of failure to manage a patient's airway speaks to the need for superior training and experience in airway management (Kennedy, Cannon, Warner, & Cook, 2014). To increase knowledge of airway management skills for practitioners, medical centers can implement airway task-trainers to enhance learning at a more affordable price as compared to full-body simulators.

A large variety of task trainers are currently available and can be used for airway skills, bag-and-mask ventilation, direct laryngoscopy, placement of supraglottic devices, fiberoptic intubation, and one-lung ventilation. Trainers for these skills have differing anatomy but commonly include anatomic representations of the head, neck, and upper torso (Figure 1). Most of the available trainers also include mobility of the neck and jaw of the models to allow students to learn proper positioning of the head and neck during placement of oral and nasal airways and mask ventilation. Task trainers such as these are great tools for teaching the basics of airway skills in the setting of normal anatomy without complications.

More sophisticated airway task trainers have also been developed in order to teach the necessary skills of airway management. These trainers commonly allow for alteration to the normal anatomy of the model such that the tongue can be inflated and the airway can be made to mimic swelling. The jaw and neck of these models can also be adjusted to restrict mobility to teach students "can't-intubate"/"can't-ventilate" patient scenarios. While the challenge of recreating the many possible anatomical changes that result in a difficult airway can be challenging, these models demonstrate common causes of problematic airways and allow learners to gain valuable experience with working through the difficult airway algorithm (Torsher & Craigo, 2014).

Figure 1. Part task trainer with normal airway anatomy that can be used for acquisition of basic airway management skills
Source: Photo courtesy of Courtney McCain

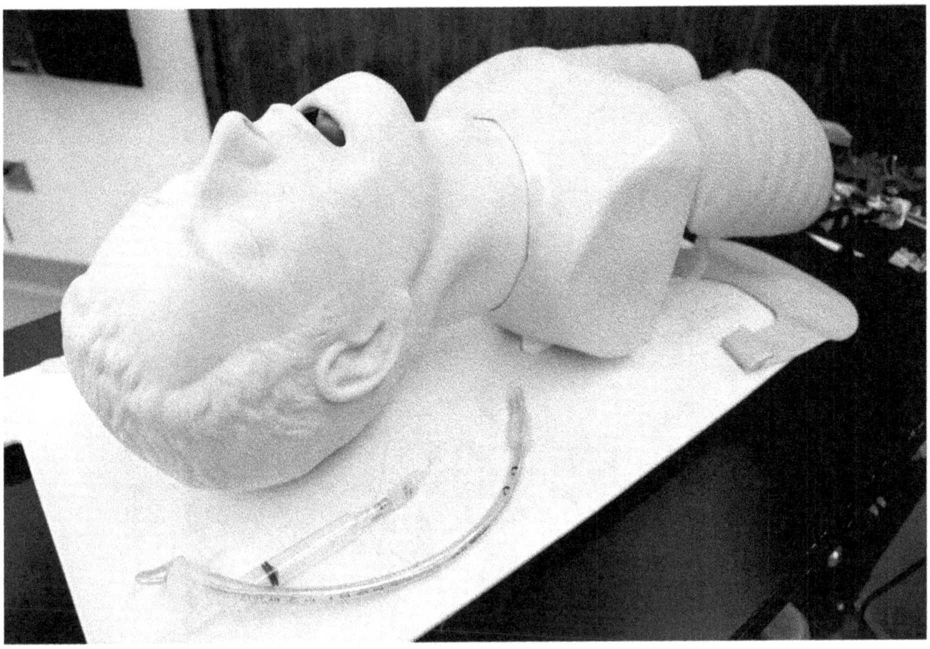

Whole-body simulation mannequins can also be utilized for teaching airway management; however, these systems are costly and more cumbersome to set-up—making them comparatively less suitable if applied to only basic airway management (Torsher & Craigo, 2014). Potential benefits of using a whole-body simulator include the ability to simulate the effects of multiple attempts at airway acquisition, such as hemodynamic instability and hypoxia.

It should be noted that all of these trainers can be used with video laryngoscopes for practice using the device as well as for increased student knowledge of airway anatomy and proper endotracheal tube placement (Figure 2). The laryngoscope can also be used with most anatomically-correct task trainers to enhance students' knowledge of underlying anatomical considerations.

Simulation through the use of part-task trainers, as described above, provides a safe environment for airway management learning that allows for multiple attempts to practice both technical skills and crisis management. The benefits of simulation-based airway management training was shown in a meta-analysis by Kennedy, Cannon, Warner, and Cook in 2014. According to this meta-analysis, simulation-based airway management training was shown to be effective with learners exhibiting increased

Figure 2. Video laryngoscope use with upper airway part task trainer allowing for visualization of airway anatomy and proper endotracheal tube placement
Source: Photo courtesy of Courtney McCain

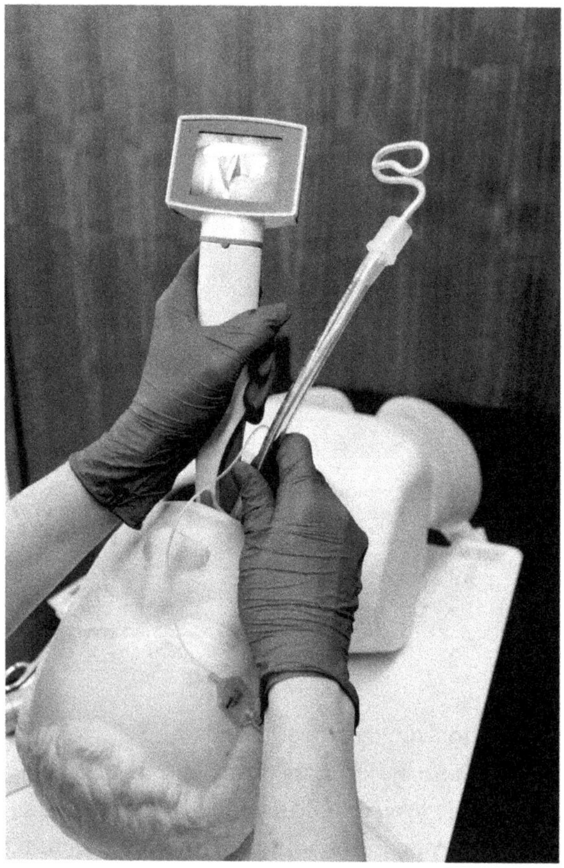

crisis management skills as well as improved learning satisfaction and patient effects when compared to no intervention and non-simulation education such as lectures, video instruction, and self-study (Kennedy et al., 2014). Furthermore, Naik and Brien showed that a simulation-based warm-up resulted in learners being better able to rapidly and efficiently complete endotracheal intubation in the operating room, resulting in decreased operating times and improved patient safety (Naik & Brien, 2013).

Although part-task trainers and whole-body high-fidelity trainers have been developed with considerable anatomical consideration, there remain some limitations to these trainers when compared to practice on patients. One such limitation is the possibility of increased difficulty in creating a seal with supraglottic devices such as a laryngeal mask airway (Torsher & Craigo, 2014). Other limitations include the decreased realism compared to learning in a clinical setting with patients as well as the cost associated with obtaining the trainers themselves.

Bronchoscopy Trainers

Bronchoscopy and the technique of guiding the thin camera scope to its desired location within the lungs require both proper recognition of anatomy as well as proficient ability to manipulate the scope. While the development of the video laryngoscope has decreased the use of bronchoscopy for management of the difficult airway, knowledge of the technique remains necessary in both the operating room and intensive care setting. Bronchoscopy trainers continue to be a valuable resource for learners who desire to master efficient scope operation for securing difficult airways, visualization of airway anatomy, broncheoalveolar lavage, and specimen retrieval (Torsher & Craigo, 2014).

Although sufficient practice is necessary to master the skill of fiberoptic orotracheal intubation (FOI), the number of patients with difficult airways requiring the skill is limited, leading to the necessity of simulation education for adequate FOI experience during training (Naik et al. 2001). Bronchoscopy simulation trainers are available as 3-dimentional models and screen-based high-fidelity systems. 3-dimentional systems commonly include accurate proximal airway anatomy to the level of the carina followed distally by a system of sequentially smaller branching tubes. These smaller branching tubes are easily constructed and allow learners to practice scope camera orientation and the skill of driving the scope (Torsher & Craigo, 2014). Screen-based high-fidelity bronchoscopic trainers are also available for use learning the skill of FOI. These systems consist of a controller that resembles a bronchoscope and a computer screen-based system that shows simulated images of the anatomy encountered based on the manipulation of the controller. Advantages to these simulation systems include the ability of the system to depict detailed anatomy as well as convenience of using the simulator (Torsher & Craigo, 2014).

Interestingly, there does not appear to be enhanced skill acquisition of securing the airway with sophisticated bronchoscopic simulators in terms of time to complete a task compared with less sophisticated models (Crabtree, Chandra, Weiss, Joo, & Naik, 2008). Likewise, it has been shown that the skills learned with FOI simulation training using a simple model transferred with greater efficacy into the operating room setting than learning the skill though conventional didactic instruction (Naik et al. 2001). A meta-analysis completed by Kennedy, Maldonado, and Cook in 2013 also demonstrated that a plastic part-task trainer model use to simulate the bronchial tree was more effective than was a non-anatomic wooden model, and that a rubber-plastic model was favored over a virtual-reality simulator (Kennedy et al., 2013).

Kennedy's study also found through comparison of various training approaches that a longer simulation training program or one with more structures was comparatively more effective for bronchoscopic learning (Kennedy et al., 2013).

Central Line Placement Trainers

Proficiency in central line venous catheterization is an important skill for anesthesiologists, critical care, emergency medicine, and internal medicine professionals alike for improved patient care. However, although central venous catheterization monitoring is an essential tool, the procedure comes with several risks. It is estimated that anywhere from 5% to 26% of patients experience an infectious complication related to their central venous catheter (Gerolemou et al., 2014). Besides infectious complications such as catheter-associated bloodstream infection and sepsis, other potential adverse events include arterial puncture, excessive blood loss, pneumothorax, and even death. The serious nature of these complications highlight the need for proficiency in both sterile technique as well as in actual placement of central venous catheters. Additionally, the likelihood of these adverse events has been seen to decrease independently with increasing operator experience level, ultrasound guidance, proper sterile technique, and appropriate needle placement, which are all skills that through educational simulation have been shown to improve (Evans et al., 2010).

Part-task simulation models provide a safe way for residents and medical students alike to learn proper technique for central venous catheterization. These models often take the form of the neck and torso and include accurate underlying bony architecture and vascular system with internal jugular, subclavein, and potentially even femoral cannulation capabilities. In addition, trainers that feature accurate replication of the trachea, nerves, and surrounding muscles with reflective properties can be used to teach ultrasound-guided central line placement (Torsher & Craigo, 2014)(Figure 3). While central venous cannulation was historically done aided only by the identification of surrounding palpable anatomic structures and arterial pulsations, ultrasound is now commonly employed to help increase procedure success through visualization of the target, identify anatomical variations, and decrease complications related to needle placement. The skills necessary for the successful cannulation include correct patient positioning, preparation, and sterilization as well as tray setup, identification of landmarks, puncture of the vessel, dilation of the tissue path, and confirmation of guidewire placement. The patient's vitals and comfort must also be monitored throughout the procedure, as cardiac arrhythmias are a possible adverse effect due to direct stimulation of the right heart by the guidewire (Stuart et al. 1990).

Figure 3. Example of part-task simulator that can be used for central venous catheterization with accurate neurovascular representation allowing for use of ultrasound-guided placement of the catheter
Source: Photo courtesy of Courtney McCain

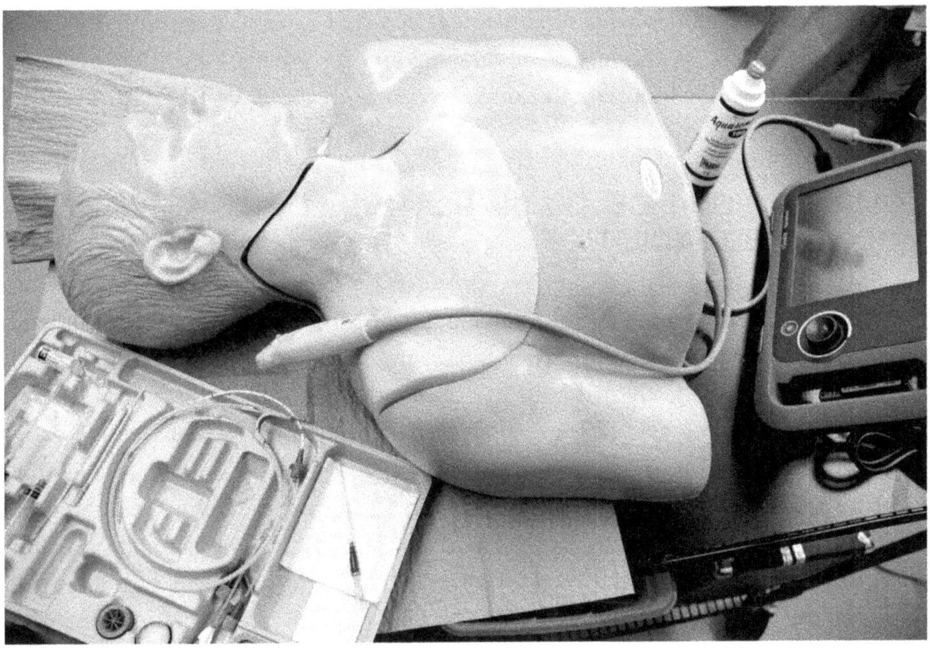

As with other examples of simulation education use before procedures are attempted on patients, the pressure-free environment of simulated central line cannulation allows learners to master basic skills and setup of the procedure without concern for adverse events immediately impacting an actual patient. Once learners are ready to advance to bedside teaching with an actual patient, they can concentrate on more advanced skills such as identification of anatomical variations without concern over familiarity with the basics of the procedure (Torsher & Craigo, 2014). Furthermore, Evans et al. (2010) was able to show that simulation training of ultrasound-guided central venous catheter insertion skills on a partial task trainer improved the success of the procedure in subsequent clinical practice. Evans determined this through a prospective, controlled, single-blind study observing the clinical success of central line placement of 195 first- and second-year residents after being randomized into a group taught the procedure with competency-based simulation training versus training based on the bedside apprenticeship model. The results of the study showed that simulation training was both independently and significantly associated with greater success at first cannulation in the clinical setting (Evans et al., 2010). Peltan, Shiga, Gordon, and Currier (2015) also found that simulation central venous cannulation training in addition to standard lecture and video-based training improved protocol adherence and resident competency, and reduced rates of complications such as central-line associated blood stream infections and arterial puncture. Based on these studies, part task trainers are a valuable tool for greater educational efficacy for residents as well as for patient safety.

COMPLEX HIGH-FIDELITY SIMULATION MODELS AND FACILITIES

Complex whole-body simulation models have become the mainstay for academic programs desiring a versatile educational simulation experience. Beginning in the 1990's, anesthesiology residents and medical students have used high-fidelity simulators to the effect of quicker responses, better performance, and less deviation from accepted procedure protocol (Chopra et al, 1994). Patient simulators are now used to train physicians of many specialties, nurses, and emergency care personnel for both basic and advanced clinical skills (Good, 2003). Most complex simulators feature head, neck, trunk, pelvis, and limbs with ever-increasing advances in realism and ability to portray different disease processes. The simulation mannequins commonly have speakers that allow for a stethoscope to auscultate the heart and lungs, a chest that rises with each respiratory cycle, and palpable pulses over the carotid, radial, and femoral arteries. Normal or abnormal heart sounds can be controlled by the instructor either in the room or in a control booth (Figure 4). Clinical scenarios can also be automatically programmed in many mannequin systems that include changing heart sounds and pulses. The mannequins feature accompanying synchronized monitors with vitals and electrocardiogram capabilities (Figure 5). Of great interest to anesthesia education, the airway of the mannequins can feature a lung model capable of simulating spontaneous breaths and is compatible with assisted and controlled mechanical ventilation with endotracheal intubation. Some mannequins even feature lung models that allow for oxygen consumption, exhalation of carbon dioxide, and take up or exhale of anesthetic gases (Good, 2003). The sophistication of these lung models allows for the simulation mannequins to be compatible with spirometers, mechanical ventilation systems, and gas analyzers for learners to obtain realistic measurements from corresponding data displays. This capability allows for simulation scenarios such as anesthesia machine malfunction, contaminated air supply, intravenous air embolism, status asthmaticus, failed intubation with inability to ventilate, and malignant hyperthermia. For simulation of "can't-intubate-can't-

Figure 4. Complex whole-body simulation model with in-room control system for scenario variation
Source: Photo courtesy of Courtney McCain

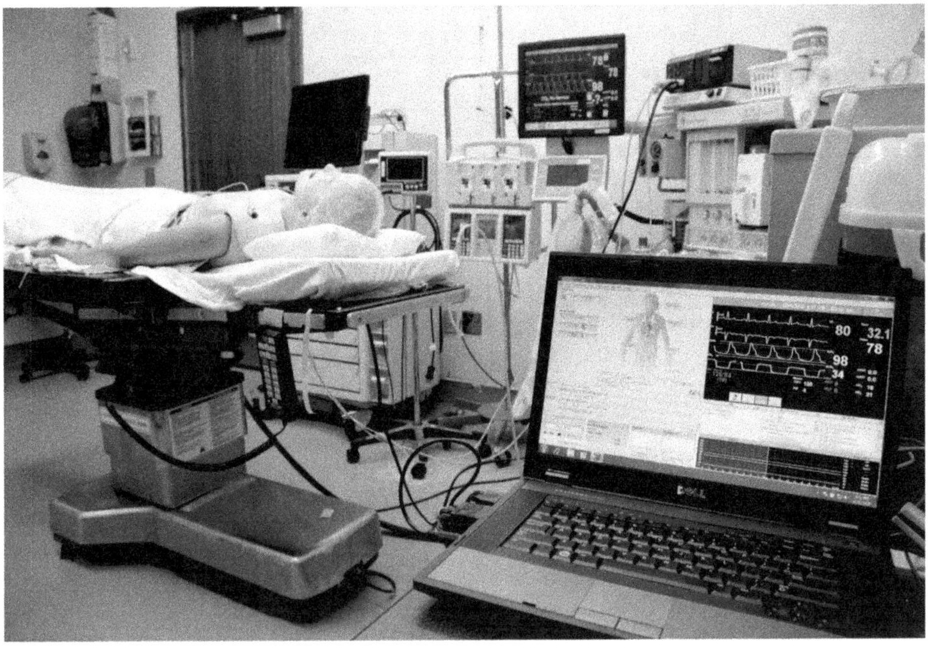

ventilate" scenarios, transtracheal jet ventilation and emergency cricothyrotomy can be practiced as the model can allow for transtracheal needle, catheter, or tube placement (Good, 2003).

Additional features include the production of invasive arterial, central venous, and pulmonary artery (PA) pressure, and pulmonary capillary wedge pressure waveforms through the placement of a pulmonary artery catheter with corresponding displays. The cardiac and respiratory cycles can also be controlled by the instructor to change in association with the real-time influences of the advancing pulmonary catheter (Good, 2003). Likewise, cardiac output can be obtained from these modules through simulation of the thermodilution technique by mimicking the injection of cold saline into the right atrium and observing temperature change over time measured by a catheter in the pulmonary artery (ibid.). Needles can also be introduced into the second intercostal space to allow for management of tension pneumothorax. Along the same lines, chest tubes can be placed in the lateral chest wall with resulting collection of fluid or blood in advanced systems. Not to be overlooked, electrical cardioversion and defibrillation can also be performed using standard hospital equipment by way of electrical posts mounted on the chest of most mannequins. Advances in high-

Figure 5. Complex whole-body simulation model with accompanying synchronized monitors displaying vitals
Source: Photo courtesy of Courtney McCain

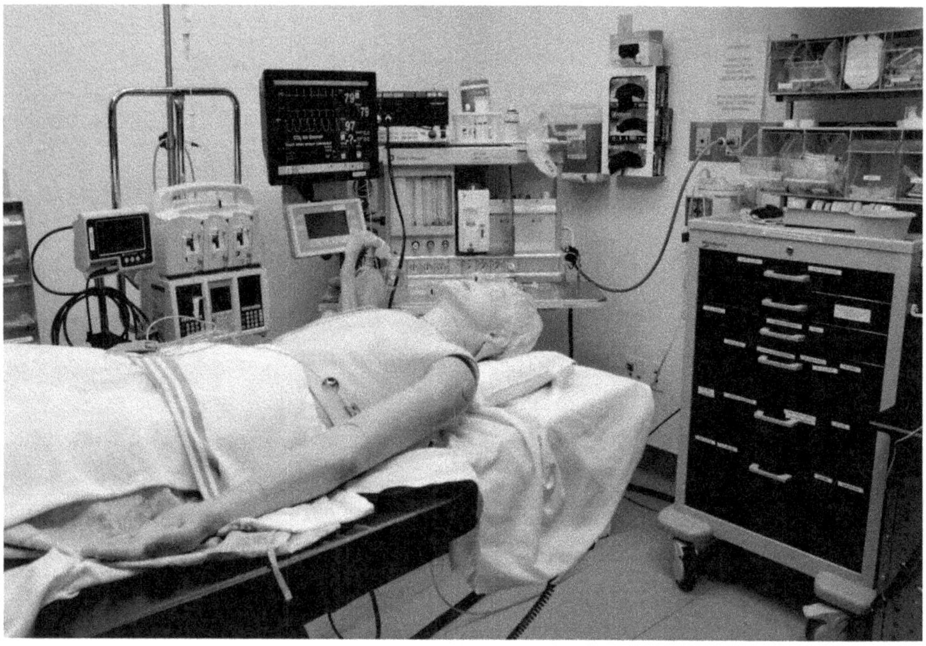

fidelity simulation mannequins, such as these, continue to evolve to incorporate new technology for an ever-expanding repertoire of learning opportunities.

Many health systems are seeking simulation facilities that can provide learning opportunities for almost every domain of health care. These facilities feature high-fidelity simulation models in realistic settings such as simulated patient rooms with bathrooms, labor and delivery rooms, functioning operating rooms, and intensive care settings. These rooms are also commonly designed to mimic the room layout at the given facility and are outfitted with identical accessories and location of recourses. In order to monitor the simulation exercise in each room, these centers employ audiovisual equipment for recording simulation exercises with control rooms for live monitoring of the educational exercises (Figure 6). Personnel in these control rooms can change elements of the scenario and initiate physiological resolution once the correct intervention has been completed. The rooms also facilitate inter-professional learning as techs, emergency personnel, nurses, and physicians can come together to practice scenarios with an emphasis on teamwork and good communication.

Debriefing rooms, collaborative workspace, and classrooms are other components incorporated into simulation facilities. While these facilities represent a great

Figure 6. Simulation center control room with audio and visual capabilities
Source: Photo courtesy of Courtney McCain

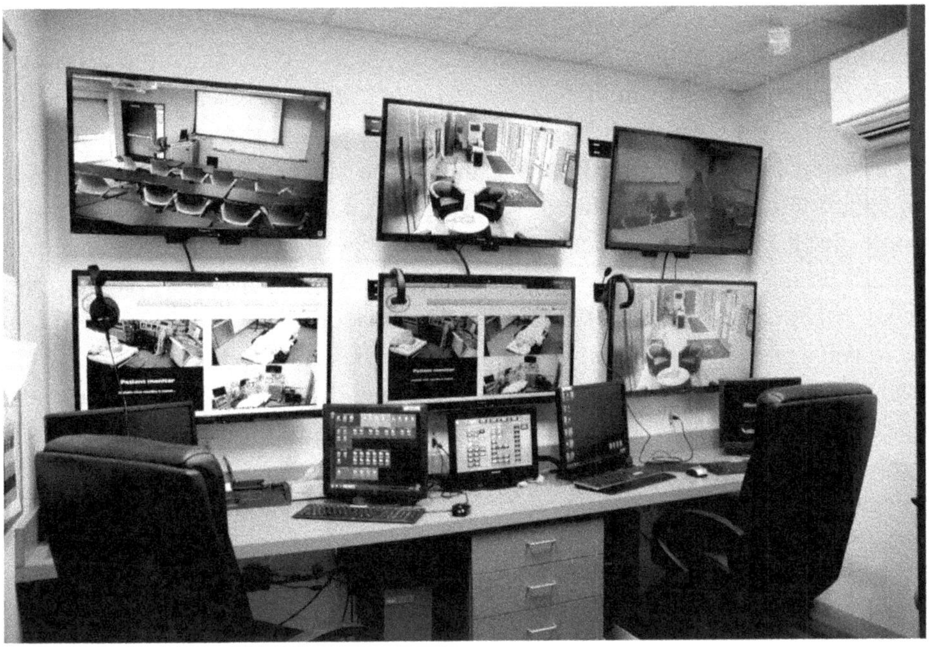

educational resource for learning for all medical professionals they are also a significant investment. The initial cost for a freestanding simulation center in 2008 was estimated to cost anywhere from $200,000 to $1.6 million USD, not including $15,000 USD for annual maintenance as well as the cost to staff the facility and building expenses (Tuoriniemi & Schott-Baer, 2008). As patient simulator technology continues to advance combined with the growing trend of freestanding simulation centers, it is reasonable to imagine greater expenditure related to simulation education, but also the value gained from a hands-on educational experience.

SIMULATION SCENARIO STRUCTURE

According to Pazin et al (2007), successful simulation sessions are comprised of four core components. The first of these is "exposure" and consists of the participants being briefed on the patient and case ahead. This is followed by "sequence," which is accomplished by creating sessions with escalating complexity to help participants build upon consolidated knowledge as one might experience in a real-life clinical scenario. The third element is "feedback," referring to the continuous exchange of information between the scenario facilitator and the trainee during and after the simulation. The final component is "repetition," as repeat exposure to new knowledge increases information retention (Filho & Romano, 2007). However perhaps the most important element of the simulation education focuses on a structured debriefing session following each simulation scenario, or "feedback" according to Pazin's components. The debriefing session is used for feedback and commonly involves a physician facilitator and all participants of the scenario. Debriefing serves as an opportunity for the team to work through a guided reflection of the scenario. Topics discussed include outcomes, goals, inadequacies, quality of communication, teamwork, and – most importantly – how the experience affects future practice (Jones et al., 2015). Most sessions also identify the impact of the experience; clarify the facts, concepts, and principals; identify different views formed by participants; and evaluate how emotion was involved in the experience (Chang, 2013). Open-ended questions, positive reinforcement, and the use of cognitive aids are hallmarks of debriefing sessions (ibid.). The positive environment of these sessions allows trainees to gain insight toward a better understanding of the event, possible mistakes that were made, appropriate interventions, and its application to future experiences in the clinical setting – free from fear of criticism (Jones et al., 2015).

EDUCATIONAL ADVANTAGES OF SIMULATION TECHNOLOGY

As alluded to throughout this chapter, patient simulation has dramatically augmented medical education in the field of anesthesia, as well as across many specialties. This increased focus on using simulation as a tool to allow learners to acquire basic and advanced clinical skills has been shown to be an effective and safe alternative to previous methods used. The efficacy and utility of simulation in anesthesia training has been largely attributed to four main advantages (Good, 2003):

1. The training agenda can be determined by the needs of the learner, focusing on a whole procedure or breaking it down into specific components. The learner has the opportunity to practice these as often as necessary.
2. In a controlled environment, where mistakes do not put a patient at risk such as in a clinical setting, learners have "permission to fail" – and they get the opportunity to learn from their failures.
3. Simulators provide a great objective tool to measure the learners' performance, doing so using built-in tracking functions to highlight a learners' strengths and weaknesses with regards to a specific simulation.
4. Collaborative and individual learning can both be utilized with the simulation's ability to provide immediate feedback in digital form.

In 2006, a *New England Journal of Medicine* article entitled "Teaching Surgical Skills- Changes in the Wind" was published (Reznick & MacRae, 2006). The authors discussed the Fits and Posner Multi-stage theory regarding the three stages of learning and how it related to training physician's procedural skills. The authors argued that simulation allowed for each of these three stages to occur, ensuring that the learners successfully mastered the concepts taught with the simulations.

1. **Cognition:** The first stage, Cognition, is defined as developing an understanding of the task. The learner should be able to make a clear description and demonstration of what is trying to be accomplished.
2. **Integration:** The second stage, Integration, combines the knowledge obtained from the cognition into learning the motor skills for each task.
3. **Autonomous:** Finally, in the Autonomous stage, the learner no longer needs to think about how to execute the task—and can focus on other aspects of the procedure (Chang, 2013).

With this method of teaching, rare and complex clinical problems can be simulated in a way that provides a low-stress environment with no risk to a live patient. Previously, issues arose in that these clinical encounters did not occur with sufficient frequency to allow for trainees to get the exposure needed. When these encounters did occur, the severity of the cases required the taking of immediate measures to provide adequate patient care as opposed to there being an opportunity for a trainee to learn (Good, 2003). Simulation eliminates this problem. Trainees have the opportunity to run and react to cases including a patient experiencing anaphylaxis; cardiopulmonary arrest; tension pneumothorax; pulmonary embolism; or cardiogenic, hemorrhagic, and septic shock. Simulations of cases that are comparatively more specific to training anesthesiologists include malignant hyperthermia, a contaminated oxygen supply, intravenous air embolism, and a malfunction of the anesthesia gas delivery system (Good, 2003).

Another benefit uncovered by the recent incorporation of simulation into anesthesia training has been the enrichment of non-technical skills. Non-technical skills can be defined as cognitive, social, and personal resource skills that complement technical skills and contribute to safe and efficient task performance (Chang, 2013; Flin & Maran, 2004) The enrichment of this includes providing skills to trainees to interact in an effective manner according to a team-based model of practice. Patient simulation allows for the entire interdisciplinary health care team to practice responding to a specific clinical encounter and establish each of their roles in a safe, controlled environment (Good, 2003). This provides an opportunity to develop interpersonal skills – including communication, teamwork, and leadership – among the entire group. While simulation has improved group communication and has been an invaluable tool for enrichment of the interdisciplinary model of team-based care, it has also shown to improve individual behavioral skills needed by new practicing physicians.

Medical practice is characterized by a constant pursuit of perfection. During medical school and residency, trainees strive for an error-free practice in an environment where mistakes are not well accepted. As discussed above, simulation has helped minimize the impact of some of the common errors encountered by new trainees, serving as a tool to develop error management skills. Error management involves understanding the nature and causes of error in order to avoid further mistakes (Fernandez & Williams, 2009; Jones et al., 2015). This model is based on a training modality used by new pilots titled “Crew Resource Management.” With this concept, pilots are trained both on how to change conditions to induce errors and also on non-technical skills that can prevent them. These skills include optimal communication and teamwork (Helmreich, 2000; Jones et al., 2015). Simulation has proved an overdue stride by the medical field to embrace learning-based on mistakes, improving core competences such as knowledge, communication skills, teamwork, patient care, clinical skill, and professionalism (Sukalich, Elliott, & Ruffner 2014). Those in favor of simulation argue that simulation-based education provides behavioral techniques including coping skills that allow trainees to recover from errors in medical practice (Jones et al., 2015; Ziv, Ben-David, & Ziv, 2005).

Finally, one less explored benefit to simulation-based teaching is the elimination of past ethical dilemmas faced by teachers and trainees alike. Previously, two of the only opportunities that trainees had to practice advanced, less-commonly used skills had been either with animal models or with recently deceased patients. While these practices are still used, some argue that simulation eliminates this ethical ‘gray area” thus ensuring respect to patient autonomy. Whereas medical students and residents were taught important lessons in physiology and pharmacology with live animals, modern-day simulators can be programmed with sophisticated responses that emulate drug and physiologic responses, eliminating the need for practice on live animals (Good, 2003). Instead of using recently deceased patients to practice airway management skills, simulators have the ability to provide real-time changes in heart rate, blood pressure, and oxygen saturations not possible with deceased patients (Good, 2003). Simulation provides the opportunity for trainees to learn these valuable skills while eliminating the ethical dilemmas previously faced (Jones et al., 2015).

BARRIERS TO THE USE OF SIMULATION FOR EDUCATION

While simulation-based education has been widely accepted as an integral part of anesthesia training throughout the country, barriers exist that have prohibited this method from complete acceptance. As with most barriers associated with education, cost is a major limitation. As to be expected with such advanced technology, the cost to start and maintain a simulation program is very substantial. A significant issue for cost analysis in education and training is the absence of generally-accepted standardized cost models. In a 2011 survey conducted by the AAMC, 68 medical schools and 42 teaching hospitals provided data on their annual operating budget for medical simulation labs. Of this group, 57% of teaching hospitals and only 22% of medical schools reported having a budget of $250,000 or less. 15% of the medical schools and 11% of the teaching hospitals reported an annual budget in the $1-million- to $2-million-dollar range (Passiment, et al., 2011). The remaining responders reported annual costs somewhere between these two groups. These costs are significant and are not sustainable for all academic centers.

Another limitation often reported by trainees who have used medical simulation models is a lack of clinical realism. Although this gets better with continued advancement in technology, problems still exist. One example of such issue is seen with personnel who perform interventions that rely on a change in skin color as a way to measure success. (Good, 2003; Tuoriniemi & Schott-Baer, 2008). This has been addressed with newer simulators using colored lights as a way to signify a change; however, it is an imperfect solution. One way that operators of simulation labs combat this lack of clinical realism is by using a combination of patient simulators and standardized patients. Trainees perform a history and physical exam on a standardized patient, use a simulation model to perform the necessary appropriate interventions, and can then follow up with the standardized patient once the task is completed. This allows the trainee to follow the patient through their hospital course while enhancing the clinical realism of the scenario (Good, 2003).

One final barrier seen with simulation models is providing the time and resources necessary to training faculty on how to implement this simulation-based curriculum. Teaching physicians must learn how to teach the trainees using the simulators, as well as how to operate the simulators to portray the appropriate clinical scenario they desire. This is much different than teaching the skills to trainees on a live patient in a true clinical setting. Simulation companies have tried to make the transition easier by using fool-proof operating systems and user-friendly interfaces; however, issues still arise (Good, 2003). As discussed in the Simulation Scenario Structure section, there is a proper way to conduct a scenario; and instructors must also be trained on how to hold a productive and effective simulation. Although these barriers remain prevalent in simulation-based education, most training programs have found that the benefits outweigh the limitations.

CONCLUSION

The field of simulation technology for use in anesthesia education has grown markedly since the first contemporary simulation model was developed in 1960. Today, simulation part-task trainers as well as complex high-fidelity models are produced commercially with the capability of simulating a vast array of technically procedures and patient management techniques. The ever-evolving nature of simulation in medical education is driven by its potential to improve performance in knowledge, patient care, teamwork, communication, and clinical skills as well as professionalism (Good, 2003; Jones et al., 2015). Beyond just use for educational purposes, simulation technology is becoming an integral part for the assessment of skills and competency in anesthesia. This fact is highlighted by the American Board of Anesthesiology's (ABA's) decision to incorporate the OSCE (Objective Structured Clinical Examination) starting in March 2018 in addition to the traditional oral examination for board certification (The American Board of Anesthesiology, 2016). The OSCE will incorporate standardized patients as well as simulation technology in order to assess technical skills including interpretation of monitors in event scenarios, management of ventilator modes, and proficiency using echocardiogram and ultrasonography for patient care (The American Board of Anesthesiology, 2016). Due to the proven success of simulation technology for use in medical education (as described in this chapter) and its future role in skill assessment, it is clear that simulation will continue to play an integral part in anesthesia education in the years to come.

REFERENCES

Abrahamson, S., Denson, J. S., & Wolf, R. M. (1969). Effectiveness of a simulator in training anesthesiology residents. *Journal of Medical Education*, *44*, 515–519. doi:10.1136/qhc.13.5.395 PMID:5789592

Chang, C.-H. (2013). Medical simulation is needed in anesthesia training to achieve patient's safety. *Korean Journal of Anesthesiology*, *64*(3), 204–211. doi:10.4097/kjae.2013.64.3.204 PMID:23560184

Chopra, V., Gesink, B. J., de Jong, J., Bovill, J. G., Spierdijk, J., & Brand, R. (1994). Does training on an anesthesia simulator lead to improvement in performance? *British Journal of Anaesthesia*, *73*(3), 293–297. doi:10.1093/bja/73.3.293 PMID:7946851

Cooper, J. B., & Taqueti, V. R. (2008). A brief history of the development of mannequin simulators for clinical education and training. *Postgraduate Medical Journal, 84*(997), 563–570. doi:10.1136/qshc.2004.009886 PMID:19103813

Crabtree, N. A., Chandra, D. B., Weiss, I. D., Joo, H. S., & Naik, V. N. (2008). Fibreoptic airway training: Correlation of simulator performance and clinical skill. *Canadian Journal of Anaesthesia, 55*(2), 100–104. doi:10.1007/BF03016321 PMID:18245069

Dorey, S. (2010). *Link Aviation, A History. Susan Dorey Designs.* Accessed from www.susandoreydesigns.com/genealogy/clirehugh/LinkAviationHistory.pdf

Drake, J. (1998). Commercial simulation market drives industry's future growth. *National Defense Magazine.* Accessed November 12, 2007 from http://www.nationaldefensemagazine.org

Evans, L. V., Dodge, K. L., Shah, T. D., Kaplan, L. J., Siegel, M. D., Moore, C. L., ... D'Onofrio, G. (2010). Simulation training in central venous catheter insertion: Improved performance in clinical practice. *Academic Medicine, 85*(9), 1462–1469. doi:10.1097/ACM.0b013e3181eac9a3 PMID:20736674

Fernandez, E., & Williams, D. G. (2009). Training and the European working time directive: A 7 year review of paediatric anesthetic trainee caseload data. *British Journal of Anaesthesia, 103*(4), 566–569. doi:10.1093/bja/aep170 PMID:19556272

Filho, A. P., & Romano, M. M. D. (2007). Simulacao: Aspectos conceituais. *Rev Fac Med Ribeirao Preto, 40*(2), 167–170.

Flin, R., & Maran, N. (2004). Identifying and training non-technical skills for teams in acute medicine. *Quality & Safety in Health Care, 13*(Suppl. 1), i80–i84. doi:10.1136/qshc.2004.009993 PMID:15465960

Gerolemou, L., Fidellagra, A., Rose, K., Cooper, S., & Venturanza, M. (2014). Simulation-based training for nurses in sterile techniques during central vein catheterization. *American Journal of Critical Care, 23*(1), 40–48. doi:10.4037/ajcc2014860 PMID:24382616

Good, M. L. (2003). Patient simulation for training basic and advanced clinical skills. *Medical Education, 37*(1), 14–21. doi:10.1046/j.1365-2923.37.s1.6.x PMID:14641634

Helmreich, R. L. (2000). On error management: Lessons from aviation. *BMJ (Clinical Research Ed.)*, *320*(7237), 781–785. doi:10.1136/bmj.320.7237.781 PMID:10720367

James, J. T. (2013). A new, evidence-based estimate of patient harms associated with hospital care. *Journal of Patient Safety*, *9*(3), 122–128. doi:10.1097/PTS.0b013e3182948a69 PMID:23860193

Jones, F., Passos-Neto, C. E., & Braghiroli, O. F. M. (2015). Simulation in medical education: Brief history and methodology. *J PPCR*, *1*(2), 56–63.

Kennedy, C. C., Cannon, E. K., Warner, D. O., & Cook, D. A. (2014). Advanced airway management simulation training in medical education: A systematic review and meta-analysis. *Critical Care Medicine*, *42*(1), 169–178. doi:10.1097/CCM.0b013e31829a721f PMID:24220691

Kennedy, C. C., Maldonado, F., & Cook, D. A. (2013). Simulation-based bronchoscopy training: Systemic review and meta-analysis. *Chest*, *144*(1), 183–192. doi:10.1378/chest.12-1786 PMID:23370487

Kohn, L. T., Corrigan, J. M., & Donaldson, M. S. (1999). *To err is human: Building a safer health system*. Washington, DC: National Academy Press.

L3 Link. (2017). *Innovation heritage*. Accessed October 15, 2017 from http://www.link.com/about#our-innovation-heritage

Laerdal Medical. (2006). *The girl from the River Seine (History in brief)*. Accessed September 24, 2017 from http://www.laerdal.com/about/default.htm

Loftin, B. (2002). Med school 1.0: Can computer simulation aid physician training. *Quest*, *5*(5), 16–19.

Michael S. Gordon Center for Research in Medical Education. (2007). *History/Overview*. Accessed September 24, 2017 from http://www.crme.med.miami.edu/history.html

Myers, B. A. (1998). A brief history of human computer interaction technology. *Interactions (New York, N.Y.)*, *5*(2), 44–54. doi:10.1145/274430.274436

Naik, V. N., & Brien, S. E. (2013). Review article: Simulation: A means to address and improve patient safety. *Canadian Journal of Anaesthesia*, *60*(2), 192–200. doi:10.100712630-012-9860-z PMID:23239487

Naik, V. N., Matsumoto, E. D., Houston, P. L., Hamstra, S. J., Yeung, R. Y.-M., Mallon, J. S., & Martire, T. M. (2001). Fiberoptic orotracheal intubation on anesthetized patients: Do manipulation skills learned on a simple model transfer into the operating room? *Anesthesiology*, *95*(2), 343–348. doi:10.1097/00000542-200108000-00014 PMID:11506104

Owen, H. (2012, April). Early use of simulation in medical education. *Simulation in Healthcare*, *7*(2), 102–116. doi:10.1097/SIH.0b013e3182415a91 PMID:22374231

Passiment, M., Sacks, H., & Huang, G. (2011, Sept.). *Medical simulation in medical education: Results of an AAMc survey*. Association of American Medical Colleges. Accessed from https://www.aamc.org/download/259760/data/

Peltan, I. D., Shiga, T., Gordon, J. A., & Currier, P. F. (2015). Simulation improves procedural protocol adherence during central venous catheter placement: A randomized-controlled trial. *Simulation in Healthcare*, *10*(5), 270–276. doi:10.1097/SIH.0000000000000096 PMID:26154250

Reznick, R. K., & MacRae, H. (2006). Teaching surgical skills — changes in the wind. *The New England Journal of Medicine*, *355*(25), 2664–2669. doi:10.1056/NEJMra054785 PMID:17182991

Rosen, K. R. (2008). The history of medical simulation. *Journal of Critical Care*, *23*(2), 157–166. doi:10.1016/j.jcrc.2007.12.004 PMID:18538206

Satava, R. M. (2001). Accomplishments and challenges of surgical simulation: Dawning of the next-generation surgical education. *Surgical Endoscopy*, *15*(3), 232–241. doi:10.1007004640000369 PMID:11344421

Strachan, I. W. (2000). Technology leaps all around propel advances in simulators. *National Defense Magazine*. Accessed November 19, 2007 from http://www.nationaldefensemagazine.org

Stuart, R. K., Shikora, S. A., Akerman, P., Lowell, J. A., Baxter, J. K., Apovian, C., ... Bistrian, B. R. (1990). Incidence of arrhythmia with central venous catheter insertion and exchange. *JPEN. Journal of Parenteral and Enteral Nutrition*, *14*(2), 152–155. doi:10.1177/0148607190014002152 PMID:2112623

Sukalich, S., Elliott, J. O., & Ruffner, G. (2014). Teaching medical error disclosure to residents using patient-centered simulation training. *Acad Med J Assoc Am Med Coll*, *89*(1), 136–144. doi:10.1097/ACM.0000000000000046 PMID:24280843

Tegtmeyer, K., Ibsen, L., & Goldstein, B. (2001). Computer-assisted learning in critical care: From ENIAC to HAL. *Critical Care Medicine, 29*(8Suppl), N177–N182. doi:10.1097/00003246-200108001-00006 PMID:11496040

The American Board of Anesthesiology. (2016). *Standardized Oral Examination (SOE) and Objective Structured Clinical Examination (OSCE)*. Raleigh, NC: ABA. Accessed from http://www.theaba.org/TRAINING-PROGRAMS/APPLIED-(Staged-Exam)/About-APPLIED-(Staged-Exam)

Torsher, L., & Craigo, P. (2014). Simulation in anesthesiology. In A. I. Levine & ... (Eds.), *The Comprehensive Textbook of Healthcare Simulation* (pp. 257–285). New York: Springer.

Tuoriniemi, P., & Schott-Baer, D. (2008). Implementing a high-fidelity simulation program in a community college setting. *Nursing Education Perspectives, 29*(2), 105–109. doi:10.1097/00024776-200803000-00012 PMID:18459626

Yang, D., Wei, Y. K., Xue, F. S., Deng, X. M., & Zhi, J. (2016). Simulation-based airway management training: Application and looking forward. *Journal of Anesthesia, 30*(2), 284–289. doi:10.100700540-015-2116-7 PMID:26671260

Ziv, A., Ben-David, S., & Ziv, M. (2005). Simulation[-]based medical education: An opportunity to learn from errors. *Medical Teacher, 27*(3), 193–199. doi:10.1080/01421590500126718 PMID:16011941

KEY TERMS AND DEFINITIONS

Bronchoscopy: A technique of visualizing the inside of the airways via an endoscopic camera for diagnostic and therapeutic purposes. A bronchoscope is inserted either through the mouth, nose, or tracheostomy and then progressed into the airways.

Cricothyrotomy: A procedure that established an airway for oxygenation and ventilation by placing a tube through an incision in the cricothyroid membrane.

Electrocardiogram: A record or display shoeing the electrical activity of the heart over a period of time. The reading is obtained using electrodes placed on the skin and attached to a monitor.

Endotracheal Intubation: The medical procedure where a flexible plastic tube is placed into the trachea via the mouth or nose to maintain an open airway and allow for assisted patient ventilation.

High-Fidelity Simulation: Simulations systems that attempt to be as realistic as possible with multiple elements that allow for training of a large number of tasks. These simulation systems also simulate the relationship or interactions between their different elements.

Part Task Trainer: A training device that is designed for education of only a particular task. These trainers allow for repeated practice of a specific skill.

Thermodilution Technique: Method for determining cardiac output of the heart by measuring the thermal deficit created by a cold solution moving through the right atrium and ventricle to the pulmonary artery by means of a temperature sensitive catheter. Measurements of the temperature change over time are charted on a curve and cardiac output is inversely proportional to the area under this curve.

Chapter 4
The Use of Mobile ECG Monitoring Devices in Embolic Stroke Associated With Atrial Fibrillation

Nikita Maniar
University of Missouri – Kansas City School of Medicine, USA

Charles Donohoe
University of Missouri – Kansas City School of Medicine, USA

Ellen Lau Troudt
University of Missouri – Kansas City School of Medicine, USA

ABSTRACT

Stroke prevention is a primary aim in clinical neurology. Atrial fibrillation (AF), the most common cardiac arrhythmia affecting 35 million people worldwide, carries a 5x risk of devastating stroke largely preventable with anticoagulation. The AliveCor Kardia™ mobile application for iPhones and Kardia Band™, a wristband for the Apple Watch, are approved by the Food and Drug Administration (FDA). These clinically validated mobile electrocardiograms (ECGs) utilize an artificial intelligence algorithm to provide instant analysis for detecting AF. The preliminary experience using this novel technology at a safety net, teaching hospital was very positive. AliveCor's™ was easy to use by neurologists, residents, medical students and nursing personnel and, in combination with pulse palpation, consistently detected AF that was confirmed by a cardiologist with standard ECG. With this new technology, the identification of AF that previously went unrecognized and often asymptomatic has

DOI: 10.4018/978-1-5225-6289-4.ch004

prompted significant changes in patient therapy (additional cardiology evaluation and administration of anticonvulsants). AliveCor™ improved the ability to identify AF in elderly patients with and without a prior history of stroke. Although detection of paroxysmal, persistent and chronic AF was achieved, stratification of the risk versus benefit of anticoagulation therapy in individual patients became more difficult. The anticipated epidemic of AF will be easier to detect with technological advances like AliveCor™, which provides accurate analysis compared to current anticoagulation risk population-based assessment tools. One assessment tool, the CHA2DS2-VASc, depicts a predictive value for stroke in patients with AF with a P value equal to 0.58, making it merely significant. More precise physiologic biomarkers of thrombus formation using blood or cardiac imaging are needed to segregate subgroups of this expanding population of patients found to be in AF.

INTRODUCTION

The AliveCor Kardia™ is a portable ECG (iECG) for the iPhone, Android and iPad that incorporates electrodes for wireless cardiac telemetry monitoring. It was approved by the FDA in 2013 (AliveCor® KardiaMobile EKG Monitor, 2018). It provides a 30 second single (lead 1) rhythm strip when held in the right and left hands. A real-time display of the electrocardiogram is created by conversion of an electrical signal into ultrasound which is captured by the smartphone microphone. Approved automated algorithms provide immediate rhythm analysis of suspected atrial fibrillation (Figures 1 and 2).

Figure 1. AliveCor KardiaMobile for cellphone
Source: From Alivecor by AliveCor, Inc, 2018 (https://store.alivecor.com). Copyright 2018 by AliveCor. Reprinted with permission

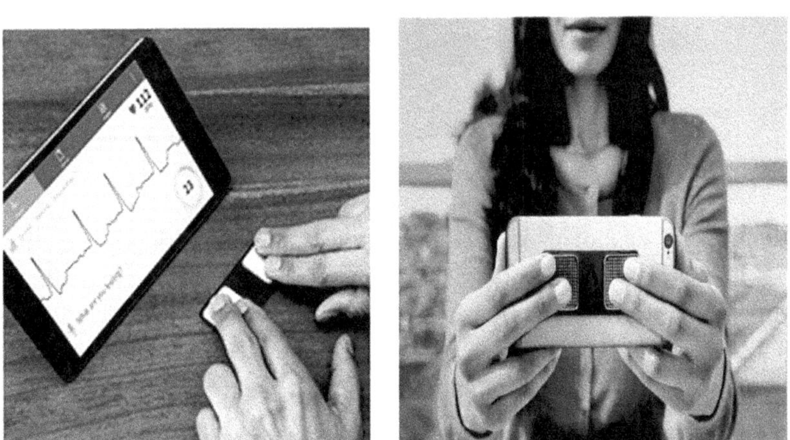

Figure 2. AliveCor KardiaBand: replaces Apple Watch wristband
Source: From Alivecor by AliveCor, Inc, 2018 (https://store.alivecor.com). Copyright 2018 by AliveCor. Reprinted with permission

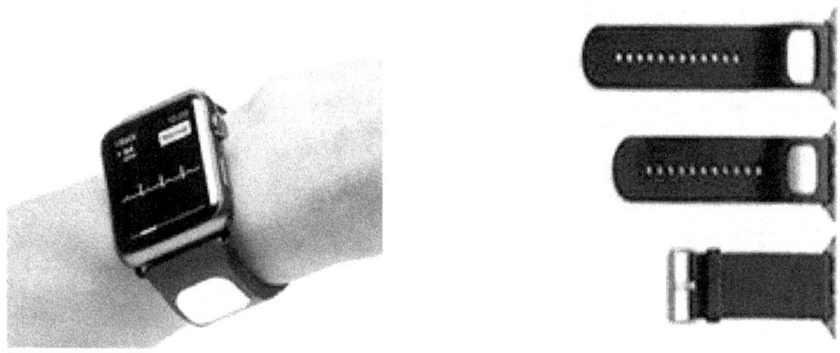

Figure 3. Available handheld EKG monitors
Source: Images courtesy of Dr. James W. Grier

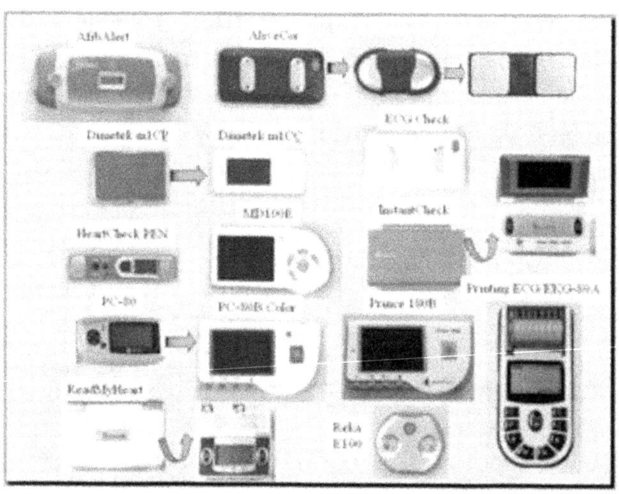

Although not designed as a continuous rhythm monitor, the relatively low cost ($100) and high-level outpatient acceptance make an attractive alternative to conventional Holter monitors and implantable loop recorders in high risk individuals who require prolonged monitoring for AF. The use of this device requires minimal training and the cell phone application is succinct and intuitive. We adapted the previous methodology (Halcox, Wareham, Cardew, Gilmore, Barry, Phillips, &

Figure 4. Design of EKG sensor in KardiaBand: Conversion of an ultrasound to an electrical signal EKG

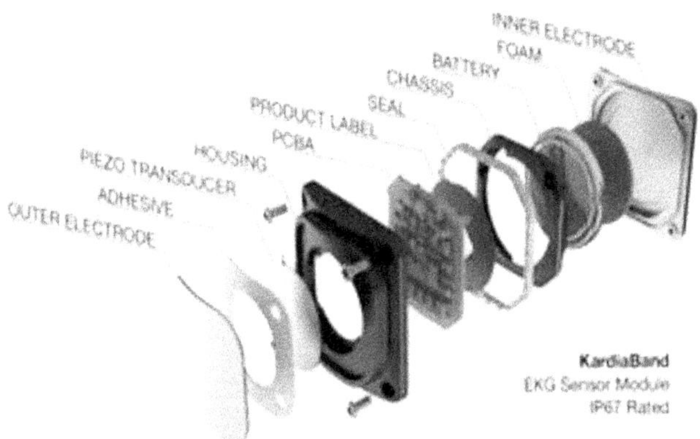

Figure 5. AliveCor KardiaMobile Lead I rhythm strip obtained by placing the fingers of the left and right hands on the electrodes
Source: From Dr. Richard Bogle (https://www.richardbogle.com/). Copyright 2018 by Richard Bogle MD. Reprinted with permission.

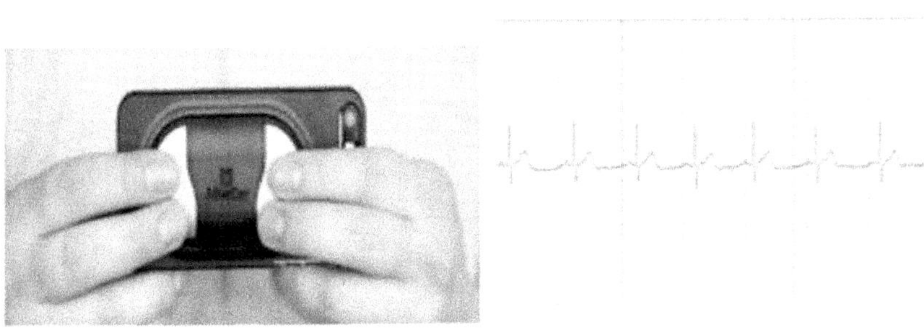

Gravenor, 2017) of screening ambulatory patients over 65 years of age who are at an increased risk of stroke. Each individual was screened twice a week using the Kardia™ ECG plus additional transmissions if the patient became symptomatic (dizziness, palpitations, shortness of breath).

In Case 1, a 71-year-old retired male physician with a prior history of hypertension and obstructive sleep apnea was one of initial trial patients evaluated with AliveCor Kardia™ (Figure 8). He was completely asymptomatic without palpitations, shortness of breath or exercise intolerance. His initial 30 second iECG was interpreted as 'possible atrial fibrillation' which was later confirmed on formal EKG. Echocardiogram demonstrated a normal ejection fraction but moderate left

Figure 6. AliveCor KardiaMobile Lead II obtained with the left electrode on the left knee and the right electrode held with the right hand. Note the larger more distinct P waves in Lead II.
Source: From Dr. Richard Bogle (https://www.richardbogle.com/). Copyright 2018 by Richard Bogle MD. Reprinted with permission.

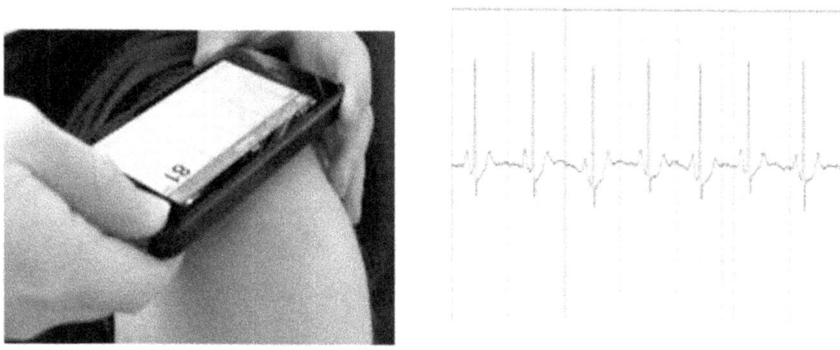

Figure 7. AliveCor can provide Lead I or Lead II recording depending on the position of the electrodes

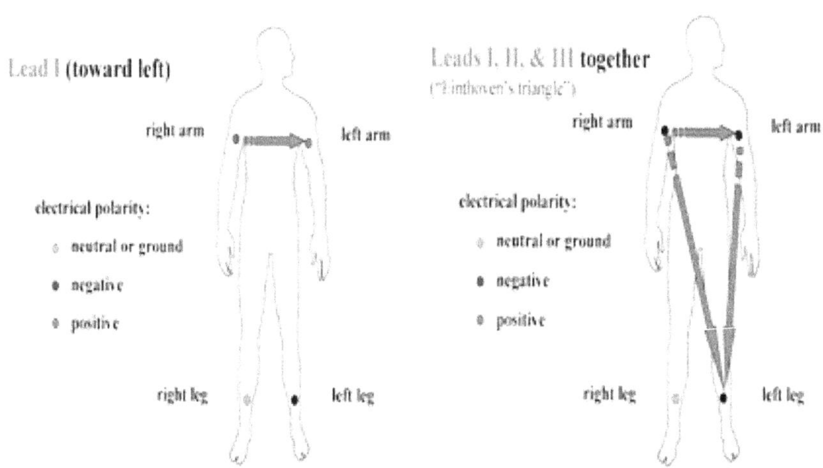

**For a more accurate representation see the electronic version.*

atrial enlargement. Consultation was conducted with a cardiologist and a non-vitamin K oral anticoagulant was prescribed.

In case 2, a 76-year-old African-American obese, male was evaluated in the neurology clinic for episodic dysequilibrium, ataxia, fatigue and shortness of breath. During measurement of his vital signs, his pulse was found irregular. AliveCor Kardia™ was used by a nursing assistant to obtain a 30 second lead one iECG

Figure 8. Case 1

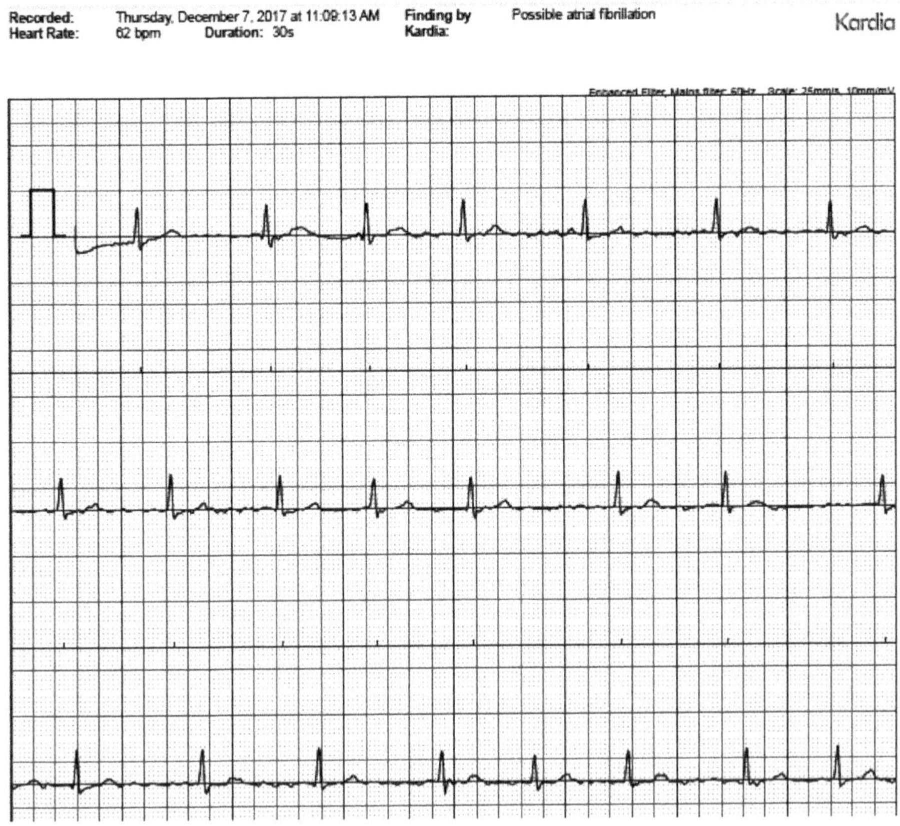

(Figure 9) interpreted as 'possible atrial fibrillation' and later confirmed by formal ECG. Echocardiogram was notable for severe left atrial enlargement and brain MRI (Figure 10) suggested a pattern of embolic infarction (areas of restricted diffusion in multiple vascular territories). The patient was started on oral anticoagulation utilizing a non-vitamin K agent. He has continued to use the device to monitor his heart rate which persists in atrial fibrillation with the rate between 70 and 90 bpm.

The AliveCor Kardia™ algorithm for atrial fibrillation is not perfect. Below are several examples where premature atrial contractions (PACs) and premature ventricular contractions (PVCs) can be misread as possible atrial fibrillation. These examples demonstrate false positive 'possible atrial fibrillation' interpretations seen with premature contractions and the mandatory need for re-interpretation

Figure 9. Case 2

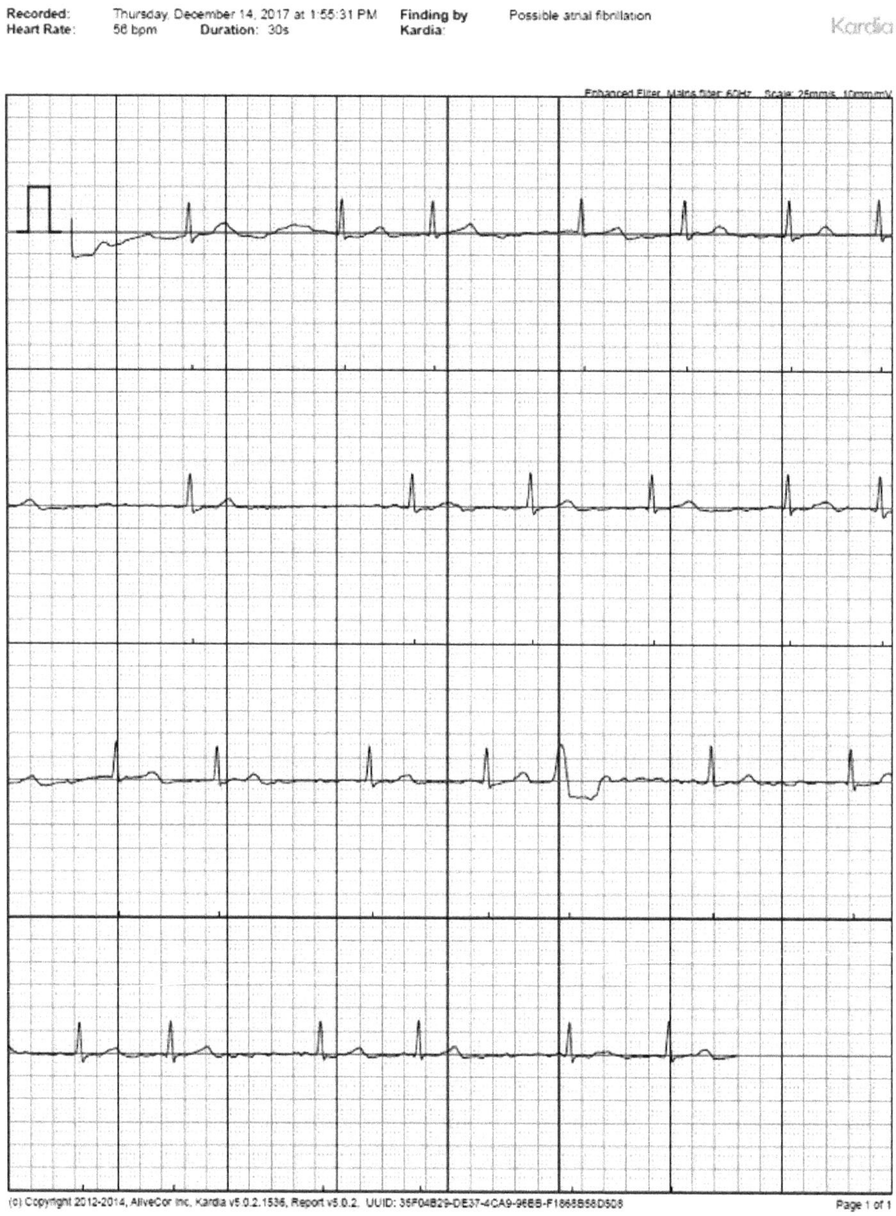

Figure 10. B1000 DWI demonstrates areas of restricted diffusion in multiple vascular territories consistent with acute cardioemboli infarction associated with atrial fibrillation
Source: Provided by Anthony Pearson, MD, The Skeptical Cardiologist, Chesterfield, Mo.

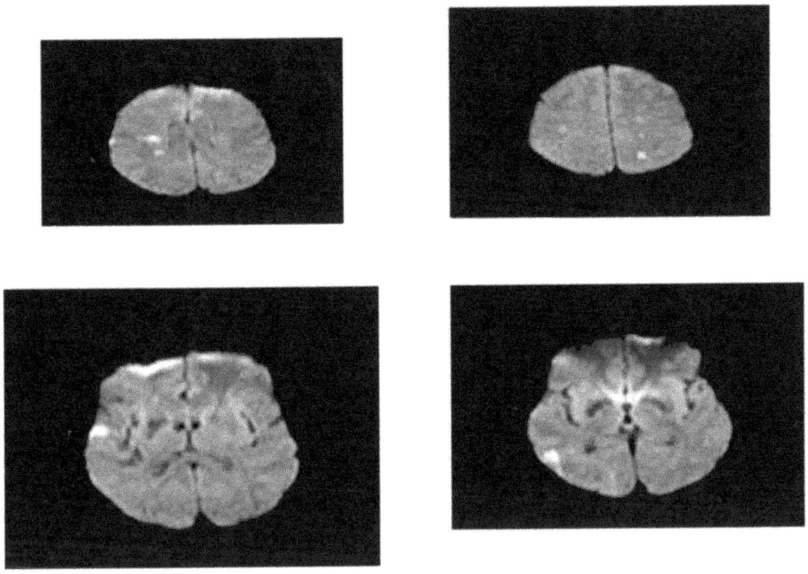

by an experienced cardiologist. The AliveCor Kardia™ algorithm is not alone in misinterpretation of the ECG. The vast majority of ECGs performed in the United States are provided with a computerized algorithm which medical personnel rely upon prior to review by a cardiologist. One study demonstrated that computerized ECG interpretation is correct only 54% of the time when dealing with rhythms other than normal sinus rhythm.

CONCLUSION

Advances in cellphone based technologies such as the AliveCor Kardia™ will increase the identification of paroxysmal, persistent and chronic atrial fibrillation and foster patient involvement in their own care. Our century old concept of atrial fibrillation as a primary rhythm disturbance causing clot formation in the left atrium is being updated to include its role as an important downstream marker for heterogeneous conditions which increase the risk of both embolic and non-embolic stroke, carotid atherosclerosis and cerebral small vessel disease.

Figure 11. AliveCor is good but not perfect

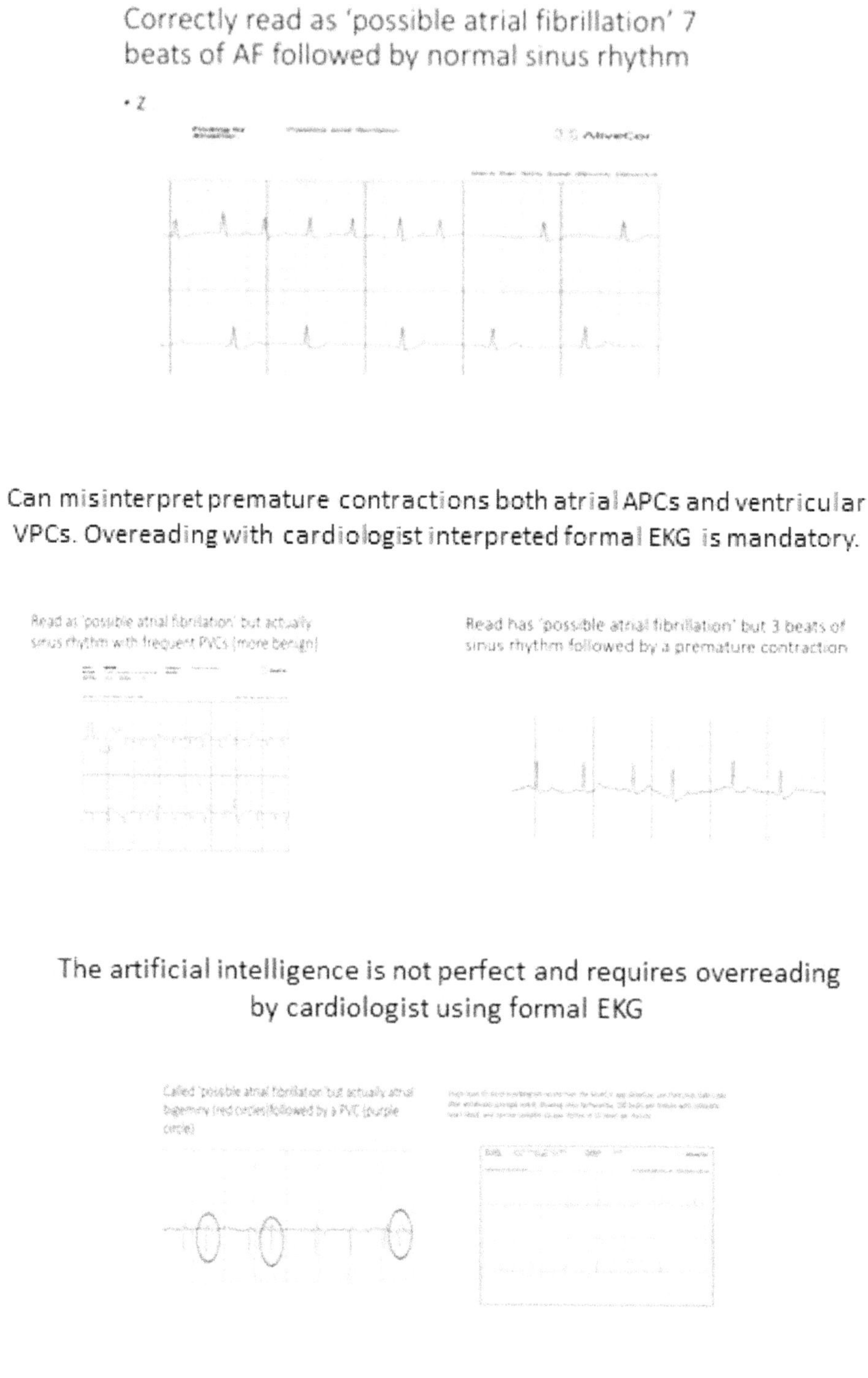

As the detection and monitoring of this common arrhythmia becomes widely accessible to patients with cell phones, the focus will shift from detection to aggressively modifying the myriad of stroke risk factors and preventing atrial fibrillation. With the aging of the population, stroke neurologists managing an epidemic of atrial fibrillation will await identification of either blood or cardiac imaging biomarkers that stratify the risk of stroke in an individual patient beyond our current population based on assessment tools such as CHA2DS2-VASc (Figure 12).

Our experience as neurologists using this cellphone based ECG monitor to screen for atrial fibrillation in a safety net teaching hospital has been extremely positive with multiple practical benefits. AliveCor Kardia™ is inexpensive, reliable and easy to use. Its introduction into our Neurology department has resulted in real life, therapy changing decisions in the care of our patients at risk for stroke, promoted interest in ECG monitoring by our medical students and residents and exposed the need for remediation of our rusty skills in ECG interpretation. We anticipate future benefits to emerge from the big data obtained from this innovative device that may answer essential questions critical to the individual management of the increasing number of patients with atrial fibrillation effected by this emerging public health crisis.

Major Points

1. Atrial fibrillation AF, an evolving public health epidemic affecting 35 million people worldwide, is the most common arrhythmia and is associated with all forms of stroke beyond cardioembolic, congestive heart failure, systemic embolism and death. Because many patients have subclinical AF, there is a

Figure 12. Population based risk assessment of atrial fibrillation CHA2DS2-VASc Score

	Condition	Points
C	Congestive heart failure (or Left ventricular systolic dysfunction)	1
H	Hypertension: blood pressure consistently above 140/90 mmHg (or treated hypertension on medication)	1
A_2	Age ≥75 years	2
D	Diabetes Mellitus	1
S_2	Prior Stroke or TIA or thromboembolism	2
V	Vascular disease (e.g. peripheral artery disease, myocardial infarction, aortic plaque)	1
A	Age 65–74 years	1
Sc	Sex category (i.e. female sex)	1

Annual Stroke Risk[12]		
CHA_2DS_2-VASc Score	Stroke Risk %	95% CI
0	0	-
1	1.3	-
2	2.2	-
3	3.2	-
4	4.0	-
5	6.7	-
6	9.8	-
7	9.6	-
8	12.5	-
9	15.2	-

need for an affordable, patient accessible device to replace annual ECG testing, Holter monitoring and implantable loop recorders.

2. Our experience as clinical neurologists found AliveCor Kardia™ to be an inexpensive, easy-to-use, FDA approved and HIPPA compliant device capable of detecting and monitoring atrial fibrillation on a cell phone. It can be used by neurologists, residents, nurses, medical assistants and patients to facilitate the detection of paroxysmal, persistent and chronic atrial fibrillation in both symptomatic and asymptomatic patients.
3. The basic AliveCor Kardia™ costs about 100 US dollars which includes the device with instant analysis. We recommend purchase of the premium service ($9.99 per month or $99 per) year that allows unlimited storage and history of prior recordings, furnishing summary reports with longitudinal data of blood-pressure monitoring and tracking of weight and medications use
4. In our neurology clinic, screening patients previously found to be in sinus rhythm with a prior stroke or at risk for stroke begins with pulse palpation, blood pressure measurement and use of AliveCor Kardia™ to obtain a 30 second ECG rhythm strip iECG. Patients whose tracings are interpreted as 'possible atrial fibrillation' are referred for a mandatory standard 12 lead ECG read by a cardiologist. If atrial fibrillation is confirmed they are sent for formal cardiology consultation. Long term monitoring in select patients undergo twice weekly AliveCor Kardia™ iECGs for 3-6 months and an additional iECG if they become symptomatic (palpitations, dizziness, faintness or excessive fatigue upon exercising).
5. Atrial fibrillation is more than a rhythm disturbance but a heterogeneous marker for vascular disease beyond embolic stroke including large vessel non-embolic stroke, carotid atherosclerosis and small vessel disease. When AF is found modifiable risks including obesity, hypertension, sleep apnea are primary therapeutic targets.
6. Cellphone devices like AliveCor Kardia™ will ultimately identify increasing numbers of patients in atrial fibrillation. This will intensify the need for a new metric that stratifies the risk/benefit ratio for an individual patient considering long term anticoagulation, one based on physiologic correlates of left atrial thrombus formation rather than epidemiological population measures (CHA2DS2-VASc).
7. The access to data provided by AliveCor Kardia™ offers promise in answering not only what subgroup of patients in atrial fibrillation would benefit from anticoagulation but also in developing proven strategies from preventing paroxysmal atrial fibrillation before it becomes permanent.

Practical Points

1. The AliveCor Kardia™ algorithm has a sensitivity approaching 95% making it a suitable 'rule out' for atrial fibrillation. (Szu, Hsu, Moon, Landa, Nakajima, & Hata, 2013)
2. Tracings read as abnormal should always be over read by a cardiologist.
3. Technical problems we encountered in acquiring good iECG tracings and practical suggestions to improve an 'unclassified' or 'no diagnosis' designation include:
    a. Switching cellphone setting to airplane mode thereby reducing ambient radio frequency interference.
    b. Moisten (not wash) the electrodes with an alcohol wipe.
    c. Rest hands in lap and relax before acquiring a tracing.
    d. Keep silent and as still as possible during the acquisition.
4. Detecting atrial fibrillation with AliveCor™ in an individual patient is easier than providing evidence based treatment.
5. Aggressively modify risk factors such as obesity, hypertension, obstructive sleep apnea and stress.

REFERENCES

AliveCor® KardiaMobile EKG Monitor. (2018). *AliveCor*. Retrieved Sept. 12 2018 from www.alivecor.com/getkardiamobile/

Graff, B., Gąsecki, D., Rojek, A., Boutouyrie, P., Nyka, W., Laurent, S., & Narkiewicz, K. (2013). Heart rate variability and functional outcome in ischemic stroke. *Journal of Hypertension, 31*(8), 1629–1636. doi:10.1097/HJH.0b013e328361e48b PMID:23751963

Gregoski, M. J., Mueller, M., Vertegel, A., Shaporev, A., Jackson, B. B., Frenzel, R. M., ... Treiber, F. A. (2012). Development and validation of a smartphone heart rate acquisition application for health promotion and wellness telehealth applications. *International Journal of Telemedicine and Applications, 2012*, 1–7. doi:10.1155/2012/696324 PMID:22272197

Halcox, J. P., Wareham, K., Cardew, A., Gilmore, M., Barry, J. P., Phillips, C., & Gravenor, M. B. (2017). Assessment of remote heart rhythm sampling using the AliveCor heart monitor to screen for atrial fibrillation: The REHEARSE-AF study. *Circulation, 136*(19), 1784–1794. doi:10.1161/CIRCULATIONAHA.117.030583 PMID:28851729

Izzard, L. C., & Bhalla, A. (2015). Post-stroke cardiac complications. *Management of Post-Stroke Complications,* 21-31. doi:4_3 doi:10.1007/978-3-319-17855

Kai, L., Zhang, X., Wang, Y., Suibiao, H., Ning, G., Wangyong, P., ... Chen, H. (2011). A system of portable ECG monitoring based on Bluetooth mobile phone. *2011 IEEE International Symposium on IT in Medicine and Education.* doi:10.1109/itime.2011.6132113

Mitchell, A. R., & Page, P. L. (2015). Living with the handheld ECG. *BMJ Innovations, 1*(2), 46–48. doi:10.1136/bmjinnov-2014-000029

Morillo, C. A., Banerjee, A., Perel, P., Wood, D., & Jouven, X. (2017). Atrial fibrillation: The current epidemic. *Journal of Geriatric Cardiology, 14*(3), 195–203. 5411.2017.03.011 doi:10.11909/j.issn.1671

Piatkowska, A., Nowicka, A., Szymanowska, M., Kandziora, M., & Wierzchowiecki, M. (2005). *Evaluation of prognostic value of heart rate variability (HRV) and heart rate turbulence (HRT) in patients with congestive heart failure* EP. Europace Oxford Academic. Retrieved September 12, 2018 from https://academic.oup.com/europace/article/7/Supplement_1/137/696396

Rahman, T., & Amirfar, V. A. (2016). AliveCor Mobile ECG: A smartphone with heart. *Pharmacy Today, 22*(3), 56. doi:10.1016/j.ptdy.2016.02.026

Szu, H., Hsu, C., Moon, G., Landa, J., Nakajima, H., & Hata, Y. (2013). Smartphone homecare monitoring of hearts. *Applied Computational Intelligence and Soft Computing, 2013*, 1–10. doi:10.1155/2013/983515

Walsh, J. A. III, Topol, E. J., & Steinhubl, S. R. (2014). Novel wireless devices for cardiac monitoring. *Circulation, 130*(7), 573–581. doi:10.1161/CIRCULATIONAHA.114.009024 PMID:25114186

Chapter 5
Optimizing Medical Education With Instructional Technology:
Technology to Optimize Teaching Human Anatomy

George C. Chang Chien
Ventura County Medical Center, USA

Armen Haroutunian
Advocate Illinois Masonic Medical Center, USA

Bryant England
Advocate Illinois Masonic Medical Center, USA

Kenneth D. Candido
Advocate Illinois Masonic Medical Center, USA

ABSTRACT

Technological advancements and imaging evolution in contemporary medicine continue to change the ways medical education and clinical care are delivered. Historical methods of learning anatomy through human cadaveric dissection may be supplanted by three-dimensional renderings, injection models, and virtual reality simulations. The cost effectiveness of new imaging and study modalities may demonstrate major advantages in the logistics of information delivery, cost containment, and skills development in the current healthcare environment.

DOI: 10.4018/978-1-5225-6289-4.ch005

INTRODUCTION

Cadaveric dissection is widely considered the gold standard for learning gross anatomy of the human body. In medical schools, 2-dimensional artwork as an adjunct to dissection in anatomy lab is not only an integral part of learning about the three-dimensional anatomy and the concept of anatomic variations, but also a time-honored essential of the medical education curriculum bounded by heavy ethical and moral considerations. Through dissection, a student can experience the respective tissues and structures of the human body. However, restrictions related to specimen collection, availability of sufficient teaching funds, resources, as well as arguments related to learning outcomes has produced a shift toward other ancillary learning modalities. With the arrival of the 21st century, non-cadaveric models and phantoms, computer imaging, and affordable technological advancements have changed the standard of teaching and are beginning to implement themselves in schooling and professional curricula (Brown, Adhikari, Marx, Lander, & Todd, 2012).

TRADITIONAL APPROACH

Traditionally, cadaveric dissection has been at the foundation of the paradigm for teaching human anatomy. It provides the student a first exposure to the human body and helps them overcome their inhibitions (McLachlan, Bligh, Bradley, & Searle, 2004). Through the emotionally-charged task of human cadaver dissection, the principles of anatomically-based learning become instilled and allows students to implement values that can act as a foundation for future clinical care. The initial exposure to death also acts to desensitize the students. Dissection allows for improvement of manual dexterity while providing a pathway towards understanding the 3-dimensional structures and reinforces the didactic knowledge acquired in lectures. Working in the anatomy lab also allows for collaboration and teamwork between and among student partners.

Dissection also has many disadvantages. Dissection of a cadaver does not necessarily translate to the performance of surgical procedures on a living body, because by nature a cadaver is not responsive to movements such as percussion and palpation. Dissection does not promote understanding of cross-sectional views, which is often represented by different types of imaging encountered in clinical practice. There are questions regarding whether or not preclinical exposure has any educational benefit due to the lack of problem-based learning. The financial burden of cadaveric preparation and maintenance of a laboratory with staffing can question its cost-effectiveness. Infectious pathogens such as mycobacterium, Hepatitis, HIV, and Creutzfeldt-Jakob disease pose a hazard to those handling tissue specimens. Indeed, slow-virus disease has plagued pathologists and anatomists for centuries, albeit the actual pathogens responsible for these conditions and syndromes has only more recently been recognized (Demiryürek, Bayramoğlu, & Ustaçelebi, 2002). There is also concern with a decrease in trained anatomists to provide education. Lastly, there is consideration as to whether or not cadaveric dissection is an appropriate introduction to death and the resultant emotional stress and mental burden that may be a sequela of that process (McLachlan et al., 2004).

MOVEMENT TOWARD DYNAMIC IMAGINING AS A TOOL TO SUPPLANT GROSS DISSECTION

The use of ultrasonography has expanded across different medical specialties over the course of the decade and has a very well-established role in clinical practice, for both diagnostic purposes and for procedural guidance (Fakoya, 2013). Recently, the role of the ultrasound has expanded past clinical use and has made its way to supplementing teaching gross human anatomy dissections in many medical curricula. The real-time and dynamic use appeals to the current generation of students and residents because it is technologically advanced compared to traditional static teaching methods (Brown et al., 2012). Advances in technology with smaller and more portable and compact units increase the accessibility for in-patient and out-patient imaging. Thus, non-invasiveness, lack of ionizing radiation exposure, portability and high resolution have resulted in its increasing use in anesthesiology, emergency medicine, surgery, internal medicine, and obstetrics and gynecology (Fakoya, 2013).

The ultrasound (US) is safe and allows real-time, dynamic visualization of structures with high resolution imaging in a non-invasive manner. The resolution enables the detection of tendon tears, calcifications, and foreign bodies that are readily apparent with ultrasound at an earlier stage than with X-ray, Cat Scans (CT), or Magnetic Resonance Imaging (MRI) use. The portability has allowed for bedside use and has enabled clinicians to make timely diagnoses with higher specificity and sensitivity. The use of the ultrasound has improved the safety of key procedures including venous catheter placement and thoracentesis. Operating costs are low and there is no risk of ionizing radiation emission (Fakoya, 2013). It is safe for patients with cardiac pacemakers and metal implants. Importantly, US imaging can be performed in patients in a comfortable position. The cost-effectiveness of an ultrasound is also very appealing as it is cheaper than fluoroscopy and the machine can pay for itself within three to four months with a good volume of cases. Currently, many cases that require an ultrasound are being reimbursed (Callard, 2018).

In pain management, ultrasound is used to facilitate the performance of procedures with increased safety and fidelity. It can serve to find difficult nerves such as an entrapped lateral cutaneous nerve of the thigh (Korbe, Udoji, Ness, & Udoji, 2015). Ultrasound guidance has been recently used to identify myofascial trigger points as well as reducing complications associated with the injection procedure, including the development of hematomas and pneumothoraces. Concerns over blind needle placement and manual palpation have generated novel approaches using US guidance (Finlayson, 2017). In the perioperative setting, point of care US use has been used to evaluate gastric volumes in patients at risk for aspiration, difficult laryngoscopies secondary to temporomandibular joint dysfunction, determination of accidental endobronchial intubation, and for monitoring cardiac pathologies. (Haskins, Boublik, & Wu, 2017). Currently, The Society of Critical Care Anesthesiologists (SCCA) have identified goals and objectives with the use of US in fellowship training. In the meantime, there is an increasing demand to expand the use of ultrasound for the residents in training.

Limitations of US include technical, anatomic, and operator factors. Technical factors include poor image resolution with increasing depths of targeted structures, and formation of an acoustic shadow or artifact imposed by bone. This can create difficult needle visualization at deep layers. Anatomic factors include large patient body habitus. Operator factors include lack of skill and experience (Graham & Barry, 2013).

ALTERNATIVE APPROACHES TO USE OF ULTRASOUND FOR ANATOMY TEACHING

Many institutions are now adopting new approaches to learning anatomy beyond the cadaver lab (White, 2018). Virtual anatomy tables and interactive touchscreens with a library of clinical images including MRI, CT-scanning, X-ray, ultrasonography, and pathology slides allows for visualization of human anatomy through multiple perspectives. Recently, BioDigital, Inc., creators of the BioDigital Human Platform announced the world's first 3-D human visualization platform. The application uses innovative, web-based technology to view anatomy, disease states and health data. Recent collaboration with Johns Hopkins Medicine allows users to explore 3,000 anatomical objects and key muscle movements in interactive 3-D. Users can rotate and zoom-in on all objects; select and dissect anatomy objects to customize their view; add or remove layers of anatomical complexity; and draw and annotate directly on models to save for future reference.

A multi-approach model with virtual-reality imaging, examination of living anatomy on peers and models, medical imaging focused on problem based learning, and real-time 3 dynamic imagining is instrumental in learning anatomy. The millennials of the 21st century are often called "joystick generation" or "generation Z" that are quick to adapt to "high-tech" tools (such as smartphones, tablets, gaming devices, personal computers and laptops), emulated by the ultrasound. Some institutions have begun to integrate an ultrasound curriculum into their medical schools that includes both didactics and hands-on training sessions (Fakoya, 2013). Virtual reality simulators are very promising, but high costs currently prevent most programs from implementing this resource. Nonetheless, repetition and visibility of structures that are difficult to expose on a cadaver allow for more effective learning.

Models for injection training (including synthetic, animal, and food products) have now evolved, shifting the focus away from human cadavers. Synthetic products include a large variety of clinical skill trainers for intramuscular injections, subcutaneous injections, intraosseous injections, intravenous injections, spinal and epidural injections, as well as trainers for different patient age groups (neonatal, pediatric and adult injection trainers). Animal models including both rabbit and rat models have been used to examine the efficacy of the botulinum toxin type A injection for treatment of hypertrophic scars as well as for observing its impact on esophageal anastomoses. These same animal models have been used for the practice of various neuraxial injection techniques. Food products (poultry and tofu) have been used to study technical aspects by surgical specialties to help increase dexterity and maximize surgical technique.

Studies demonstrated the ability to enhance basic skills with low, medium, and high-fidelity models of varying costs. It was concluded that medium and high-fidelity models are better reserved for more experienced students secondary to limiting overall expenses and time consumption. However, 3D printing shows much promise in increasing model availability and decreasing the cost of high-fidelity models. Examples of low-fidelity models used included empty normal saline bags with foam inserts (Liu, Glass, Glover, Power, & Watcha, 2013). The major advantage was the elimination of patient care, repetitive exposure, and real-time availability allowing for more accurate feedback (Chang et al., 2017). This may translate to a reduction in the rate of complications and opportunities for troubleshooting in a controlled environment.

For anesthesiologists, regional anesthesia has shown consistent outcomes with varying fidelity models. Residents in training had enhanced technical development and identification skills. More importantly, participants were observed to make fewer errors in judgement and analysis.

CLINICAL APPLICATION

The use of ultrasound and 3D technology has become an essential tool in the clinical practice of anesthesiology and pain medicine. In pain medicine, the authors have used ultrasound in a variety of procedures, including stellate ganglion blocks, nerve root blocks, and joint injections. Despite the inability to see through bony structures, its proven superiority over blind procedures and combination with fluoroscopic techniques can be useful (Korbe et al., 2015). Procedures that utilize the ultrasound include: neuraxial injections (facet blocks, medial branch blocks, epidural injections), joint injections (sacroiliac joint, knee, shoulder, wrist, greater trochanteric bursa, intra-articular hip injections, and peripheral/nerve injections (intercostal nerve, lateral femoral cutaneous nerve, stellate ganglion block, greater occipital nerve block, branches of the brachial and lumbosacral plexus). Injections in the shoulder, hip, and knee have greater success when ultrasound is utilized. Additionally, ilioinguinal, iliohypogastric, and genitofemoral blocks have greater accuracy and efficacy when performed with ultrasound (korbe et al., 2015).

More recently, the use of ultrasound for minimally invasive peripheral nerve stimulation has become a topic of interest. Ultrasound-guided percutaneous placement of peripheral nerve stimulators allows targeting of deep nerves to help treat painful peripheral nerve syndromes while avoiding the morbidity and mortality of an open procedure, as well as avoiding stimulation to other areas non-painful areas. For example, tibial and peroneal nerve stimulation procedures are traditionally performed in an open fashion, but recent case reports describe successful ultrasound guided percutaneous placement of these nerve stimulators (Chan, Brown, Park, & Winfree, 2010). This minimally invasive technique could be theoretically applied to any peripheral nerve, and future studies may eventually validate the wide scope of its application.

CONCLUSION

Technological advancements and imaging evolution in contemporary medicine continue to change the ways medical education and clinical care are delivered. Historical methods of learning anatomy through human cadaveric dissection may be supplanted by 3-dimensional renderings, injection models, and virtual reality simulations. The cost effectiveness of new imaging and study modalities may demonstrate major advantages in the logistics of information delivery, cost containment, and skills development in the current healthcare environment.

REFERENCES

Brown, B., Adhikari, S., Marx, J., Lander, L., & Todd, G. L. (2012). Introduction of ultrasound into gross anatomy curriculum: Perceptions of medical students. *The Journal of Emergency Medicine*, *43*(6), 1098–1102. doi:10.1016/j.jemermed.2012.01.041 PMID:22459597

Callard, A. (2011). *5 Points on Ultrasound for Pain Management.* Retrieved January 20, 2018, from https://www.beckersspine.com/pain/item/9956-5-points-on-ultrasound-for-pain-management

Chan, I., Brown, A.R., Park, K., & Winfree, C.J. (2010). Ultrasound-guided, percutaneous peripheral nerve stimulation: Technical note. *Neurosurgery, 67*(3), 136-9. doi:10.1227/01.NEU.0000383137.33503.EB

Chang, D. R., Lin, R. P., Bowe, S., Bunegin, L., Weitzel, E. K., McMains, K. C., ... Chen, P. G. (2017). Fabrication and Validation of a Low-Cost, Medium-Fidelity Silicone Injection Molded Endoscopic Sinus Surgery Simulation Model. *Larygoscope*, *127*(4), 781–786. doi:10.1002/lary.26370 PMID:28000224

Demiryürek, D., Bayramoğlu, A., & Ustaçelebi, S. (2002). Infective agents in fixed human cadavers: A brief review and suggested guidelines. *Anat Rec., 269*(4), 194-7.

Fakoya, F.A. (2013). Integrating ultrasound technology into teaching gross anatomy: point of order! *Medical Education Online*. doi:. doi:10.3402/meo.v18i0.20888

Finlayson, R. J. (2017). Ultrasound Guidance for Trigger Point Injections: Gold Standard or Fool's Gold? *Regional Anesthesia and Pain Medicine*, *42*(3), 279–280. doi:10.1097/AAP.0000000000000599 PMID:28419045

Haskins, S. C., Boublik, J., & Wu, C. L. (2017). Point-of-Care Ultrasound for the Regional Anesthesiologist and Pain Specialist: A Series Introduction. *Regional Anesthesia and Pain Medicine*, *42*(3), 281–282. doi:10.1097/AAP.0000000000000570 PMID:28419046

Korbe, S., Udoji, E. N., Ness, T. J., & Udoji, M. A. (2015). Ultrasound-guided interventional procedures for chronic pain management. *Pain Management*, *5*(6), 465–482. doi:10.2217/pmt.15.46 PMID:26402316

Liu, Y., Glass, N. L., Glover, C. D., Power, R. W., & Watcha, M. F. (2013). Comparison of the development of performance skills in ultrasound-guided regional anesthesia simulations with different phantom models. *Simulation in Healthcare*, *8*(6), 368–375. doi:10.1097/SIH.0b013e318299dae2 PMID:24096912

McLachlan, J. C., Bligh, J., Bradley, P., & Searle, J. (2004, April). Teaching anatomy without cadavers. *Medical Education*, *38*(4), 418–424. doi:10.1046/j.1365-2923.2004.01795.x PMID:15025643

Simpson, G., & Nicholls, B. (2013). Use of ultrasound in chronic pain medicine. Part 1: Neuraxial and sympathetic blocks. *Continuing Education in Anaesthesia, Critical Care & Pain*, *13*(5), 145–151. doi:10.1093/bjaceaccp/mkt013

White, T. (n.d.). *Body image: Computerized table lets students do virtual dissection*. Retrieved January 20, 2018, from Https://med.stanford.edu/news/all-news/2011/05/body-image-computerized-table-lets-students-do-virtual-dissection.html

Chapter 6
Modern Technology in Dermatopathology Education

Kristin M. Torre
University of Connecticut, USA

Michael J. Murphy
University of Connecticut, USA

Jane M. Grant-Kels
University of Connecticut, USA

ABSTRACT

Technological advancement is steadily reshaping the field of medical education. In histopathology and especially dermatopathology training, the transition from glass slide microscopy (GSM) to virtual microscopy (VM) is serving as an instructional tool for medical students, residents, fellows, and experienced physicians. Online slide atlases and digitalized content are being utilized by educators and trainees to enhance and assess both individual and collaborative learning. With the expansion of mobile technology, new avenues are emerging for image attainment, in addition to remote instruction and consultation in resource-limited areas. Various computer-based applications ("apps") and social media sites also serve as digital assets in education and training and allow for rapid dissemination and sharing of information around the world.

INTRODUCTION

Advancements in technology are inevitably changing the landscape of medical education. Textbooks and paper exams are being replaced by digital content across multiple educational realms. Undergraduate medical education, post-graduate residency and fellowship training, and experienced physicians are all facing this

DOI: 10.4018/978-1-5225-6289-4.ch006

shift towards electronic material for teaching and clinical work. The advent of the electronic medical record, online academic resources, and virtual microscopy are just a few examples of recently implemented technological milestones. Virtual microscopy has gained popularity as a method of digitalizing glass microscope slides for high-resolution interactive viewing. Herein, we will focus on modern technology and its application to education in dermatopathology (DP), in addition to the undergraduate teaching of histopathology. Within these fields, the transition from glass slide microscopy (GSM) to virtual microscopy (VM) has been successfully incorporated into all levels of education through online databases, atlases, and digital slide sets. Digital expansion has also created opportunities in mobile microscopy and other computer-based applications for instruction and telepathology services. Image sharing through the internet and networking sites has not only been shown to be beneficial for educational purposes, but also for collaborative research and widespread dissemination of information. New technologic advances that efficiently and easily convert stained tissue on glass slides to digital images have made these educational innovations possible.

Education using digital microscopy is steadily being incorporated into the specialty of DP. Understanding histopathology is critical for both clinicians and pathologists in the diagnosis and management of numerous dermatologic disease processes. Relevant training is essential for dermatology, pathology, and DP fellows. The importance of DP to the education of a dermatologist is exemplified by the fact that 19% of the American Board of Dermatology (ABD) certifying exam in 2017 was dedicated to DP (American Board of Dermatology, 2017). As a result, dermatology residencies commit a great deal of educational time to DP. To highlight the importance of histopathological correlation for dermatology-trained clinicians, a previous study estimated that 25% of the residency curriculum is reserved for DP teaching; however, a more recent study found that number to be closer to 30% (Hinshaw, Hsu, Lee, & Stratman, 2009). In this latter study, only 19.2% of the programs surveyed reported utilizing computer-based learning, with preferential use of GSM for educational purposes (Hinshaw et al., 2009). Although DP instruction has evolved over the years as a result of technological progress, opportunity for further growth exists. Virtual technology in this field is presently underutilized, despite the vast potential for its future implementation and teaching roles.

BREAKING THE GLASS: THE TRANSITION FROM TRADITIONAL MICROSCOPY TO VIRTUAL MICROSCOPY

Glass slide microscopy has been the gold standard for both diagnostic and educational purposes for over two centuries. However, advances in modern technology have led to the emergence of VM, which is the "software-assisted manipulation of high-definition digital images of tissue sections to stimulate the experience of examining glass slides under a standard optical microscope" (Mooney & Hedblad, 2012, p. 40). As a result of whole slide imaging (WSI) techniques introduced almost 20 years ago, these virtual images can now be viewed on desktop computers and even mobile devices. Technologically advanced scanners convert processed and stained tissue on glass slides into high-resolution images using commercially available software. Slides can be scanned at multiple magnifications, generally to 40x with some up to 100x, in a relatively short amount of time given the high-resolution of the images (1 hour per 100 slides for advanced scanners) (Higgins, 2015; Pantanowitz et al., 2011). On average, scanning speeds vary from less than a minute per slide to 1-3 minutes per slide depending on magnification and plane of focus requirements (Farahani, Parwani, & Pantanowitz, 2015). Slides can be navigated in all directions (i.e., X, Y) and some scanners enable scanning in more than one focus plane (Z-stacking), therefore allowing for the creation of three-dimensional images which is useful for review of cytological specimens, frozen sections, and other thick samples (Al-Janabi, Huisman, & Van Diest, 2012; Farahani et al., 2015). Images can be examined and manipulated using a mouse or joystick, permitting multiple functions including zooming features. WSI has numerous advantages compared with conventional GSM, including the following: (Al-Janabi et al., 2012; Farahani et al., 2015; Higgins, 2015; Mooney & Hedblad, 2012; Pantanowitz et al., 2011; Saco, Bombi, Garcia, Ramirez, & Ordi, 2016; Shahriari, Grant-Kels, & Murphy, 2017).

- Image viewers can show an "overview" thumbnail image in the corner of a higher-power scan, allowing for better orientation and ease of navigation through the image
- Multiple slides can be arranged and displayed side-by-side to compare different stains or magnifications
- Images of small tissue specimens can be archived, and digital imaging eliminates the problem of having insufficient tissue to generate further slides
- Multiple students or examiners can view the exact same image at the same time
- The quality of images using WSI does not deteriorate over time
- WSI images can be integrated into the patient's electronic medical record for complete clinical care
- Large storage rooms are not needed for glass slides nor do slides need to be constantly retrieved for review, teaching, research, and quality assurance
- Digital slides do not get lost or broken
- Fluorescence in situ hybridization (FISH)/immunofluorescence images do not lose their fluorescence over time

- WSI eliminates the need for multiple microscopes and continuous maintenance, leading to a reduction in overall costs over time
- Software viewers have tools to acquire measurements and annotate directly on the virtual images
- Images can be viewed remotely with a virtual software program for education, consultation, and telepathology purposes
- The slides are always in focus as the scanner does the initial focusing
- There are numerous benefits in the education and assessment of medical students, residents, and fellows, which will be discussed in subsequent sections

Due to the extensive versatility of VM, it is currently being employed in academic and professional settings for examinations and competency evaluations, image analysis, archiving of data, research and publications, quality assurance, and remote consultation services (Shahriari et al., 2017).

Despite the numerous advantages of WSI technology, it does not remain without its challenges. Glass microscope slides have been the standard for years, and therefore the transition to VM represents a fundamental change in practice for many pathologists and dermatopathologists, whereas for undergraduate and post-graduate students this shift towards use of digital technology is generally more accepted. Currently, one of the greatest challenges for VM is creating one affordable universal method for generating virtual slide images. Presently, there are various software programs and scanners in use (Higgins, 2015). A number of available WSI scanners are listed in Table 1. Cost of acquisition remains high, over $160,000, for some virtual scanners and software; however, over multiple years such an investment in VM may prove cost-effective (Berger, Townsend-Kraft, Murphy, & Elaba, 2017). Additional costs include data storage, data maintenance, and firewall installation. Some concerns noted by users include technical issues such as difficulty scanning tissue folds, bubbles, and samples that are inadequately stained. In addition, legal considerations such as Federal Drug Administration (FDA) regulation of WSI systems, teleconsultation licensing, and malpractice coverage across state and international borders are important (Pantanowitz et al., 2011). Given this technology is relatively new, these barriers and challenges must be addressed in order for VM to gain wider approval in both educational and clinical settings.

A concern with any new technology is how it compares to the gold standard in practice. Various studies have addressed this issue, and found that there is no significant difference in diagnostic accuracy among dermatopathologists and pathologists when using VM versus GSM; this is critical for its widespread acceptance (Al Habeeb, Evans, & Ghazarian, 2012; Al-Janabi et al., 2012; Koch et al., 2009; Lee, Jedrych, Pantanowitz, & Ho, 2017; Leinweber et al., 2006; Massone et al., 2007; Mooney,

Table 1. Commercial whole-slide imaging (WSI) scanners

WSI Model	Vendor
Axio Scan.ZI	Zeiss
D2	Mikroscan
iScan Coreo, iScan HT	Ventana
Lamina	PerkinElmer
NanoZoomer RS, HT, XR	Hamamatsu
Pannoramic SCAN II, 250 Flash	3DHistech
PathScope	DigiPath
Precice 500, Precice 600x	Unic
Aperio Ariol, AT2, AT Turbo, CS2, CSO, FL, LV1, SCN400, VERSA	Leica
TISSUEscope 4000, 4000XT, HS	Huron
Ultra-Fast Scanner	Philips
VisionTek	Sakura Finetek
VL4, VL120	Omnyx
VS120-SL	Olympus

Source: Adapted from "Whole slide imaging in pathology: advantages, limitations, and emerging perspectives," Farahani et al. (2015, p. 24)

Hood, Lampros, Kempf, & Jemec, 2011; Nielsen et al., 2010; Pantanowitz et al., 2011; Thorstenson, Molin, & Lundstrom, 2014). Notably, a recent report found that diagnosis using WSI was equivalent to traditional GSM of 499 cases in a statistically powerful study of dermatopathologists (Kent et al., 2017). Similarly, studies have found no difference in diagnostic ability among residents and medical students using digital images compared to glass slides. Furthermore, many students prefer the former and believe it to be a useful educational tool (Berger et al., 2017; Koch et al., 2009; Scoville & Buskirk, 2007).

MODERN MICROSCOPY AND MEDICAL SCHOOL

A version of the optical microscope has been around since the 17th century (Boyce, 2015). Since the inception of medical education, microscopes have helped provide students with a foundational understanding of normal histology and disease pathology to better serve them in clinical practice. Today in the 21st century, curriculum reform has been sweeping across medical schools throughout the United States and encouraging the transition to small group, interactive team-based learning (Triola & Holloway, 2011). With computers becoming more cost-effective than microscopes, many medical schools have adopted VM into their histopathology curriculum and some have replaced traditional glass slides completely (Koch et al., 2009). Institutions have started generating robust libraries of digital images. For example, the University of Iowa has more than 400 digital pathology slides in their online *Virtual Slidebox* for education of medical students. According to a 2009 study among allopathic and osteopathic medical schools, 44% indicated full transition to VM compared to only 14% in 2002 (Drake, McBride, Lachman, & Pawlina, 2009). That number is likely to be even higher today.

Education was among the first applications of WSI, with the replacement of live viewing of glass slides and static digital images (Al-Janabi et al., 2012). Studies have shown that students react favorably to incorporation of VM into medical curricula, often preferring VM to traditional microscopes (Alotaibi & ALQahtani, 2016; Blake, Lavoie, & Millette, 2003; Krippendorf & Lough, 2005; Kumar et al., 2004; Nelson, Ziv, & Bandali, 2012; Ordi et al., 2015; Weaker & Herbert, 2009). Students in the modern era are familiar with digital technology which is the likely explanation for their overwhelming acceptance of this new technology (Saco et al., 2016). They report the benefits of sharp digital images and ease of navigation, opportunities for both independent and collaborative study, and efficient use of time learning histology and pathology rather than the logistics of microscope operation (Alotaibi & ALQahtani, 2016; Blake et al., 2003; Boutonnat et al., 2006; Cotter, 2001). Regarding efficiency, the streamlined workflow of VM systems has reduced laboratory sessions by as much as one hour in one study, without compromising content being taught (Triola & Holloway, 2011). Comments from users of VM include: "[VM] doesn't hurt my eyes; clear images that are always in focus; faster to use; more convenient" (Kumar et al., 2004).

For educators, it is important for technological innovations to not only positively impact the learning environment, but also to be beneficial to student performance. A study of first-year medical students investigated their scores and found no significant difference between VM versus GSM (Scoville & Buskirk, 2007). Other studies have found similar results (Kumar et al., 2004; Ordi et al., 2015). A report from Johns Hopkins University found their students performed better in areas where VM was utilized in the curriculum (Goldberg & Dintzis, 2007). Furthermore, a recent meta-analysis indicated that the use of VM is modestly superior compared to GSM when looking at student performance scores, and VM is overwhelmingly preferred by learners (Wilson et al., 2016). Digital microscopy is favored for many reasons as the advantages of this innovative technology are numerous.

The most appreciated feature of VM in medical education is remote access at any time and from any location (Al-Janabi et al., 2012; Mooney et al., 2011; Ordi et al., 2015; Pantanowitz et al., 2011; Saco et al., 2016). One study found that over half of digital slide searches were made on holidays and one-third after working hours (Saco et al., 2016), whereas another identified rates of 58% on holidays and 42% after 6 pm (Ordi et al., 2015). These findings demonstrate that VM allows for greater flexibility in learning and takes into account students' individual schedules. Aside from home use at any time of the day, provided that students have access to the VM software, digital microscopy can be employed in any classroom with internet availability. Multiple users can examine the exact same case material simultaneously, thereby promoting standardization of materials for all learners. Students no longer have to worry about breaking valuable specimens or carrying around boxes of glass slides. Other benefits include the side-by-side slide feature which allows viewing of normal, abnormal, and special stains simultaneously, in addition to the thumbnail feature in the corner of the slide which orients students navigating through the digital image (Nelson et al., 2012). By digitalizing microscopy, students can be provided access to images they would not normally have the opportunity to be exposed to using traditional microscopy. These images include exotic and rare specimens, cytology slides, and small biopsies with minimal tissue (Farahani et al., 2015; Mooney & Hedblad, 2012).

With the increased focus on collaborative scholarship in medical education, one irreplaceable benefit of VM is the opportunity for team-based group learning (Mione, Valcke, & Cornelissen, 2013). Students can work together while viewing the same images, and the software programs used allow for image capture, annotation, sharing, and upload to programs such as Google Drive, Dropbox, and Wiki pages for collective learning (Leifer, 2015). Digital slides can also be stored and shared for free, through websites such as PathXChange, Pathobin, and Whole Slide Imaging Repository (Morrison & Gardner, 2015a). VM is more interactive and educators can utilize annotation, circles, and arrows to highlight specific areas on slides (Foster, 2010; Nelson et al., 2012). Additionally, instructors can create clickable "hotspots", indicated with markers to highlight areas of interest which contain further case information and descriptions (Dziegielewski, Velan, & Kumar, 2003). The incorporation of clinical vignettes, video tutorials, and annotated slides with case questions has been shown to stimulate knowledge and enthusiasm for learning, in addition to improved understanding of pathologic disease processes (Boyce, 2015; Horn, Czarnecki, & Lele, 2012). Clinical photos, radiographs, gross pathology images, and other ancillary studies (such as cytogenetics) can be incorporated into the digital file to provide students with a complete clinical picture (Foster, 2010). VM has also been employed for medical school histology and histopathology examinations with favorable results, as previously described.

New innovation inevitably comes with challenges and certain disadvantages. GSM has been the gold standard for centuries and adoption of new methods can be met with resistance. One main concern according to some educators is that students do not learn how to use microscopes during their undergraduate education if only

VM is utilized. However, proponents of VM argue that educational value should be measured by the students' understanding of clinical-pathological correlation and mechanisms of disease, regardless of the instrument used (Al-Janabi et al., 2012; Saco et al., 2016). Others have expressed dissatisfaction with current viewing speeds and lag times for loading large images (Farahani et al., 2015). For VM to be fully incorporated into medical education, a well-functioning IT infrastructure, high-speed internet, and high-capacity server are critical (Saco et al., 2016). These requirements are not absolute, however, and for schools that lack support for streaming images via the internet or the monetary funds, pocket-sized external hard drives and CD-ROMS have been employed to distribute software and digital images to students (Blake et al., 2003; Weaker & Herbert, 2009). Undoubtedly, undergraduate medical education has led the way in adoption and implementation of VM for educational purposes.

GRADUATE TRAINING WITH VIRTUAL MICROSCOPY

For residents in pathology, dermatology, and DP fellows, training in histopathology has largely been achieved through the study of textbook atlases and glass slide cases (Shahriari et al., 2017). With an increasing focus on VM in education, printed materials are being transformed into online formats, and digital images are available in online DP libraries for easy access. Similar to the way VM is revolutionizing histology and histopathology in medical education, it is beginning to do the same in the residency training of pathologists, dermatologists, and fellows, albeit at a slower pace. Advantages similar to the ones outlined for undergraduate medical education also apply to graduate training. With numerous benefits of WSI, there has been a shift towards integrating VM with traditional glass slides into residency curricula. The UConn Health Department of Dermatology has developed its own virtual DP atlas with over 1000 digital whole slide images for education of medical students, residents, fellows, and experienced physicians. The database is used for DP learning as well as examination preparation. Virtual libraries are particularly useful in planning for resident in-service and maintenance of certification (MOC)/ recertifying examinations which now use virtual images as exam questions. Images in the UConn Health atlas were originally scanned using a commercially available WSI system. However, additional images are expected to be added to the database using a low-cost, upright microscope-based WSI system called "InstantScope", recently developed and validated at the University of Connecticut as seen in Figure 1 (Guo, Liao, Bian, Heng, & Zheng, 2015). Other various institutions, organizations, and professional bodies, as shown in Table 2, have created their own personal digital slide sets and online atlases which are free-of-cost to users all over the world. Many of these resources have annotated images, clinical photos, and self-assessments for

Figure 1. "InstantScope"- Low-cost, upright microscope-based whole slide imaging system developed and validated at UConn Health

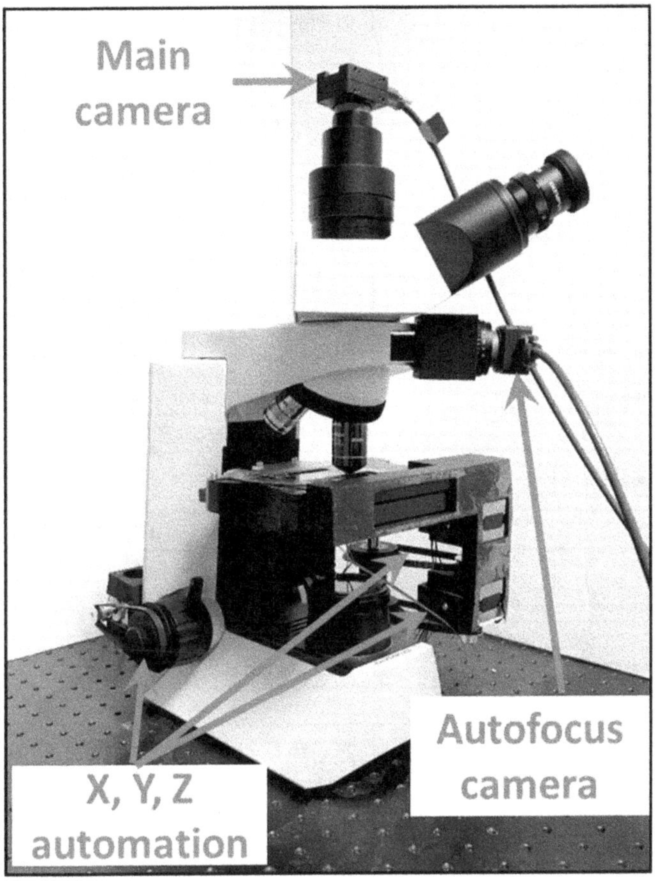

enhanced learning. PathPresenter is an example of a free online atlas with over 2400 virtual images with features for learning such as video tutorials, side-by-side images for comparison, and a section with high-yield annotated educational cases (https://pathpresenter.com). For a more exhaustive list of online resources with both static and whole slide images, learners can refer to the Whole Slide Imaging Repository of the Digital Pathology Association (https://digitalpathologyassociation.org/whole-slide-imaging-repository). An additional resource is the Digital Pathology Blog, an online VM website for both educators and learners (www.tissuepathology.com). Other technological innovations in DP education include a simulation-based training site (SlideTutor), which is a case-based system to teach histopathologic diagnosis and sign-out report writing to trainees (Hinshaw, 2012; http://slidetutor.upmc.edu). Of note, continuing medical education credits can also be earned through VM platforms.

Table 2. Dermatopathology online virtual/digital educational resources

Resource	Website
American Society of Dermatopathology (ASDP) Interactive Case Study of the Month	(http://www.asdp.org/education/case-study-of-the-month/case-archive)
Atlas of Dermatopathology	(https://atlases.muni.cz/en/index.html)
Clearpath "app"	(http://www.dermpathlab.com/clearpath/)
College of Pathologists (CAP) Case of the Month	(http://www.cap.org)
College of Pathologists (CAP) Online Dermatopathology—DPATH	(http://www.cap.org)
Derm In-Review (Dermpath Study Tool)	(http://dermatologyinreview.com)
Dermatopathology Interactive Atlas	(http://www.dermpathatlas.com)
Dermatopathology Institute Slide Atlas	(http://www.dermpathmd.com/dermatopathology_slide_atlas.htm) (Static Images)
Dermpath University	(http://www.dermpathdiagnostics.com/university/digitaldermpath)
Dermpedia	(http://www.dermpedia.org)
Digital Pathology Association	(https://digitalpathologyassociation.org/whole-slide-imaging-repository)
Digital Pathology Blog	(https://tissuepathology.com)
Enjoy Pathology	(http://www.enjoypath.com)
Juan Rosai's Collection of Surgical Pathology Seminars	(http://www.rosaicollection.org)
MyDermPath+ "app"	(http://mydermpath.com)
Nordic Institute of Virtual Dermatopathology	(http://www.nivdp.com)
Pathology Outlines Case of the Week	(http://www.pathologyoutlines.com)
Pathorama—University of Basel	(http://pathorama.ch)
PathPresenter	(https://pathpresenter.com)
RecutClub	(https://www.recutclub.com)
Uniformed Services University—Department of Pathology	(https://images.nlm.nih.gov/pathlab)
United States and Canadian Association of Pathology (USCAP) Virtual Slide Box	(http://www.uscapknowledgehub.org)
University of British Columbia—Slide Box	(http://histo.anat.ubc.ca)
University of Iowa Virtual Slidebox	(http://www.mbfbioscience.com/iowavirtualslidebox)
University of Leeds	(http://www.virtualpathology.leeds.ac.uk)
University of Michigan Virtual Slide Box	(https://www.pathology.med.umich.edu/slides/index.php)
University of Western Ontario—Virtual Slide Box	(http://slidebox.uwo.ca)
Virtual Dermpath	(http://www.virtualdermpath.com)
Virtual Histology Laboratory	(http://www.histologyguide.org/slide-box/slide-box.html)
WebPathology	(http://www.webpathology.com)

Source: Adapted from "Dermatopathology education in the era of modern technology," Shahriari et al. (2017, p. 767)

A review of DP curricula found that barriers to education include lack of cases, microscopes, disappearing slide sets, inconvenient laboratory location, and availability of educators (Saco et al., 2016). VM online atlases with annotations and case descriptions help to solve these problems for training programs that report such obstacles (Hinshaw, 2012, 2009). In response to these noted challenges, the American Society of Dermatopathology has been converting their glass slide collection to a digital format, which will be available online when completed (Mooney & Hedblad, 2012; http://www.asdp.org/education/). Given the nature of histopathology, it is paramount that new technology used for education, and even diagnosis, is validated and shown to be at least equivalent to the gold standard of GSM. There have been two peer-reviewed published studies that examined diagnostic precision of VM compared to glass slides among dermatology and pathology residents (Berger et al., 2017; Koch et al., 2009). Both studies found no significant difference in accuracy when comparing the two modalities, although residents preferred GSM (Berger et al., 2017; Koch et al., 2009). Trends were consistent across all resident levels, revealing that prior experience with VM was not necessary to make accurate diagnoses (Koch et al., 2009). In one study, 23% of respondents reported using VM in their residency education via departmental virtual slide collections (39%), internet image libraries (71%), and additional virtual compilations (11%) (Koch et al., 2009). Challenges reported include decreased ease of viewing and mobility of virtual slides; therefore, only 44% of trainees in this study deemed VM to be as effective for testing functions (Koch et al., 2009). Additionally, another group of investigators found that 33% of dermatology and pathology residents in their study had employed VM more than once in the preceding 6 months, and 81% reported using it more frequently for studying purposes (Gertz et al., 2015). Reported disadvantages included slow loading speeds, inadequate resolution, freezing of the screen, and problems starting the software (Berger et al., 2017; Gertz et al., 2015; Koch et al., 2009). However, 80% of participants felt that VM is still useful in the setting of DP education (Koch et al., 2009). In contrast, another paper reported that diagnostic accuracy among dermatology residents was better with GSM than VM in an examination setting (Brick et al., 2013). There was no difference in the diagnostic accuracy of first-year trainees or those with prior exposure to VM more than twice per month (Brick et al., 2013). Residents at more formative stages in their training reported more comfort with VM compared to their senior counterparts (Koch et al., 2009). Earlier exposure to VM and frequent use for education and self-study may lead to better performance with this technology in the future (Brick et al., 2013). Of interest, one study found that there was no overall personal preference among examinees for GSM versus VM (Brick et al., 2013).

For graduate trainees, VM has percolated into high stakes assessments such as resident in-service and board certification examinations which will likely incentivize programs to implement this technology in their teaching curricula. Currently, the Dermatology Board Certification Examination contains a mixture of glass slides, static digital images, and WSI (Shahriari et al., 2017). Notably, the American Board of Dermatology has recently increased the ratio of virtual images to glass images on the exam (Shahriari et al., 2017). One noted benefit of VM is the ability to decentralize locations for the certification exam, as microscopes would not be necessary (Gertz et al., 2015). In pathology, digital slides are used to assess the diagnostic skills of trainees on the resident in-service exams and in Board Examinations of the American Board of Pathology (Boyce, 2015). A study of pathology residents found a strong correlation between performance on VM competency testing and future in-service exam scores, highlighting that VM may be helpful in evaluating trainee progress (Bruch et al., 2009). Similar studies for dermatology residents are needed. The utilization of VM overall will depend on trainees' resistance or willingness to embrace new technology while in training. Although today's students are labeled as "early adopters" of technological innovation, referring to their increased comfort and acceptance of technology, only a small proportion of residents have used VM (Gertz et al., 2015). Further studies are needed to determine the broader role and potential benefits of VM in graduate education and assessment.

SLIDE TRACKING TECHNOLOGY

Aside from its educational capabilities, VM can also be used as a research tool to assess learning in DP and pathology. Assessing the extent of learning can be achieved by studying how trainees interact with the digital slides through tracking programs. Since the foundation of histopathology relies on image viewing, it is critical to master visual perception, processing, and pattern recognition skills while training (Shahriari et al., 2017). Eye-tracking cameras can follow eye movements during the diagnostic process to understand the logical sequence to correct diagnosis (Saco et al., 2016). Movement through digital slides can be recorded, replayed, mapped, and compared between individuals (Hamilton, Wang, & McCullough, 2012). The software can track how students move through images in 4 dimensions: x and y axes, zoom (z axis), and time. For trainees, the goal is to follow more targeted and effective pathways while achieving diagnostic accuracy. Studies have shown a strong relationship between diagnostic track and diagnostic error, opening the potential for eye-tracking and slide-tracking technology to increase diagnostic efficiency and accuracy (Brunye et al., 2014; Treanor, Lim, Magee, Bulpitt, & Quirke, 2009). This technology can monitor and evaluate student progress and provide automated feedback in educational settings (Brunye et al., 2014). It can also help elucidate why students choose the right or wrong answer when viewing digital images, and therefore improve learning through guided instruction and feedback (Brunye et al., 2014; Crowley, Naus, Stewart, & Friedman, 2003; Houghton, Smoller, Leonard, Stevenson, & Dornan, 2015; Jaarsma, Jarodzka, Nap, van Merrienboer, & Boshuizen, 2014, 2015; Krupinski, Graham, & Weinstein, 2013; Treanor et al., 2009; Walkowski, Lundin M, Szymas, & Lundin J, 2014). Static images do not afford this monitoring and training feature or objective metrics. These innovative technologies can impartially highlight differences between the search patterns and eye movements of novices and practicing experienced pathologists.

There are numerous steps along the diagnostic pathway: search, detection, recognition, identification, and processing of findings to make an appropriate diagnosis (Crowley et al., 2003; Jaarsma et al., 2014; Shahriari et al., 2017). Whereas novices follow a search-then-detect pattern of slide viewing, involving extensive searching through the entire slide, experts follow a detect-then-search process, allowing for rapid detection of diagnostically relevant features (Brunye et al., 2014; Jaarsma et al., 2014; Mello-Thoms et al., 2012). Although both can eventually find the diagnostically important areas, trainees take more time to do so and spend less time examining the relevant areas (Jaarsma et al., 2014). Experts show different eye movements, employ lower magnification, spend less time on irrelevant features, use less panning and zoom movements, and make faster and more accurate diagnoses (Brunye et al., 2014; Jaarsma et al., 2015). Eye-tracking and slide-movement technology can aid in the shift from "dispersed and time-consuming" to more "targeted and effective" slide viewing (Brunye et al., 2014). Education can be steered to enhance review and interpretation of images while also addressing areas of student weakness (Shahriari et al., 2017).

MOBILE TECHNOLOGY IN EDUCATION

Educational Benefits

Despite the new era of whole slide scanners and microscope-mounted digital cameras, the most common barrier to adoption of these technologies is the acquisition cost of hardware and supplies (Farahani et al., 2015; Morrison & Gardner, 2015a). The use of mobile camera-based technology and "apps" on handheld devices, including "smartphones" and tablets, is enhancing the way medical students, residents, and physicians are learning pathology (Hartman, 2016; Lehman & Gibson, 2013;

Morrison & Gardner, 2014; Zhou, Yu, Xue, & Elston, 2016). Numerous advantages of using mobile devices include: portability, low cost, efficiency and intuitiveness of the device, and flexibility of the technology (Hartman, 2016). In addition to mobile applications, interactive virtual reality technology, such as Oculus Rift, may have future training utility in digital pathology (Farahani et al., 2016). Besides educational roles, mobile phones can be employed as image acquisition devices or attached to stand-alone microscopes to capture digital images.

Advancements in mobile technology and an increasing focus on improved educational methods have led to the development of dermatology- and pathology-specific mobile applications ("apps"). With increasing image resolution of smartphone cameras, it is now possible to use devices for image capture and subsequent diagnostic purposes. However, less than 1% of currently available dermatology apps are pathology-specific (Brewer et al., 2013). Given the visual nature of dermatology and pathology, image-based applications are beneficial due to the importance of pattern recognition (Hanna, Parwani, Pantanowitz, Punjabi, & Singh, 2015). Education in dermatopathology, and pathology in general, relied largely on glass slides and textbooks before the recent development of whole slide imaging. These digital slides can be transferred to DP-based apps which are easily accessible and readily available for viewing in any location (Bronfenbrener, 2014; Hanna et al., 2015; Shahriari et al., 2017).

Various DP apps for educational and consultation purposes have been developed and made available for iOS and Android smartphone users. MyDermPath+ is a smartphone app and corresponding website which has stored and categorized digital images with attached useful information such as diagnosis, differential diagnosis, special studies, and clinical management (https://itunes.apple.com/us/app/mydermpath/id455500880?mt=8). It is a comprehensive DP database with over 1000 diagnoses, including less common pathologies, and a user-friendly interface including a diagnosis searchability feature (Bronfenbrener, 2014; Shahriari et al., 2017). This free app also has educational quizzes available to assess user knowledge (Shahriari et al., 2017). Another app only available on iPads is Clearpath which is an extensive DP database with interactive virtual images (http://www.dermpathlab.com/clearpath/). The modern interface and search function allows users to browse over 250 images with zoom capabilities; additionally, there is a timed quiz mode for knowledge check. Other mobile educational apps include the live video-streaming application called Periscope, which is free for smartphone users (https://www.periscope.tv/about). It allows for real-time presentation of various topics and lectures that can be shared with multiple users around the world. Pathologists have employed the app as a tool for teaching purposes; this platform could also supplement DP education, allowing for remote learning (Fuller, Mukhopadhyay, & Gardner, 2016).

MICROSCOPES AND MOBILE PHONES

In addition to educational roles, smartphones are also being utilized to directly capture images from microscope oculars, both with and without the use of a mounting device as in Figure 2 (Lehman & Gibson, 2013; Morrison & Gardner, 2015b; Roy et al., 2014). Mobile camera resolution has advanced such that image quality is similar to standard capture methods (Roy et al., 2014). Additionally, smartphones are portable and pervasive in today's world, allowing for easy use with any standard microscope. Of importance, students in educational settings have shown enhanced participation, engagement, and group discussion in pathology laboratory sessions when smartphone technology is employed (Umudum, 2015). The term "smart teledermatopathology" was created by Lehman and Gibson (2013) to describe the combined use of a smartphone, microscope with adapter, electronic tablet, and high-speed internet. Their "store-and-forward method" of image capture at low, medium, and high power magnifications includes a smartphone attached to the eyepiece of a microscope via an adapter (Lehman & Gibson, 2013). Digital images can then be sent to electronic tablets where recipients can view the interactive slides, making the technology useful for educational purposes. Real-time video recording is also possible with this aforementioned method; however, image quality and resolution can be suboptimal (Lehman & Gibson, 2013).

Other methods that do not require a camera adapter have been published, allowing for overall reduced equipment costs. The method called "m-microscopy" involves the joining of the user's thumb and index finger around the microscope eyepiece to block external light interference when using a mobile phone for image acquisition (Bellina & Missoni, 2009). Recently, a hands-free and adapter-free technique, which involves moving the smartphone camera close to one eyepiece until the image comes into focus (usually a distance of 1 cm apart) has been described and evaluated in the clinical setting (Morrison & Gardner, 2015b; Zhou et al., 2016). These new image acquisition techniques allow for easy use and cost-effective methods of teaching and clinical consultation, particularly in areas lacking resources and specialists such as dermatopathologists. Lastly, other researchers are looking into the possibility of mobile phones doubling as microscopes themselves. One group conducted a study using a 3-mm sapphire ball lens apparatus over the smartphone camera to scan DP specimen slides (Jahan-Tigh, Chinn, & Rapini, 2016). Their results showed high sensitivity and specificity for diagnosing basal cell carcinoma and squamous cell carcinoma; however, melanoma diagnosis had low sensitivity (60%) when evaluating 15 samples (Jahan-Tigh et al., 2016). The technology employed in this aforementioned study is inexpensive and costs approximately US $14; therefore,

Figure 2. Image acquisition of skin specimens with a mobile device
Source: Used with permission from Akanksha Gupta, MD

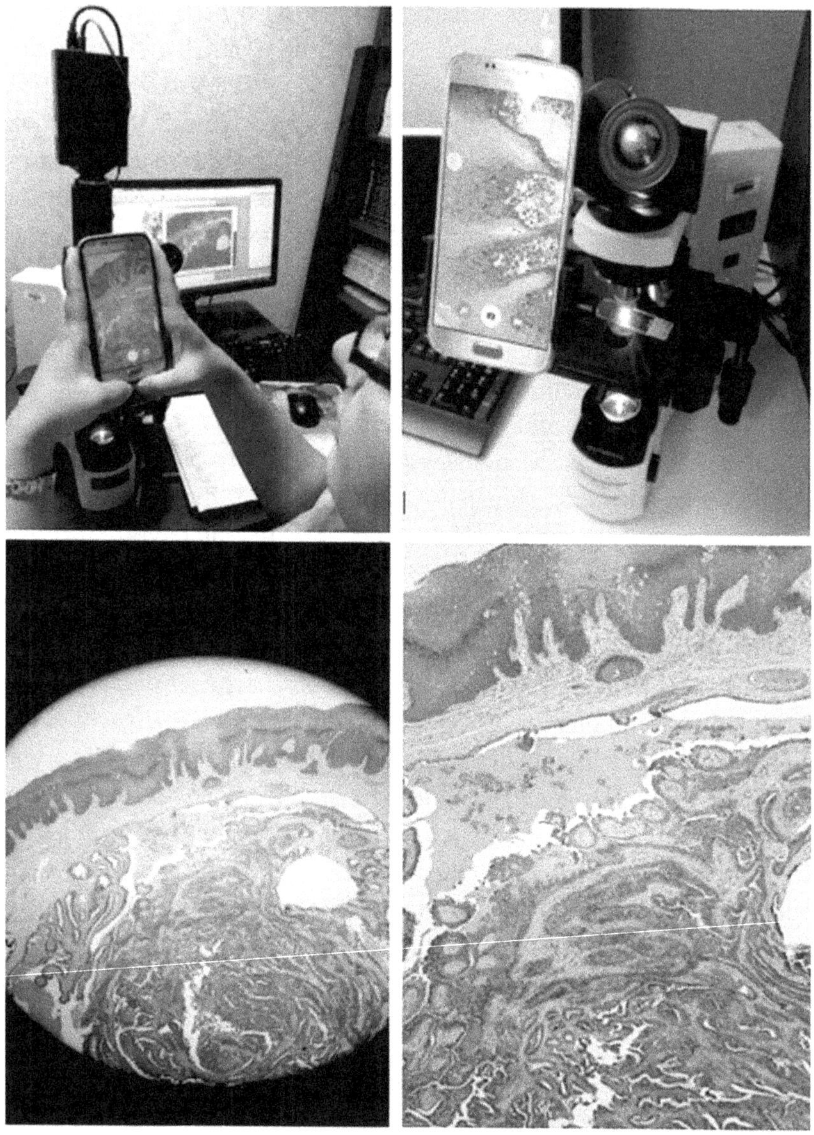

it is useful for obtaining and sharing DP information in resource-limited settings (Jahan-Tigh et al., 2016). Although this technology is relatively new and there is no data available for its role in education, further developments in imaging processing and diagnostic accuracy will likely lead to increased usage for both clinical and training purposes, especially in areas lacking support and resources.

ONLINE INFORMATION AND IMAGE SHARING

The internet is home to a wide array of educational materials for numerous disciplines. Users can interact with other people worldwide and upload material for information and image sharing. These platforms can be employed in promoting pathology and DP education. In 2017, one group outlined three categories of online content: (1) message boards and email list-servs; (2) websites for pathologist-generated material; and (3) social media websites such as Facebook, Instagram, Twitter, and Periscope (Gonzalez et al., 2017). With high-speed internet, there is limitless potential for knowledge sharing and access to scientific materials that were previously only available in print form. Online DP and pathology journals and websites have increased the rapid dissemination of educational material for medical students, residents, and practicing physicians. Various resources include: PathologyOutlines.com, WebPath, and Dermpedia. The former two are diagnosis-based study tools, whereas the latter is a free site for trainees and physicians to share interesting cases and information online (https://library.med.utah.edu/WebPath/webpath.html; www.dermpedia.org). The Pathology Resident Wiki and Libre Pathology are resources with pathologist-generated content for further learning and sharing of data (http://pathinfo.wikia.com/wiki/Pathology_Resident_Wiki; https://librepathology.org/). Global information exchange is now possible through these sites and online communities with clinical-pathological conferences, grand rounds, seminars, and educational courses (Shahriari et al., 2017). Other resources, such as Dermpath-l which is an international mailing list for people interested in DP, connect people from different institutions around the world and allow for the exchange of ideas and knowledge (http://lists.umanitoba.ca/mailman/listinfo/dermpath-l). Another DP educational website, MDlive, contains medical presentations and a lecture series, including a DP Master Series for remote and supplemental learning (http://www.mdlive.net/dermpath_sch.htm).

SOCIAL MEDIA

Social media has provided an avenue for rapid distribution of information and exchange of ideas among people worldwide. Facebook, Twitter, and Instagram are utilized by pathologists and dermatopathologists for a variety of purposes including discussion groups, presentation of unique cases, and educational seminars. One Facebook group in particular, the Dermatopathology Group, has 27,884 members as of 2017 and over 800 cases posted (facebook.com/groups/dermatopathology). The American Society of Dermatopathology and International Society of Dermatopathology, which both have Twitter accounts, as well as ASDP Instagram and JAAD Facebook, frequently provide updates for followers and present current cases and topics in dermatology, pathology, and dermatopathology (https://www.instagram.com/asdpdermpath/; https://www.facebook.com/JAADjournals/). Social media is also frequently used during conferences, especially Twitter, for "live-tweeting" of events and cases (Isom, Walsh, & Gardner, 2017). On Twitter from November 2016 to May 2017, there were 33,403 #dermpath tweets made by 1,973 users (Madke & Gardner, 2017). Teaching institutions, such as Columbia University, Johns Hopkins University, and many others have pathology-dedicated Twitter and Facebook accounts (Isom et al., 2017). Additionally, within the Pathology Resident Wiki page, there is a list of pathology-related Facebook groups in the Social Media Guide for Pathologists (http://pathinfo.wikia.com/wiki/Social_Media_Guide_for_Pathologists). These groups have the capability to reach a wider audience and encourage collaboration and participation among members. Discussion of cases and varying opinions allow for enhanced learning; however, it is of utmost importance to protect patient privacy (Crane & Gardner, 2016).

Besides powerful networking and collaboration, social media encourages dissemination of DP knowledge. One such tool is iSlide, an interactive e-learning system which contains digital DP and pathology slides coupled with a Facebook application (Lee et al., 2015). Online learning is possible through user annotation and comments on slides shared within the "iSlide Community" Facebook group (https://www.facebook.com/iSlide-Community-232031680144669/). Through this platform, educators off-site are able to instruct students and participate in online discussions, allowing for expanded educational opportunities.

EDUCATION IN NEW TECHNOLOGIES

In the era of modern technology, new devices for the diagnosis of melanoma and other cutaneous lesions have been developed and determined to be efficacious in clinical practice (Winkelmann et al., 2017). These techniques include high-frequency ultrasound, optical coherence tomography, and reflectance confocal microscopy (RCM). Among these, RCM is leading the way due to its superior resolution for diagnostic purposes (Gonzalez, 2008). RCM enables the non-invasive in vivo examination, diagnosis, and risk-stratification of skin lesions in real-time. The device, including a handheld version, uses a near-infrared 830-nm laser to image horizontal skin sections up to 300 micrometers in depth, generally to the level of the superficial dermis. Sensitivity and specificity of RCM for melanoma detection has been determined to be 91-100% and 68-98%, respectively (Que, Grant-Kels, Longo, & Pellacani, 2016). Various advantages of this new technology include its usefulness for visualizing in vivo non-pigmented lesions, lesions in cosmetically sensitive areas, and avoidance of an unnecessary biopsy if benign-appearing on imaging (Winkelmann et al., 2017). As with any new technology, disadvantages include high cost of the device, difficulty with insurance coverage, and a lack of knowledge about this imaging modality (Que et al., 2015; Winkelmann et al., 2017). The greatest current obstacle to broader use in clinical practice is the need for education in image interpretation (Gonzalez, 2008). The basics of RCM are occasionally taught at continuing medical education courses and conferences; however, a training curriculum in the United States has not yet been formally developed (Que, 2015, 2016). Instruction in this technology is critical for more widespread implementation in practice. By incorporating relevant training into dermatology residency, more practicing clinicians will be able to use RCM and therefore potentially spare their patients unnecessary biopsies. With the rising incidence of melanoma and non-melanoma skin cancers, further research and education using these devices is important, given the early indication of enhanced clinical efficiency and improved patient outcomes.

CONCLUSION

Technological advancement is changing the field of DP and the training of future clinicians and pathologists. Prior to these developments, DP education relied on glass slide microscopy, textbook atlases, and on-site dermatopathologists for teaching. Today, the adoption and implementation of VM in histology, pathology, DP, and other subspecialties now serves to train medical students, residents, and fellows. Digital databases and online atlases are utilized as interactive educational tools which can be deployed at any time in any location. The expansion of mobile apps and online resources has also contributed to the educational revolution by giving students flexibility in their training. Trainees can work at their own pace and perform "knowledge checks" via interactive online assessments. DP learning has also spread to social media sites, such as Facebook and Twitter, allowing for widespread dissemination of information and image sharing among users. Instant access to specialists around the world enhances education for all participants and fosters discussion of various cases and topics. Importantly, technology provides an avenue for resource-limited areas to receive quality care and access to trained experts that would otherwise be unattainable. Overall, technology is steadily moving the field of DP forward and providing students with a collaborative, interactive, and practical format for learning histopathology in an ever-changing digital world.

REFERENCES

Al Habeeb, A., Evans, A., & Ghazarian, D. (2012). Virtual microscopy using whole-slide imaging as an enabler for teledermatopathology: A paired consultant validation study. *Journal of Pathology Informatics*, *3*(1), 2. doi:10.4103/2153-3539.93399 PMID:22439122

Al-Janabi, S., Huisman, A., & Van Diest, P. J. (2012). Digital pathology: Current status and future perspectives. *Histopathology*, *61*(1), 1–9. doi:10.1111/j.1365-2559.2011.03814.x PMID:21477260

Alotaibi, O., & ALQahtani, D. (2016). Measuring dental students' preference: A comparison of light microscopy and virtual microscopy as teaching tools in oral histology and pathology. *The Saudi Dental Journal*, *28*(4), 169–173. doi:10.1016/j.sdentj.2015.11.002 PMID:27872547

American Board of Dermatology. (2017). *Certification examination details.* Retrieved from https://www.abderm.org/residents-and-fellows/primary-certification-examination/certification-examination-details.aspx

Bellina, L., & Missoni, E. (2009). Mobile cell-phones (M-phones) in telemicroscopy: Increasing connectivity of isolated laboratories. *Diagnostic Pathology*, *4*(1), 19–22. doi:10.1186/1746-1596-4-19 PMID:19545373

Berger, W. A., Townsend-Kraft, M., Murphy, M. J., & Elaba, Z. (2017). Randomized comparison of virtual microscopy and glass microscopy among dermatology and pathology residents during a simulated in-training examination. *Journal of Cutaneous Pathology*, *44*(4), 409–410. doi:10.1111/cup.12896 PMID:28150326

Blake, C. A., Lavoie, H. A., & Millette, C. F. (2003). Teaching medical histology at the University of South Carolina school of medicine: Transition to virtual slides and virtual microscopes. *Anatomical Record. Part B, New Anatomist*, *275*(1), 196–206. doi:10.1002/ar.b.10037 PMID:14628320

Boutonnat, J., Paulin, C., Faure, C., Colle, P. E., Ronot, X., & Seigneurin, D. (2006). A pilot study in two French medical schools for teaching histology using virtual microscopy. *Morphologie*, *90*(288), 21–25. doi:10.1016/S1286-0115(06)74314-4 PMID:16929817

Boyce, B. F. (2015). Whole slide imaging: Uses and limitations for surgical pathology and teaching. *Biotechnic & Histochemistry*, *90*(5), 321–330. doi:10.3109/10520295.2015.1033463 PMID:25901738

Brewer, A. C., Endly, D. C., Henley, J., Amir, M., Sampson, B. P., Moreau, J. F., & Dellavalle, R. P. (2013). Mobile applications in dermatology. *JAMA Dermatology*, *149*(11), 1300–1304. doi:10.1001/jamadermatol.2013.5517 PMID:24067948

Brick, K. E., Sluzevich, J. C., Cappel, M. A., DiCaudo, D. J., Comfere, N. I., & Wieland, C. N. (2013). Comparison of virtual microscopy and glass slide microscopy among dermatology residents during a simulated in-training examination. *Journal of Cutaneous Pathology*, *40*(9), 807–811. doi:10.1111/cup.12189 PMID:23808673

Bronfenbrener, R. (2014). Learning dermatopathology in the digital age. *Cutis*, *94*(4), E22–E24. PMID:25372265

Bruch, L. A., De Young, B. R., Kreiter, C. D., Haugen, T. H., Leaven, T. C., & Dee, F. R. (2009). Competency assessment of residents in surgical pathology using virtual microscopy. *Human Pathology*, *40*(8), 1122–1128. doi:10.1016/j.humpath.2009.04.009 PMID:19552936

Brunye, T.T., Carney, P.A., Allison, K.H., Shapiro, L.G., Weaver, D.L., & Elmore, J.G. (2014). Eye movements as an index of pathologist visual expertise: a pilot study. *PLoS One, 9*(8), 1-7.

Cotter, J. R. (2001). Laboratory instruction in histology at the University at Buffalo: Recent replacement of microscope exercises with computer applications. *The Anatomical Record*, *265*(5), 212–221. doi:10.1002/ar.10010 PMID:11745105

Crane, G. M., & Gardner, J. M. (2016). Pathology image-sharing on social media: Recommendations for protecting privacy while motivating education. *AMA Journal of Ethics*, *18*(8), 817–825. doi:10.1001/journalofethics.2016.18.8.stas1-1608 PMID:27550566

Crowley, R. S., Naus, G. J., Stewart, J., & Friedman, C. P. (2003). Development of visual diagnostic expertise in pathology: An information-processing study. *Journal of the American Medical Informatics Association*, *10*(1), 39–51. doi:10.1197/jamia.M1123 PMID:12509356

Drake, R. L., McBride, J. M., Lachman, N., & Pawlina, W. (2009). Medical education in the anatomical sciences: The winds of change continue to blow. *Anatomical Sciences Education*, *2*(6), 253–259. doi:10.1002/ase.117 PMID:19890982

Dziegielewski, M., Velan, G. M., & Kumar, R. K. (2003). Teaching pathology using 'hotspotted' digital images. *Medical Education*, *37*(11), 1047–1048. doi:10.1046/j.1365-2923.2003.01646.x PMID:14629446

Farahani, N., Parwani, A. V., & Pantanowitz, L. (2015). Whole slide imaging in pathology: Advantages, limitations, and emerging perspectives. *Pathology and Laboratory Medicine International: PLMI*, *7*, 23–33.

Farahani, N., Post, R., Duboy, J., Ahmed, I., Kolowitz, B. J., Krinchai, T., ... Pantanowitz, L. (2016). Exploring virtual reality technology and the Oculus Rift for the examination of digital pathology slides. *Journal of Pathology Informatics*, *7*(1), 22–26. doi:10.4103/2153-3539.181766 PMID:27217972

Foster, K. (2010). Medical education in the digital age: Digital whole slide imaging as an e-learning tool. *Journal of Pathology Informatics*, *1*(1), 14–16. doi:10.4103/2153-3539.68331 PMID:20922031

Fuller, M. Y., Mukhopadhyay, S., & Gardner, J. M. (2016). Using the periscope live video-streaming application for global pathology education: A brief introduction. *Archives of Pathology & Laboratory Medicine*, *140*(11), 1273–1280. doi:10.5858/arpa.2016-0268-SA PMID:27441785

Gertz, R., Longley, B. J., Bennett, D., Ranheim, E., Rajamanickam, V., Kawahara, T., & Endo, J. (2015). Integrating virtual dermatopathology as part of formative and summative assessment of residents: A feasibility pilot study. *Journal of Cutaneous Pathology*, *42*(10), 779–781. doi:10.1111/cup.12503 PMID:25990466

Goldberg, H. R., & Dintzis, R. (2007). The positive impact of team-based virtual microscopy on student learning in physiology and histology. *Advances in Physiology Education*, *31*(3), 261–265. doi:10.1152/advan.00125.2006 PMID:17848592

Gonzalez, R. S., Amer, S. M., Yahia, N. B., D'Almeida Costa, F., Noatay, M., Qiao, J. H., ... Gardner, J. M. (2017). Facebook discussion groups provide a robust worldwide platform for free pathology education. *Archives of Pathology & Laboratory Medicine*, *141*(5), 690–695. doi:10.5858/arpa.2016-0369-OA PMID:27763789

Gonzalez, S. (2008). Clinical applications of reflectance confocal microscopy in the management of cutaneous tumors. *Actas Dermo-Sifilograficas*, *99*(7), 528–531. doi:10.1016/S0001-7310(08)74737-9 PMID:18682165

Guo, K., Liao, J., Bian, Z., Heng, X., & Zheng, G. (2015). InstantScope: A low-cost whole slide imaging system with instant focal plane detection. *Biomedical Optics Express*, *6*(9), 3210–3216. doi:10.1364/BOE.6.003210 PMID:26417493

Hamilton, P. W., Wang, Y., & McCullough, S. J. (2012). Virtual microscopy and digital pathology in training and education. *APMIS*, *120*(4), 305–315. doi:10.1111/j.1600-0463.2011.02869.x PMID:22429213

Hanna, M. G., Parwani, A. V., Pantanowitz, L., Punjabi, V., & Singh, R. (2015). Smartphone applications: A contemporary resource for dermatopathology. *Journal of Pathology Informatics*, *6*(1), 44–48. doi:10.4103/2153-3539.161612 PMID:26284155

Hartman, D. J. (2016). Mobile technology for the practice of pathology. *Advances in Anatomic Pathology*, *23*(2), 118–124. doi:10.1097/PAP.0000000000000093 PMID:26849818

Higgins, C. (2015). Applications and challenges of digital pathology and whole slide imaging. *Biotechnic & Histochemistry*, *90*(5), 341–347. doi:10.3109/10520295.2015.1044566 PMID:25978139

Hinshaw, M., Hsu, P., Lee, L. Y., & Stratman, E. (2009). The current state of dermatopathology education: A survey of the Association of Professors of Dermatology. *Journal of Cutaneous Pathology*, *36*(6), 620–628. doi:10.1111/j.1600-0560.2008.01128.x PMID:19515041

Hinshaw, M. A. (2012). Dermatopathology education: An update. *Dermatologic Clinics*, *30*(4), 815–826. doi:10.1016/j.det.2012.06.003 PMID:23021060

Horn, A. J., Czarnecki, D., & Lele, S. M. (2012). Interactive case vignettes utilizing simulated pathologist-clinician encounters with whole slide imaging and video tutorials of whole slide scans improve student understanding of disease processes. *Journal of Pathology Informatics*, *3*(1), 34–38. doi:10.4103/2153-3539.101786 PMID:23243552

Houghton, J. P., Smoller, B. R., Leonard, N., Stevenson, M. R., & Dornan, T. (2015). Diagnostic performance on briefly presented digital pathology images. *Journal of Pathology Informatics*, *6*(1), 56–61. doi:10.4103/2153-3539.168517 PMID:26605121

Isom, J., Walsh, M., & Gardner, J. (2017). Social media and pathology: Where are we now and why does it matter? *Advances in Anatomic Pathology*, *24*(5), 294–303. doi:10.1097/PAP.0000000000000159 PMID:28719442

Jaarsma, T., Jarodzka, H., Nap, M., van Merrienboer, J. J., & Boshuizen, H. P. (2014). Expertise under the microscope: Processing histopathological slides. *Medical Education*, *48*(3), 292–300. doi:10.1111/medu.12385 PMID:24528464

Jaarsma, T., Jarodzka, H., Nap, M., van Merrienboer, J. J., & Boshuizen, H. P. (2015). Expertise in clinical pathology: Combining the visual and cognitive perspective. *Advances in Health Sciences Education: Theory and Practice*, *20*(4), 1089–1106. doi:10.100710459-015-9589-x PMID:25677013

Jahan-Tigh, R. R., Chinn, G. M., & Rapini, R. P. (2016). A comparative study between smartphone-based microscopy and conventional light microscopy in 1021 dermatopathology specimens. *Archives of Pathology & Laboratory Medicine*, *140*(1), 86–90. doi:10.5858/arpa.2014-0593-OA PMID:26717060

Kent, M., Olsen, T., Feeser, T., Tesno, K. C., Moad, J. C., Conroy, M. P., ... Bottomley, M. A. (2017). Diagnostic accuracy of virtual pathology vs traditional microscopy in a large dermatopathology study. *JAMA Dermatology*, E1–E7. PMID:29049424

Koch, L. H., Lampros, J. N., Delong, L. K., Chen, S. C., Woosley, J. T., & Hood, A. F. (2009). Randomized comparison of virtual microscopy and traditional glass microscopy in diagnostic accuracy among dermatology and pathology residents. *Human Pathology*, *40*(5), 662–667. doi:10.1016/j.humpath.2008.10.009 PMID:19144382

Krippendorf, B. B., & Lough, J. (2005). Complete and rapid switch from light microscopy to virtual microscopy for teaching medical histology. *Anatomical Record. Part B, New Anatomist*, *285*(1), 19–25. doi:10.1002/ar.b.20066 PMID:16032757

Krupinski, E. A., Graham, A. R., & Weinstein, R. S. (2013). Characterizing the development of visual search expertise in pathology residents viewing whole slide images. *Human Pathology*, *44*(3), 357–364. doi:10.1016/j.humpath.2012.05.024 PMID:22835956

Kumar, R. K., Velan, G. M., Korell, S. O., Kandara, M., Dee, F. R., & Wakefield, D. (2004). Virtual microscopy for learning and assessment in pathology. *The Journal of Pathology*, *204*(5), 613–618. doi:10.1002/path.1658 PMID:15470688

Lee, J. J., Jedrych, J., Pantanowitz, L., & Ho, J. (2017). Validation of digital pathology for primary histopathological diagnosis of routine, inflammatory dermatopathology cases. *The American Journal of Dermatopathology*, *0*, 1–7. PMID:28763335

Lee, P., Chen, C. F., Wan, H. T., Jian, W. S., Hsu, M. H., Syed-Abdul, S., ... Li, Y. C. (2015). iSlide: A 'big picture' interactive teledermatopathology e-learning system. *British Journal of Dermatology*, *172*(3), 692–699. doi:10.1111/bjd.13274 PMID:25040884

Lehman, J. S., & Gibson, L. E. (2013). Smart teledermatopathology: A feasibility study of novel, high-value, portable, widely accessible and intuitive telepathology methods using handheld electronic devices. *Journal of Cutaneous Pathology*, *40*(5), 513–518. doi:10.1111/cup.12108 PMID:23472602

Leifer, Z. (2015). The use of virtual microscopy and a wiki in pathology education: Tracking student use, involvement, and response. *Journal of Pathology Informatics*, *6*(1), 30–36. doi:10.4103/2153-3539.158063 PMID:26110097

Leinweber, B., Massone, C., Kodama, K., Kaddu, S., Cerroni, L., Haas, J., ... Smolle, J. (2006). Teledermatopathology: A controlled study about diagnostic validity and technical requirements for digital transmission. *The American Journal of Dermatopathology*, *28*(5), 413–416. doi:10.1097/01.dad.0000211523.95552.86 PMID:17012916

Madke, B., & Gardner, J. (2017). Enhanced worldwide dermatology–pathology interaction via facebook, twitter, and other social media platforms. *The American Journal of Dermatopathology*, *0*, 1–5. PMID:28796693

Massone, C., Soyer, P. H., Lozzi, G. P., Di Stefani, A., Leinweber, B., Gabler, G., ... Kerl, H. (2007). Feasibility and diagnostic agreement in teledermatopathology using a virtual slide system. *Human Pathology*, *38*(4), 546–554. doi:10.1016/j.humpath.2006.10.006 PMID:17270240

Mello-Thoms, C., Mello, C. A., Medvedeva, O., Castine, M., Legowski, E., Gardner, G., ... Crowley, R. (2012). Perceptual analysis of the reading of dermatopathology virtual slides by pathology residents. *Archives of Pathology & Laboratory Medicine*, *136*(5), 551–562. doi:10.5858/arpa.2010-0697-OA PMID:22540304

Mione, S., Valcke, M., & Cornelissen, M. (2013). Evaluation of virtual microscopy in medical histology teaching. *Anatomical Sciences Education*, *6*(5), 307–315. doi:10.1002/ase.1353 PMID:23463716

Mooney, E., & Hedblad, M. A. (2012). Virtual dermatopathology: Current technology and use. *Forum for Nordic Dermato-Venerology*, *17*(2), 40–43.

Mooney, E., Hood, A. F., Lampros, J., Kempf, W., & Jemec, G. B. E. (2011). Comparative diagnostic accuracy in virtual dermatopathology. *Skin Research and Technology*, *17*(2), 251–255. doi:10.1111/j.1600-0846.2010.00493.x PMID:21251087

Morrison, A. O., & Gardner, J. M. (2015a). Microscopic image photography techniques of the past, present, and future. *Archives of Pathology & Laboratory Medicine*, *139*(12), 1558–1564. doi:10.5858/arpa.2014-0315-RA PMID:25989285

Morrison, A. O., & Gardner, J. M. (2015b). The Morrison technique: A free-hand method for capturing photomicrographs using a smartphone. *Journal of Cutaneous Pathology*, *43*(5), 472–474. doi:10.1111/cup.12650 PMID:26679477

Morrison, A. S., & Gardner, J. M. (2014). Smart phone microscopic photography: A novel tool for physicians and trainees. *Archives of Pathology & Laboratory Medicine*, *138*(8), 1002. doi:10.5858/arpa.2013-0425-ED PMID:24199830

Nelson, D., Ziv, A., & Bandali, K. S. (2012). Going glass to digital: Virtual microscopy as a simulation-based revolution in pathology and laboratory science. *Journal of Clinical Pathology*, *65*(10), 877–881. doi:10.1136/jclinpath-2012-200665 PMID:22791768

Nielsen, P. S., Lindebjerg, J., Rasmussen, J., Starklint, H., Waldstrom, M., & Nielsen, B. (2010). Virtual microscopy: An evaluation of its validity and diagnostic performance in routine histologic diagnosis of skin tumors. *Human Pathology*, *41*(12), 1770–1776. doi:10.1016/j.humpath.2010.05.015 PMID:20869750

Ordi, O., Bombí, J. A., Martínez, A., Ramirez, J., Alos, L., Saco, A., ... Ordi, J. (2015). Virtual microscopy in the undergraduate teaching of pathology. *Journal of Pathology Informatics*, *6*(1), 1–6. doi:10.4103/2153-3539.150246 PMID:25722941

Pantanowitz, L., Valenstein, P. N., Evans, A. J., Kaplan, K. J., Pfeifer, J. D., Wilbur, D. C., ... Colgan, T. J. (2011). Review of the current state of whole slide imaging in pathology. *Journal of Pathology Informatics*, *2*(1), 36–45. doi:10.4103/2153-3539.83746 PMID:21886892

Que, S. K., Fraga-Braghiroli, N., Grant-Kels, J. M., Rabinovitz, H. S., Oliviero, M., & Scope, A. (2015). Through the looking glass: Basics and principles of reflectance confocal microscopy. *Journal of the American Academy of Dermatology*, *73*(2), 276–284. doi:10.1016/j.jaad.2015.04.047 PMID:26051696

Que, S. K., Grant-Kels, J. M., Longo, C., & Pellacani, G. (2016). Basics of confocal microscopy and the complexity of diagnosing skin tumors: New imaging tools in clinical practice, diagnostic workflows, cost-estimate, and new trends. *Dermatologic Clinics*, *34*(4), 367–375. doi:10.1016/j.det.2016.05.001 PMID:27692444

Roy, S., Pantanowitz, L., Amin, M., Seethala, R. R., Ishtiaque, A., Yousem, S. A., ... Hartman, D. J. (2014). Smartphone adapters for digital photomicrography. *Journal of Pathology Informatics*, *5*(1), 24–28. doi:10.4103/2153-3539.137728 PMID:25191623

Saco, A., Bombi, J. A., Garcia, A., Ramírez, J., & Ordi, J. (2016). Current status of whole-slide imaging in education. *Pathobiology*, *83*(2-3), 79–88. doi:10.1159/000442391 PMID:27101397

Scoville, S. A., & Buskirk, T. D. (2007). Traditional and virtual microscopy compared experimentally in a classroom setting. *Clinical Anatomy (New York, N.Y.)*, *20*(5), 565–570. doi:10.1002/ca.20440 PMID:17109440

Shahriari, N., Grant-Kels, J., & Murphy, M. J. (2017). Dermatopathology education in the era of modern technology. *Journal of Cutaneous Pathology*, *44*(9), 763–771. doi:10.1111/cup.12980 PMID:28612388

Thorstenson, S., Molin, J., & Lundstrom, C. (2014). Implementation of large-scale routine diagnostics using whole slide imaging in Sweden: Digital pathology experiences 2006-2013. *Journal of Pathology Informatics*, *5*(1), 14. doi:10.4103/2153-3539.129452 PMID:24843825

Treanor, D., Lim, C. H., Magee, D., Bulpitt, A., & Quirke, P. (2009). Tracking with virtual slides: A tool to study diagnostic error in histopathology. *Histopathology*, *55*(1), 37–45. doi:10.1111/j.1365-2559.2009.03325.x PMID:19614765

Triola, M. M., & Holloway, W. J. (2011). Enhanced virtual microscopy for collaborative education. *BMC Medical Education*, *11*(1), 4–10. doi:10.1186/1472-6920-11-4 PMID:21269474

Umudum, H. (2015). Smart phones and microscopic image capturing: Searching, finding, capturing, talking about, as well as sharing microscopic images of pathologic conditions form another type of learning module. *Archives of Pathology & Laboratory Medicine*, *139*(7), 847. doi:10.5858/arpa.2014-0436-LE PMID:26125424

Walkowski, S., Lundin, M., Szymas, J., & Lundin, J. (2014). Students' performance during practical examination on whole slide images using view path tracking. *Diagnostic Pathology*, *9*(1), 208–215. doi:10.118613000-014-0208-6 PMID:25358824

Weaker, F. J., & Herbert, D. C. (2009). Transition of a dental histology course from light to virtual. *Microscopy*, *73*(10), 1213–1221. PMID:19805786

Wilson, A. B., Taylor, M. A., Klein, B. A., Sugrue, M. K., Whipple, E. C., & Brokaw, J. J. (2016). Meta-analysis and review of learner performance and preference: Virtual versus optical microscopy. *Medical Education*, *50*(4), 428–440. doi:10.1111/medu.12944 PMID:26995482

Winkelmann, R. R., Farberg, A. S., Glazer, A. M., Cockerell, C. J., Sober, A. J., Siegel, D. M., ... Rigel, D. S. (2017). Integrating skin cancer-related technologies into clinical Practice. *Dermatologic Clinics*, *35*(4), 565–576. doi:10.1016/j.det.2017.06.018 PMID:28886814

Zhou, C., Yu, Y., Xue, R., & Elston, D. M. (2016). High-quality digital photomicrography utilizing a smartphone without adapter. *Journal of Cutaneous Pathology*, *43*(1), 82–84. doi:10.1111/cup.12561 PMID:26280458

ADDITIONAL READING

Brick, K. E., Comfere, N. I., Broeren, M. D., Gibson, L. E., & Wieland, C. N. (2014). The application of virtual microscopy in a dermatopathology educational setting: Assessment of attitudes among dermatopathologists. *International Journal of Dermatology*, *53*(2), 224–227. doi:10.1111/ijd.12233 PMID:24168750

Dennis, T., Start, R. D., & Cross, S. S. (2005). The use of digital imaging, video conferencing, and telepathology in histopathology: A national survey. *Journal of Clinical Pathology*, *58*(3), 254–258. doi:10.1136/jcp.2004.022012 PMID:15735155

Evans, A. J., Salama, M. E., Henricks, W. H., & Pantanowitz, L. (2017). Implementation of whole slide imaging for clinical purposes: Issues to consider from the perspective of early adopters. *Archives of Pathology & Laboratory Medicine*, *141*(7), 944–959. doi:10.5858/arpa.2016-0074-OA PMID:28440660

Helle, L., Nivala, M., & Kronqvist, P. (2013). More technology, better learning resources, better learning? Lessons from adopting virtual microscopy in undergraduate medical education. *Anatomical Sciences Education*, *6*(2), 73–80. doi:10.1002/ase.1302 PMID:22930425

Marsch, A. F., Espiritu, B., Groth, J., & Hutchens, K. A. (2014). The effectiveness of annotated (vs. non-annotated) digital pathology slides as a teaching tool during dermatology and pathology residencies. *Journal of Cutaneous Pathology*, *41*(6), 513–518. doi:10.1111/cup.12328 PMID:24620842

Payne, V. L., Medvedeva, O., Legowski, E., Castine, M., Tseytlin, E., Jukic, D., & Crowley, R. S. (2009). Effect of a limited-enforcement intelligent tutoring system in dermatopathology on student errors, goals and solution paths. *Artificial Intelligence in Medicine*, *47*(3), 175–197. doi:10.1016/j.artmed.2009.07.002 PMID:19782544

Shahriari, N., Grant-Kels, J. M., Rabinovitz, H., Oliviero, M., & Scope, A. (2018). In vivo reflectance confocal microscopy image interpretation for the dermatopathologist. *Journal of Cutaneous Pathology*, *45*(3), 187-197. doi:10.1111/cup.13084 PMID:29178501

Weinstein, R. S., Graham, A. R., Richter, L. C., Barker, G. P., Krupinski, E. A., Lopez, A. M., ... Gilbertson, J. R. (2009). Overview of telepathology, virtual microscopy, and whole slide imaging: Prospects for the future. *Human Pathology*, *40*(8), 1057–1069. doi:10.1016/j.humpath.2009.04.006 PMID:19552937

KEY TERMS AND DEFINITIONS

"Apps": Computer-based applications for educational and instructional purposes.

Dermatopathology (DP): A combined specialty of dermatology and pathology which studies cutaneous disorders and diseases at a microscopic level.

Glass Slide Microscopy (GSM): The use of glass slides for viewing specimens under a microscope. The gold-standard of histopathological analysis.

Reflectance Confocal Microscopy (RCM): A novel non-invasive imaging technique for in-vivo examination of the epidermis down to the papillary dermis in real-time.

Slide Tracking: Technology used to analyze both eye and slide movements during visualization of digital images.

Virtual Microscopy (VM): A method of digitalizing glass microscope slides for high-resolution interactive viewing.

Whole-Slide Imaging (WSI): The scanning of conventional glass slides to create digital images using various software programs.

Chapter 7
Using Competency-Based Learning to Improve Clinical Skills

Stefanie R. Ellison
University of Missouri – Kansas City School of Medicine, USA

Jordann Dhuse
University of Missouri – Kansas City School of Medicine, USA

ABSTRACT

This chapter serves to provide medical educators with an overview of competency-based education (CBME) and the clinical skills necessary for medical school graduate. Technology that supports the teaching, learning, and assessment of CBME and clinical skills is defined and examples are provided for each of the Accreditation Council for Graduate Medical Education (ACGME) core competencies. The competencies are defined, and clinical skills embedded in each are highlighted. This chapter provides a summary of the useful technological tools and provides examples of medical schools that use technology to teach and assess CBME with these tools. Online teaching or eLearning, simulation, online assessment, virtual humans, the electronic health record, gaming, procedural software, discussion boards, reflective writing, portfolios, and telemedicine programs are covered in detail.

DOI: 10.4018/978-1-5225-6289-4.ch007

INTRODUCTION

The History of Competency-Based Medical Education

Competency-based education has been in existence for decades in medical education and one can trace its roots to the 1970s (ten Cate & Billett, 2014). Over the past 15 years, it has become more consistently present in undergraduate and graduate medical curricula. The increase in competency-based education likely stems from increased accreditation requirements in undergraduate medical education and in residency training programs to assess learners' skills, increasing quality measures in physician performance, and trends to increase health system accountability (Carraccio & Englander, 2013). In addition, demands for improved safety in patient care drives the need for improved training and skills' assessment to foster consistent care (Nasca, Philibert, Brigham & Flynn, 2012). Evidence also exists to show that standardized resident training drives future clinical performance (Asch 2009; Chen 2014). The core competencies began to take shape after the Accreditation Council for Graduate Medical Education (ACGME) delineated the six core competencies in 1998 defined by the six domains of clinical competence: Patient Care, Medical Knowledge, Practice-based Learning and Improvement, Interpersonal and Communication Skills, Professionalism, and Systems-Based Practice (Swing, 2007). Development of the core competencies were an important step to help standardize the competency-based teaching and assessment movement.

Defining the competencies of a physician in practice was an important first step in assessing clinical skills in our undergraduate medical students and residents, but the devil is in the details. While core competencies can be defined, it is important to develop undergraduate and graduate medical education objectives that are detailed and measurable in order for the learner to understand precisely what they need to do to show competence in those skills. Carraccio and Englander (2016) provided recommendations for developing the learning objectives within the core competencies and called for the following in graduate CBME:

1. A standardized language;
2. The power of direct observation and assessment;
3. The need for developing meaningful measures of performance;
4. Desired outcomes as the starting point for curriculum development;
5. Dependence on the reflection of expertise;
6. Need for exploiting the role of the learner in their learning; and
7. Competent clinical systems as the environment to producing competent physicians.

Figure 1. Similarly, Canada introduced the CanMEDS framework that defines seven roles: medical expert, communicator, collaborator, manager, health advocate, scholar, and professional. Competency-based medical education (CBME) focuses on abilities, outcomes, and centers on the learner so that competency is determined by standards of performance instead of time-based training.
Source: Frank, et al. (2010)

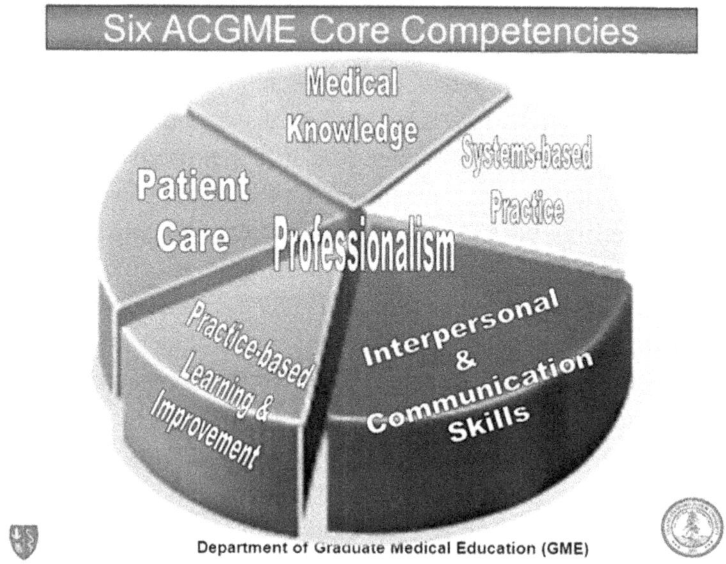

This shift in medical education to CBME is a welcome opportunity for undergraduate medical education to move from assessment of medical knowledge acquisition through standardized testing to assessment of student competence based off skills and attitudes. Adoption of CBME is an opportunity to demonstrate preparation for the independent practice of a physician, especially in the area of clinical skills (Weinberger, Pereira, Lobst, Mechaber & Bronze, 2010).

In undergraduate medical education, the adoption of CBME allows a shift toward defined competencies and expectations for medical students during their professional education. Lessons from graduate medical education have lead educators to define levels of accomplishment for the learner, tailored learning, and programmatic assessment throughout the various stages of medical school. In developing CBME curriculum and assessment, the fundamental question should be "how do we improve medical education to provide better care for patients?" (Carraccio et el., 2017).

Figure 2. Graduate medical education efforts have provided a framework for the formation of medical professionals in training and CBME has become an international phenomenon with developing frameworks in Australia, Europe, and Scotland. The international competency-based medical education (ICBME) collaborators have been working since 2009 to promote understanding of CBME to accelerate its uptake internationally.
Source: Carraccio et al. (2016)

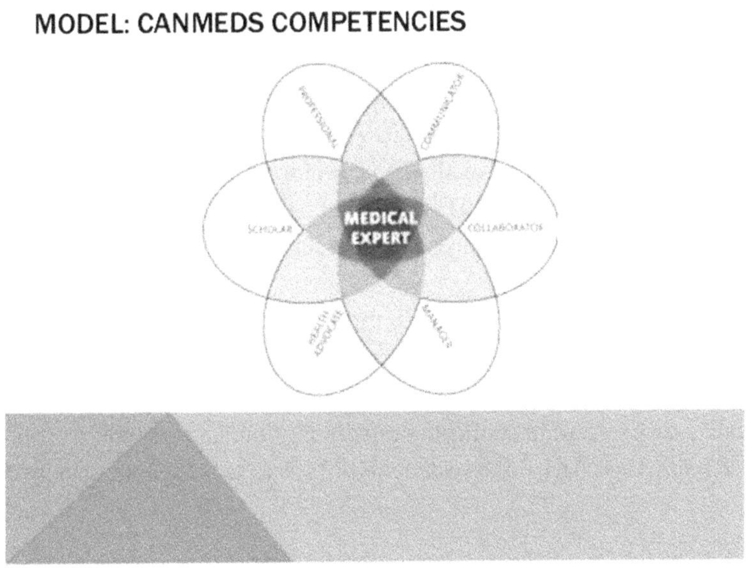

COMPETENCY-BASED UNDERGRADUATE MEDICAL EDUCATION TODAY

Assessment of competency relies on measurable objectives in knowledge, skills and attitudes. For undergraduate medical education, it makes sense to define these skills by year-specific examples of learner ability. No matter the core themes of your medical education program, you must get input from key stakeholders for establishing the curriculum, for developing teaching and assessment activities, and for measuring the competency of your learners. Competency domains should first be set and can borrow from the Accreditation of Graduate Medical Education (ACGME) Core Competencies of Patient Care and Procedural Skills (PC), Interpersonal Skills and Communication (ICS), Medical Knowledge (MK), Professionalism (P), Systems-Based Practice (SBP), and Practice-based Learning and Improvement (PBLI) (Nasca, Philibert, Brigham & Flynn, 2012).

CBME defined solely as domains of competency can be difficult to measure in our learners, especially in undergraduate medical education. For this reason,

CBME has made a notable shift to further define the skills needed for a student graduating from medical school. In the past decade, CBME has moved to teaching and assessing measurable tasks for learners and examples of this trend are found in the development of the Entrustable Professional Activities (EPAs) and the Milestones within residency programs. (Brown, Warren, & Hyderi, 2017). The background and context of this work is to provide the Undergraduate Medical Education (UME) community a common set of core behaviors that could/should be expected of all graduates from medical school to assist them in the transition of residency training. The work of this drafting panel builds on the work of the AAMC Project on the Clinical Education of Medical Students, the Milestones Project and published studies of the UME-GME transition. "EPAs are sentinel tasks (i.e., work) tailored to a specific discipline (i.e., specialty) and performed in an authentic environment (e.g., the emergency department [ED], not in a simulated fashion)" (Corbett, 2005; Carraccio, 2002). Table 1 provides a comparison of the benefits and disadvantages of using an EPA versus a competency.

The panel charge was "to delineate those activities that all entering residents should be expected to perform on day one of residency without direct supervision, regardless of specialty."

Typically, EPAs contain multiple competency objectives pulled from multiple competency domains. An EPA assessment tool uses a scale of entrustment defined as

Table 1. Comparison of the benefits and disadvantages of the two conceptual frameworks considered: competencies and EPAs

	EPAs	**Competencies**
Benefits	• EPAs are "activities," which make sense to faculty, trainees, and the public • Represent the day-to-day work of the professional • Situate competencies and milestones in the clinical context in which we live • Make assessment more practical by clustering milestones into meaningful activities • Explicitly add the notions of trust and supervision into the assessment equation	• Competencies have been the basis for assessment in the GME space for a decade • In the aggregate, define the "good physician" • Have a reasonable body of evidence around assessment of the "traditional" domains (medical knowledge and patient care) • Have been used for establishing or developing milestones of performance for at least the GME years
Disadvantages	• Were relatively recently introduced in the literature • Have had little operationalization worldwide • Were designed originally for the residency-to-practice transition	• Are abstract • Are granular and therefore often not the way we think about or observe learners

Source: AAMC Core Entrustable Professional Activities for Entering Residency Curriculum Developer's Guide 2014 www.aamc.org Page 3. www.mededportal.org/icollaborative/resource/887

the level of trust you now have in your learners based on direct observation of their performance (i.e., progression from close to indirect supervision to independence) for a given task. This measurement of entrustment is ideal for the assessment of medical students throughout the various stages of their medical school development as they move into graduate medical education. The definitions of supervision are as follows (Brown, Warren, & Hyderi, 2017):

1. **Direct Supervision:** The supervising physician is physically present with the resident and the patient.
2. **Indirect Supervision:**
   a. **Direct Supervision Immediately Available:** The supervising physician is physically within the hospital or other site of patient care, and is immediately available to provide direct supervision.
   b. **Direct Supervision Available:** The supervising physician is not physically present within the hospital or other site of patient care, but is immediately available by means of telephonic and/or electronic modalities, and is available to provide direct supervision.

Milestones describe performance at a specific stage of residency training relevant to a specific competency and specialty. Milestones are much smaller than an EPA and are not necessarily a clinical task. Milestones provide a marker of progression throughout training and provide guidance to both trainees and faculty about progression towards the overall attainment of competence within a specialty. For example, the ability to recognize and initiate care for a critical patient in the emergency department

Table 2. The AAMC core entrustable professional activities for entering residency

The 13 Core Entrustable Professional Activities for Entering Residency
EPA 1: Gather a history and perform a physical examination
EPA 2: Develop a prioritized differential diagnosis and select a working diagnosis following a patient encounter
EPA 3: Recommend and interpret common diagnostic and screening tests
EPA 4: Enter and discuss patient orders/prescriptions
EPA 5: Provide documentation of a clinical encounter in written or electronic format
EPA 6: Provide an oral presentation/summary of a patient encounter
EPA 7: Form clinical questions and retrieve evidence to advance patient care
EPA 8: Give or receive a patient handover to transition care responsibility to another health care provider or team
EPA 9: Participate as a contributing and integrated member of an interprofessional team
EPA 10: Recognize a patient requiring urgent or emergent care, initiates evaluation and treatment, and seek help
EPA 11: Obtain informed consent for tests and/or procedures that the day 1 intern is expected to perform or order without supervision
EPA 12: Perform general procedures of a physician
EPA 13: Identify system failures and contribute to a culture of safety and improvement

represents an EPA. As a milestone, it would consist of progressively increasing levels management and treatment, beginning with the recognition of an unstable patient and progressing to development of the necessary skills to stabilize the patient and can include the transfer of a critically ill patient to another service (Beeson, et al., 2012). There are overlapping features between the EPAs and milestones and approaches to integrating the two components in undergraduate medical curricula which will be highlighted by each competency section.

Curriculum Using Competency-Based Learning to Improve Clinical Skills

Organizing your curriculum using the tenets of Carraccio, Englander et al is a good first step in developing and implementing an effective competency-based learning and assessment activities of clinical skills. 1) Use a standardized language, 2) the power of direct observation and assessment, 3) develop meaningful measures of performance, 4) establish desired outcomes as the starting point for curriculum development, 5) create learning opportunities that depend on the reflection of expertise, 6) establish a need for exploiting the role of the learner in their learning, and 6) ensure competent clinical systems as the environment to producing competent physicians. Next, establish and make explicit the competencies for your learners and evaluators. All successful curriculum implementation relies on faculty development and preparation of your evaluators. Finally, technology can assist both in teaching and assessment for each of the competency objectives. A general list of technology used in competency-based medical education are:

1. Online teaching formats or eLearning
2. Simulation
3. Online assessment systems
4. Virtual humans
5. Electronic health records (EHR)
6. Gaming
7. Software systems of procedural skills
8. Discussion boards and forums
9. Blogging and wikis
10. Reflective writing
11. Portfolios
12. Telemedicine

The following is a description of the ways technology can assist teaching and assessment in each of the six ACGME core competencies and the clinical skills embedded within each competency. They can be modified to meet your needs for teaching and assessment of clinical skills.

Use of technology in enhancing teaching of competency-based teaching in the ACGME Core Competencies:

- Patient Care and Procedures
- Interpersonal and Communication Skills
- Medical Knowledge
- Systems-based Practice
- Practice-based Learning and improvement
- Professionalism

Technology for Teaching and Assessment in Patient Care and Procedures

Patient Care

The ACGME defines the Patient Care competency as "Use information technology to support patient care decisions and patient education. Perform competently all medical and invasive procedures considered essential for the area of practice. Provide health care services aimed at preventing health problems and maintaining health." Patient Care competency is a patient-centered approach to gather essential and accurate information about the patient, counsel patients and family members, make informed diagnostic and therapeutic decisions, prescribe and perform essential medical procedures, provide effective health management, maintenance, and prevention guidance. The sub-competencies also include care that is: 1) family-centered, 2) compassionate, 3) explaining in developmentally appropriate terms, 4) an effective treatment of health problems, and 5) encouraging overall health.

Online Learning, E-learning, Digital Learning, and Virtual Learning

Online learning is defined as learning that comes primarily through an internet connection and the use of a computer. Learning can occur through blended methods but uses some sort of computer platform to facilitate that learning with or without in-person contact between the teacher and student. (Brookfield, Peskill, S. 2005). E-learning is learning and teaching between the student and teacher that takes place entirely through an internet connection. Teaching materials and submission of assignments occurs through this internet connection. Digital Learning is defined a a combination of online learning and E-learning with digital modalities for communication such as digital cameras and video capabilities. Virtual Learning further builds on digital learning by allowing students to learn using the digital technology but with the option to review materials with recordings of the digital learning device (Shirley G, 2017). With these technologies it is important to mention the use of blended learning as a combination of any of the above modalities. Connecting with students online through network technologies is one of the most powerful responses to the growing need for education. With the use of the internet, there is the potential to reach greater numbers of students and allows teachers to reach students on a global scale. Many studies have reviewed the outcome of e-learning as a mode of teaching in medical education and they reveal no significant difference in learning outcomes, commonly measured as grades or exam results, between traditional and e-learning modes of delivery. (Clark, 2016; Allen, 2014).

Medical school, by design, provides opportunities in teaching and assessing students as they gain knowledge and experience in their didactic curriculum paired with clinical opportunities with patients. Technology can support learning in this competency through online teaching of the clinical skills and knowledge needed at the appropriate place in your curriculum. As an example, your clinical skills course can provide instruction on these skills through online outlines and videos that both teach and reinforce these skills. To illustrate this, Stanford School of Medicine developed Stanford Medicine 25 Promoting the Culture of Bedside Medicine. (Stanford25, www.stanfordmedicine.edu). They provide online lessons on history and physicals in a systems-based way. Your clinical skills course can use this form of online teaching to explain the approach to diagnosis through the history and physical examination to prepare medical students for workshops, skills assessments, and to see patients. Through 25 different sections presented by organ system, information is provided with pictures, audio recordings and videos of history and physical skills needed to work-up and diagnose diseases. Examples include but are not limited to the funduscopic, the cerebellar, the hand, the cardiac, and the pulmonary examinations. This is an opportunity to use technology to prepare students with the skills needed to see patients. Assessments of these skills should ideally occur during direct observation of patient care by an evaluator both trained and equipped to watch and measure performance and demonstration of skills. Setting up this technology in advance, and training your evaluators using this online format can also be helpful at defining the expected performance level for both your learners and evaluators.

Another example of Patient Care clinical skills teaching and assessment can be explained using the AAMC Core Entrustable Professional Activities (EPAs). This format can be adapted using technology to teach and assess skills fundamental to the student graduating from medical school.

First, your curriculum committee should review the AAMC Core EPAs for consideration for your curriculum and for a match to your medical education objectives. The curriculum committee members should be explicit on specific EPAs and determine where they must be taught in the curriculum. The EPA teaching content and the methods of teaching and assessment, including who should be providing direct observation and assessments, should be clearly defined. Faculty development in the EPAs is essential and training those who will make assessment and entrustment decisions must occur. How the entrustment decision be made must be defined before implementation.

To reinforce how technology can support this form of patient care teaching and assessment, let us focus on EPA 1: Gather a History and Physical. Everyone can agree that gathering a history and performing a physical examination are fundamental and germane to every medical school curriculum. The AAMC Curriculum Developer's Guide EPA 1: Gather a history and perform a physical examination includes the following: 1. Description of the activity, 2. Most relevant domains of competence; 3. Competencies within each domain critical to entrustment decisions. The following table was created using the AAMC Core Entrustable Professional Activities for Entering Residency Curriculum Developer's Guide and is an example of a modified assessment of EPA-1: Gathering a History and Physical with a scale of entrustability for evaluators to use during direct observation and in measuring student performance (Corbett, et al., 2005)

EPA-1 Gather a History and Perform a Physical Examination

Implementing EPA-1: Gather a History and Physical is an example of patient care clinical skills that technology can assist. Training of faculty on the objectives, skills and the assessment tool can occur using online teaching formats. Online teaching using an outline or video explanation fits the busy faculty or resident's schedule and allows you to reach many evaluators and track that they have viewed the objectives, skill level, and provide widespread training on the learner objectives and assessment tool. Online outlines and videos can also provide the learning objectives to your students as the assessment of skills needs to be transparent and easily explainable.

Online assessment of the EPAs is also essential. Students need direct observation of all of the EPAs and it is essential that they be provided with a private online assessment in real-time. The list of skills embedded in each EPA should be observable and a level of entrustability chosen. Written feedback on strengths and areas needing improvement are also important. Online assessment using a smartphone, a tablet, or a laptop are also especially helpful to assess and then review immediately with students and allow for feedback following direct observation. The assessment example above can be created as an online assessment that is submitted using a single sign-on

Table 3. Example of entrustment assessment for EPA-1 gather a history and perform a physical examination: score the student for the skill you are observing and their level of performance

EPA-1 *Entrustable* Behaviors	**1** Novice-Student can perform with close direct observation and continued input from supervisor **Not ready for entrustment**	**2** Advanced Learner-Student can perform with direct observation with some input from supervisor **Ready for direct supervision**	**3** Adequate-Student can perform with direct observation with minimal input from supervisor in the room **Ready for indirect supervision**	**4** Proficient-Student can perform with minimal supervision and supervisor close-by **Ready for "unsupervised" practice**	**5** Expert-Student is entrusted to perform independently with no supervisor input **Ready to supervise-"Senior Student or Resident"**
History: Individual at this level is routinely able to gather an accurate complete, accurate and organized history and can also gather a focused history in an urgent, emergent, or consultation setting					
Identifies pertinent history elements in common presenting situations, symptoms, complaints, disease states (acute and chronic)					
Identifies and uses alternate sources of information to obtain history when needed, including from family members, primary care physicians, living facilities, and pharmacies.					
Physical examination: The student learner can perform an accurate complete and accurate physical exam in a fluid sequence					
Performs a focused physical exam pertinent to the patient visit, identify and document abnormal findings, and describe such findings to team members					
Demonstrates clinical reasoning in gathering focused information relevant to a patient's care.					
Links current findings to those from previous patients.					
Uses analytic reasoning and activation of prior knowledge to guide process.					
Demonstrates patient-centered interview skills (attentive to patient verbal and nonverbal cues, patient/family culture, social determinants of health, need for interpretive or adaptive services; demonstrates active listening skills).					
Demonstrates patient-centered examination techniques that reflect respect for patient privacy, comfort, and safety (that is, explaining physical exam maneuvers, telling the patient what the physician is doing at each step, keeping patients covered during the examination).					

Source: Adapted from the AAMC Core Entrustable Professional Activities for Curriculum Development (Chen HC, van den Broek WE, ten Cat O 2005) Checklist utilized by University of Missouri Kansas City School of Medicine.

and submitted for tracking by individual students. Online assessments in the EPAs will also be essential for schools that link the EPAs to promotion and graduation. Online assessments can be tracked and monitored for the individual student for the purpose of promotion and remediation.

SIMULATION

Simulation is described in another chapter of this book. It is undeniably an excellent way to teach and assess the competency of Patient Care and Procedures. The medical education and graduate medical education literature is rich with data on the effectiveness of simulation in teaching and assessing procedures. Once you have determined the procedures required of all graduates in your undergraduate medical curriculum, it is important to determine where they are best taught and assessed. As an example, students certified in the American Heart Association (AHA) Basic Life Support (BLS) skills learn and demonstrate the skill of bag-valve-mask (BVM) ventilation and cardiopulmonary resuscitation (CPR). Students can be taught and assessed on both BVM and CPR utilizing simulation and a high-fidelity simulation (HFS) mannequin. Some models can be programmed to provide assessment information such as chest rise and rate of bagging for ventilation or depth and rate of compressions in CPR. Simulation assists with the teaching of the motor skills, deliberate practice of these procedures and can provide assessment for the individual learner. Other procedures that can be considered in undergraduate medical education should be determined with centralized oversight by your curriculum committee. Medical schools may require the AHA Advanced Cardiac Life Support (ACLS) training prior to graduation. Some of the procedural skills necessary for certification include endotracheal intubation, applying and using an automated external defibrillator, using a defibrillator for conversion of fatal heart rhythms, and identifying and treating cardiac dysrhythmias. HSF mannequins and task trainers can be programmed for practice and assessment in all of these skills.

Patient cases can be designed using the HFS for EPA 9 and can include professional learners from other programs to deliver interprofessional care. Working as an

Table 4. Simulation also suits teaching and assessment in

EPA 9: Participate as a contributing and integrated member of an interprofessional team
EPA 10: Recognize a patient requiring urgent or emergent care, initiates evaluation and treatment, and seek help
EPA 12: Perform general procedures of a physician
EPA 13: Identify system failures and contribute to a culture of safety and improvement

interprofessional team, students can work to discover answers, provide interventions and solve problems using patient simulation. Simulation teaching and assessment is also ideal for EPA 10: Recognize a patient requiring urgent of emergent care, initiates evaluation and treatment, and seek help. Critical patient cases can be programmed for the HFS such as stroke, acute myocardial infarction, and sepsis, to name a few. Simulation can provide a balance of teaching a realistic portrayal of a critically ill patient and the skills needed to recognize, initiate management, and seek help all while keeping critical patients safe. Thompson et al., (2017) provides an example of an educational design for teaching and assessment in EPA-10 for final year medical students. Five emergent patient case-scenarios were designed for the student to confront in an acute care setting. They developed high-fidelity simulations to portray the patient cases and designed a performance assessment instrument to evaluate the medical student's performance in accomplishing the critical actions related to EPA-10 competencies. Faculty facilitators completed the EPA-10 evaluation checklists in real time during the simulation and all cases evaluated *recognizing abnormal vital signs, asking for help when needed,* and *determining patient disposition.* Overall, they found that nearly 87% of students met their global assessment of ad hoc entrustment with good inter-rater reliability on pairs of faculty raters. They provide a quality design for how simulation can support evaluation for EPA-10 that includes universal critical actions, case-specific critical actions, and a global rating of ad-hoc entrustment. (Thompson et al. 2017)

Virtual Humans

Virtual humans are computer-generated characters that are visually similar to humans by their verbal responses and movements on the computer screen. This technological form of teaching provides both visual and behavioral realism. (McDonnell, 2012; von der Pütten, 2010). Software programs are available to provide instruction using virtual human patient platforms for students to engage individually or on teams to practice care on a virtual patient. The design of each case requires students to acquire important history of present illness, past medical history, social history and family history, perform a physical examination and use this information to order tests and make medical decisions. Establishing a differential diagnosis simulates the real life steps a physician takes in practice each day but with a virtual patient. The design of virtual humans supports the Patient Care competency and EPAs 1-4 (Table 5).

Virtual human cases can be completed by a single student or a team of students and as the student(s) progress through the case the virtual patient responds and data is provided similar to the electronic health record and data systems used in clinical care. Embedded in software programs are assessment opportunities at the

Table 5. EPAs 1-4

EPA 1: Gather a history and perform a physical examination **EPA 2:** Develop a prioritized differential diagnosis and select a working diagnosis following a patient encounter **EPA 3:** Recommend and interpret common diagnostic and screening tests **EPA 4:** Enter and discuss patient orders/prescriptions

conclusion of the case. Students may complete multiple choice questions, provide orders or an assessment and plan that is graded. These skills also support Patient Care and EPAs 5, 7, 9, and 10 (Table 6).

This form of virtual patient technology saves time and effort by faculty to provide bedside care and teaching, and saves students time because they can complete it at their convenience, or asynchronous to other scheduled activities. Virtual patient teaching also provides teaching and assessment on the diagnosis and management of critical diagnoses without waiting for a real clinical situation to introduce the student to the workup and management. This is ideal for teaching students an approach to identifying an urgent or emergent condition with deliberate practice while keeping patients safe. The student can learn and practice to prepare for this clinical experience during the final year of medical school and before entry into residency.

Electronic Health Records

Practicing physicians must be proficient in using the electronic medical record system in caring for patients. Students entering residency also need to have this important skill to care for patients during residencies. As our academic clinical systems have moved to an electronic health record system (EHR), medical students were having difficulty with permission to enter information in the EHR at their clinical affiliates. Thankfully, medical schools have overcome the barriers to medical student documentation in our EHRs and the AAMC reported in 2015 that students are now able to use the EHR in 140/141 or 99.3% of medical schools during their required clinical clerkship training (AAMC survey, 2012).

Table 6. EPAs 5, 7, 9, and 10

EPA 5: Provide documentation of a clinical encounter in written or electronic format **EPA 7:** Form clinical questions and retrieve evidence to advance patient care **EPA 9:** Participate as a contributing and integrated member of an interprofessional team **EPA 10:** Recognize a patient requiring urgent or emergent care, initiates evaluation and treatment, and seek help

The EHR can be a useful technological tool for teaching the Patient Care and Interpersonal and Communication Skills competencies. It is clear that the skill needs to be developed upon entering residency and is an important skill for the everyday function of a physician in practice. Objectives and entrustability for using the EHR is also defined in EPA-5 (Table 7).

The Alliance for Clinical Education (ACE) led the charge in medical training and issued a collaborative statement in 2012 that called for a new approach of medical student competency in use of the EHR (Hammoud et al., 2012). ACE recognized the importance of medical student participation in patient care which includes the ability for them to document. They propose the following guidelines:

1. Students must document in the patient's chart and their notes should be reviewed for content and format.
2. Students must have the opportunity to practice order entry in an HER.
3. Students should be exposed to the utilization of the decision aids that typically accompany EHRs.
4. Schools must develop a set of medical student competencies related to charting in the EHR and evaluate it.

The EHR itself is state-of-the-art and can provide specific teaching of health care information technology. The Institute of Medicine has strongly encouraged the use of EHR for the sake of improving quality of care and patient safety (Richardson et al., 2001). EHR curricula is innovative but must be developed to teach the essential skills needed by students while minimizing the risk of documentation in the formal medical record. Additionally, use of the EHR creates unique challenges to effective communication by creating the "triangulation of physician-patient-computer" (Wald, 2007; Rouf, 2008). Especially given that physician-patient communication plays an important role in patient satisfaction, in providing quality medical care, and providing a patient-centered approach to treatment planning (Robbins, 1993; Fremont, 2001).

A systematic longitudinal curriculum on use of the EHR is recommended. At Alpert Medical School of Brown University, they provide a systematic development of a longitudinal UME EHR curriculum within a series of six courses over four years with a focus on the narrative in patient-centered compassionate and competent care. The authors recommend that EHR training should include (Wald, et al., 2014).

Table 7. EPA-5

EPA 5: Provide documentation of a clinical encounter in written or electronic format

1. Introducing students to the presence of a computer within a clinical encounter.
2. Training students in EHR-related skills.
3. Empowering patient and relationship-centered interviewing skills while incorporating EHR skills.
4. Fostering students' appreciation for added value of integrated computer use within the clinical encounter.

Their comprehensive curriculum approach includes EHR-training modules with reflection on positives and negatives of the EHR with regards to patient care. Their final year uses a behavior grid for their fourth-year internship preparation course and focuses on integrating computer use within the clinical encounter for "information mastery". The behaviors expected are explicit and are used by learners, clinical faculty, and real patients for multi-source feedback of EHR use and reinforce the competency objectives on Interpersonal and Communication Skills.

Indiana University School of Medicine (IU) cloned its existing EHR system and de-identified patient data to create tEHR. The tEHR is used by students to experience the strengths and weaknesses of the EHR. The system was enriched with educational content with videos, text and links to other material. Students order tests and manage the EHR to demonstrate clinical reasoning and decision-making and the EHR recognizes whether the test is necessary or could cause patient harm. If a test is unnecessary, the system triggers a warning and delivers the explanation and evidence in order for the students to compare their decisions with those made by clinicians in the field who were caring for the actual patients (Jakubek & Welch, 2017). By working with the tEHR, students begin to get a sense of the value and limitations of the EHR. As result of this work the *Regenstrief EHR Clinical Learning Platform* will be disseminated by the AMA and Regenstrief to medical schools across the country. Their longitudinal curriculum is an opportunity to include the following EPAs (Table 8).

Table 8. EPAs

EPA 2: Develop a prioritized differential diagnosis and select a working diagnosis following a patient encounter
EPA 3: Recommend and interpret common diagnostic and screening tests
EPA 4: Enter and discuss patient orders/prescriptions
EPA 5: Provide documentation of a clinical encounter in written or electronic format
EPA 7: Form clinical questions and retrieve evidence to advance patient care
EPA 8: Give or receive a patient handover to transition care responsibility to another health care provider or team
EPA 9: Participate as a contributing and integrated member of an interprofessional team
EPA 13: Identify system failures and contribute to a culture of safety and improvement

Gaming

The current generation of medical students respond well to game playing as a learning tool (Pelletier, 2016). A recent definition of serious gaming can be found by Bergeron an "interactive computer application, with or without significant hardware component, that has a challenging goal, is fun to play and engaging, incorporates some scoring mechanism, and supplies the user with skills, knowledge, or attitudes useful in reality." In 2005, Stokes defined serious games as "games that are designed to entertain players as they educate, train, or change behavior." Gaming offers active and experiential learning by creating a learner centered approach to education where the learner demonstrates decision-making and critical thinking through interaction in the game (Bergeron, 2006). Gaming is most effective in medical education when it provides students with concrete experiences, opportunities to make decisions, and a safe environment to take action and provide treatment. A game spectrum classification is reported by Qin et al., (2010) (Figure 3).

Simulation and simulators is a form of gaming but has been covered in this chapter and elsewhere in this textbook. The remainder of this section will focus more on games that provide realism together with the entertainment factor of traditional computer games while creating realistic but fictitious learning environments. There are a number of programs available with undergraduate medical education, nursing education, dentistry education, prehospital education and graduate medical education especially in the areas of surgery, anesthesia, and orthopedic surgery. This section will focus on serious gaming technology that supports the teaching and assessment of clinical skills embedded in Patient Care and Procedures for undergraduate medical education.

Examples of Gaming in Undergraduate Medical Education

Kambria H. Evans, MEd, MA, and colleagues at Stanford School of Medicine developed a mobile-accessible, case-based online software program called Septris to

Figure 3. The computer game spectrum
Source: Qin et al. (2010)

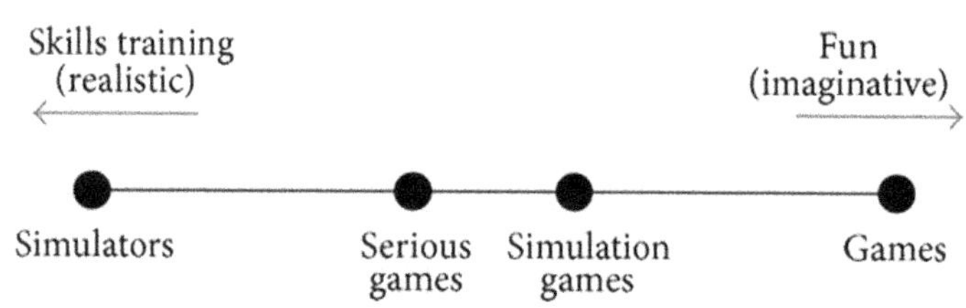

teach sepsis identification and care. (http://med.stanford.edu/septris/). Septris takes an innovative approach to teaching early sepsis identification and uses evidence-based management principles to teach learners how to treat the condition. The use of smartphones and the popularity of gaming makes this form of gaming teaching useful to the competencies of medical knowledge and patient care including critical decision making and management principles. Student and resident performance outcomes of this program demonstrated a significant improvement in users' knowledge on written testing in recognizing and managing the condition of sepsis. "There is such an opportunity here because the interest is already there," said Evans, director of education and quality improvement at Stanford (Pelletier, 2016).

Virtual Heroes 3DiTeams is a serious game developed with Duke University Medical Center and is used for their medical training of students. 3DiTeams is a realistic first person designed, multiplayer training application where the user is placed in a high-fidelity virtual hospital to address problems and patient cases (Virtual Heroes; J. M. Taekman, Segall, Hobbs &. Wright, 2007). The training is based on the Department of Defense Patient Safety Program and utilizes the Agency for Healthcare Research and Quality's Team STEPPS curriculum. The game provides opportunities for teamwork, communication on teams, and problem-solving through two phases. In the first phase, the user is introduced to teamwork and communication skills. In the second phase, the student applies these skills on a virtual patient scenario. Up to 32 players can play together in this team approach. Each player functions in a predetermined role of doctor, nurse, medical technician, or observer. The game begins with an instructor briefing on the patient. The instructor can manually control the patient's vital signs in response to the player actions or can leave the patient physiology to the pre-programmed setting of the software. Self-assessment and feedback can occur by video playback of the patient case in order for students to observe and reflect on their own behaviors as well as those of the team.

Another opportunity for serious gaming in medical education is Clinispace, a web-based application that offers immersive 3D virtual environments for teaching clinical reasoning and patient care. This program offers training experiences for many clinical conditions that present in an emergency department. The clinical space is realistic and allows learners as individuals or on teams to use objects and medical instruments to treat patients. This game can be scaled to a large class size which is necessary for medical schools. The learner performance also provides learner outcomes and assessments (Dev, Heinrichs & Youngblood, 2011).

Pulse!!© is a serious game developed for healthcare education and provides an opportunity to educate learners on a mass casualty event. Students can practice clinical skills in response to specific injuries sustained during mass casualty events. The system provides highly interactive and a detailed 3D world with patients that show accurate physiology models and the hemodynamic response of the human body to traumatic injury (Pulse!!, www.breakawaygames.com).

The aforementioned technological education tools can assist in teaching and assessing the following skills embedded in the EPAs (Table 9).

Serious Gaming Systems for Procedural Skills

Ultrasound

SonoSim LiveScan® is a commercial product that brings realism to ultrasound training by using ultrasound recorded scans of live patients and mannequins into ultrasound training cases that represent real pathological conditions. The software of SonoSim® Ultrasound Training Solution, provides didactic content and the assessment of knowledge while the LiveScan® provides real training using the ultrasound probe and maneuvers to be used anywhere. This system can teach many learners the ultrasound skills to use at the bedside and provides real images paired with patient cases. The system can also evaluate the learner's probe positioning and maneuvers and provided feedback on effectiveness of technique with knowledge assessment and performance tracking (SonoSim©, www.sonosim.com). Students learn the procedural skills of image acquisition and interpretation skills in addition to demonstrating clinical decision-making and critical thinking skills. Ultrasound is also a proven tool for clinical correlation of anatomy and physical diagnosis courses in medical education (Walrod, et al., 2017; Patten 2015). A study by Kappur, Han & Queck (2016) showed that there was statistical significant difference on normal US images of abdominal organs knowledge before and after the intervention. Walrod et al. (2017) demonstrated that first year medical student examinations of the knee and shoulder improved with the use of ultrasound when compared to those with traditional teaching of that clinical skill.

Table 9. EPAs

EPA 2: Develop a prioritized differential diagnosis and select a working diagnosis following a patient encounter
EPA 3: Recommend and interpret common diagnostic and screening tests
EPA 4: Enter and discuss patient orders/prescriptions
EPA 5: Provide documentation of a clinical encounter in written or electronic format
EPA 9: Participate as a contributing and integrated member of an interprofessional team
EPA 10: Recognize a patient requiring urgent or emergent care, initiates evaluation and treatment, and seek help
EPA 11: Obtain informed consent for tests and/or procedures that the day 1 intern is expected to perform or order without supervision
EPA 13: Identify system failures and contribute to a culture of safety and improvement

Table 10. EPAs

EPA 3: Recommend and interpret common diagnostic and screening tests requiring urgent or emergent care, initiates evaluation and treatment, and seek help
EPA 11: Obtain informed consent for tests and/or procedures that the day 1 intern is expected to perform or order without supervision
EPA 12: Perform general procedures of a physician

Discussion Boards or Forums

Discussion boards and forums for discussion are powerful forms of active and engaged learning especially for large groups of learners or distance learners. A discussion board is defined by a noticeboard or messaging board by which learners can start and continue topics of discussion with responses (Macquarrie University, 2018). Forums and discussion boards provide the sharing of new ideas while respecting the perspectives and contributions of others. Discussion boards are most effective when facilitated by a faculty member and monitored to keep the discussion on track and covering the specified learning objectives. Forums and discussion boards allow for a large number of students to attend and engage in the learning even from a distance with the assistance of a computer and in timing the discussions to be live or interactive. Self-awareness of what the individual learner brings to the discussion as well as an awareness of others, creates the opportunity to respect and appreciate what others contribute. Sufficient time for discussants to prepare and provide input is necessary (Ravindran, Kashyap, Lilis, Vivekanantham & Phoenix, 2014). Facilitators can assist with barriers to effective learning such as social, cultural, and experiential barriers between learners. Discussion boards are especially useful for the competencies of Interpersonal and Communication skills, Professionalism, and Medical Knowledge. The Blackboard Discussion Boards is an example of a discussion board that is useful for UME. Programs with online academic software programs may have access to online discussion boards. Social media such as Facebook and Twitter are also effective media tools for discussion boards and forums (George & Dellasega, 2011; Johna S, 2103).

Wikis and Blogs

The definition of a Wiki is an easily-edits set of one or more linked webpages that readers can add to or modify which can facilitate collaboration on creating content. Anyone can make additions, edits, or update in real time with the system. Multiple students can collaborate and contribute at anytime from anywhere (with internet access). It is a work in progress that can be updated fluidly over time. The contributions represent agreement on material and can have a discussion page associated with them.

The definition of a blog is an online journal with a web log that allows submissions and displays them in reverse chronological order. There are options to post as well as options to comment on posts. It is controlled by an author who determines if and when the blog is posted. It is based on opinion and is an opportunity to share knowledge, opinions and expertise (Macquarrie University, 2018).

These technological tools can provide teaching and assessment of the following EPAs (Table 11).

Reflective Writing

Writing is an essential skill of medical professionals and in the past two decades medical education has discovered the value of this opportunity and implemented more reflective writing in medical school curricula. Medicine requires the physician to develop a meaningful relationship with patients and humanistically care for them. For healing to occur, physicians must have open communication with patients and the physician-patient relationship must be carefully forged for a successful negotiation on treatment decisions. Narrative medicine is defined as medicine practiced with narrative competence. For example, assignments where the learner performs close reading of literature and reflective writing allows the student to examine their role in: physician and patient, physician and self, physician and colleagues, and physicians and society. "With narrative competence, physicians can reach and join their patients in illness." (Charon, 2017). Narrative medicine provides a framework for medical students to explore and manage the growing complexity of patient care while centering them on the relationship that occurs while caring for patients. The patient deserves and expects their physician to develop the professional attributes of honesty, integrity, empathy, and compassion. Medical students can develop these attributes by writing and reflecting on their experiences to their patients, to society, and in their quest in the practice of medicine. Students can explore their values and ideals in medicine while they share their stories as they learn the art of healing.

Table 11. EPAs

EPA 2: Develop a prioritized differential diagnosis and select a working diagnosis following a patient encounter
EPA 5: Provide documentation of a clinical encounter in written or electronic format
EPA 7: Form clinical questions and retrieve evidence to advance patient care
EPA 9: Participate as a contributing and integrated member of an interprofessional team

Reflective writing is especially helpful in teaching the competencies of Patient Care, Interpersonal and Communication Skills, Professionalism, and Practice-based Learning and Improvement. If carefully designed, reflective writing about systems of care can allow students to develop an understanding of system successes and failures and reinforce objectives in Systems-Based Practice. Technology and e-Learning Portfolios can assist the reflective writing process. Web-based academic software programs or portfolios allow for students to submit their reflective writing and faculty advisors and mentors can review these reflections for the ongoing professional development of the learner (Epstein, 2011).

Web-Based Portfolios

Web-based portfolios are opportunities for learners to document experiences and written reflection about specific areas of their own competence. Students can submit performance feedback documents, demonstrate competence in charting and documentation of patient notes, letters of reference provided by faculty, logged procedures and patient types, peer assessments, self-assessments, patient feedback and surveys, quality-improvement projects, videotaped or audiotaped discussions or consultations, literature searches and research progress, and reflective writing and objectives for learning such as a study plan or performance improvement plan (Carraccio & Englander, 2004). Portfolios are most effective when reviewed by a faculty advisor or mentor for regular review of contents and in meeting deadlines. Portfolios can be used for formative assessment; information used to monitor the learner and provide ongoing feedback, and summative assessment; an evaluation of a learner which summarizes the outcome of their learning or their final performance at the end of an educational experience. The portfolio can provide important information to and about the learner if monitored frequently enough. Competencies such as Patient Types and Procedures, written assessments and forms of Communication, Professionalism and Problem-based Learning and Improvement can be accomplished by the use of web-based portfolios. They serve as a repository for a large number of submissions and allow for students to set standards, review progress, and develop a plan for staying on track to accomplish deadlines and complete tasks. Web-based portfolio also provide educators with a research infrastructure to practice evidence-based education (Benson, 2014).

Technology for Assessments

There are currently a number of commercial assessment systems available for the evaluation of individual competencies. Medical schools can develop a competency-based assessment system linked to individual learning objectives and year-specific expectations for students. These evaluations should be available in a user-friendly software system that allows for the evaluator to provide feedback, to capture student performance through direct observation, and for the evaluator to provide detailed explanations of what they observed. The combination of competency-based assessment matched to the EPAs and measurable milestones of performance, are ideal for measuring student competence in clinical skills. These evaluations can be created in software systems and tailored for frequent direct observation of learners throughout the undergraduate curriculum and for residency training. The power of providing this evaluation platform on smartphones will make the opportunity for observation and assessment more feasible and meaningful. The ideal situation is an assessment system that clearly delineates the performed skill of the learner, is selected to a clearly communicated expectation of performance by learner level, and the opportunity to measure and reflect on skills that need to improve to achieve the competency in moving from novice, to beginner, to advanced beginner, and beyond.

This opportunity to use technology for assessments can best be demonstrated by the AAMC's Core Entrustable Professional Activities for Entering Residency Curriculum Developer's Guide. This fundamental guide demonstrates the example of the learning activity and provides a simple and effective assessment of measurable knowledge and skills of the learner for each EPA. The Entrustable Professional Activities (EPAs) as tasks or responsibilities that trainees are entrusted to perform unsupervised once they have attained sufficient specific competence, can be most effectively be observed and measured using online assessment tools.

Technology for Teaching and Assessment in Interpersonal and Communication Skills

The ACGME defines the competency of Interpersonal and Communication Skills as two parts: Communication skills are the performance of specific tasks which can be observed, such as obtaining and presenting a patient's history, or documenting information accurately in a medical record. Interpersonal skills are relationship-based and are the effect that one's communication skills have on another (NEJM Knowledge+ Team, 2018).

Competence is determined by the student's ability to communicate effectively with patients and families; demonstrate the insight to emotion and manage human interactions; communicate effectively with physicians and other health professionals; work effectively as a member of a health care team; effectively consult other professionals; and maintain comprehensive, accurate, and timely medical records (NEJM Knowledge+ Team, 2018). This competency can further be broken down into written and verbal communication.

Technology that supports this competency for written communication are Portfolios, chart audits and EHR review, feedback on written full history and physicals, essays and reflections on clinical experiences or service learning. For verbal communication, Direct Observation of oral presentations using Smartphone or online Clinical Performance Assessments, Communication in Simulation Teams, and online video and audio review and assessment of patient encounters are all effective examples of teaching and assessment in Interpersonal and Communication Skills. These forms of technology can also support teaching and assessment of the following EPAs (Table 12).

Technology for Teaching and Assessment in Medical Knowledge

The ACGME definition of Medical Knowledge is learners should continually question and investigate, and seek new knowledge. Sharing knowledge with colleagues and providing accurate diagnosis and treatment is also important (NEJM Knowledge+ Team 2018). The skills and attributes of the learner that is competent in medical knowledge has:

- An investigative and analytical approach to clinical problem solving and knowledge acquisition
- An ability to apply medical knowledge to clinical situations
- An ability to teach others

These skills should be modified from this graduate medical education level to defined undergraduate medical education program learning objectives that are year and level-specific to the medical student. The medical knowledge and skills will become more advanced with time in the undergraduate medical curriculum and observable behaviors should be explicitly stated to the students and evaluators based on their

Table 12. EPAs

EPA 1: Gather a history and perform a physical examination
EPA 4: Enter and discuss patient orders/prescriptions
EPA 5: Provide documentation of a clinical encounter in written or electronic format
EPA 6: Provide an oral presentation/summary of a patient encounter
EPA 8: Give or receive a patient handover to transition care responsibility to another health care provider or team
EPA 9: Participate as a contributing and integrated member of an interprofessional team
EPA 11: Obtain informed consent for tests and/or procedures that the day 1 intern is expected to perform or order without supervision
EPA 13: Identify system failures and contribute to a culture of safety and improvement

year in the curriculum. Technologies that support this competency are web-based Online video teaching and assessment, eLearning to deliver teaching and to assess medical knowledge through examinations, and simulation with direct observation of problem solving and the application to clinical situations. Peer-to-peer teaching expectations and opportunities to observe more senior students teaching these skills to younger students, is a useful way to observe and measure student ability to teach others for this competency.

These forms of technology can also provide teaching and assessment of the medical knowledge and clinical skills embedded in the following EPAs (Table 13).

Technology for Teaching and Assessment in Professionalism

The ACGME definition for Professionalism is the expectation that the physician will treat others with respect, compassion and dignity. The patient and patient care supersede the personal needs of the physician as they must be accountable to the needs of the patient and society as a whole. This competency also embodies the principle that diverse patient populations will be treated with respect and dignity with regard to differences in age, gender, culture, religion, race, and sexual orientation (Ludwig 2014; Arnold 2002) The learning objectives and measured outcomes for Professionalism need to include measures of professional conduct and accountability, humanism, cultural competency, and maintaining the pillars of excellence, humanism, accountability, and altruism resting on a base of legal understanding, communication and clinical competence (Stern 2006; NEJM Knowledge+ Team 2018).

It has been said that all competencies are so intimately woven with Professionalism that the accomplishment of the other competencies is meaningless without demonstrating professionalism. The call of professionalism is an arduous journey and must be a lifelong endeavor of the practicing physician. Instilling professional

Table 13. EPAs

EPA 1: Gather a history and perform a physical examination
EPA 2: Develop a prioritized differential diagnosis and select a working diagnosis following a patient encounter
EPA 3: Recommend and interpret common diagnostic and screening tests
EPA 4: Enter and discuss patient orders/prescriptions
EPA 5: Provide documentation of a clinical encounter in written or electronic format
EPA 7: Form clinical questions and retrieve evidence to advance patient care
EPA 10: Recognize a patient requiring urgent or emergent care, initiates evaluation and treatment, and seek help
EPA 11: Obtain informed consent for tests and/or procedures that the day 1 intern is expected to perform or order without supervision
EPA 13: Identify system failures and contribute to a culture of safety and improvement

Figure 4. Delivering the future of better healthcare
Source: Adapted from Measuring Medical Professionalism, David Thomas STEM 2005

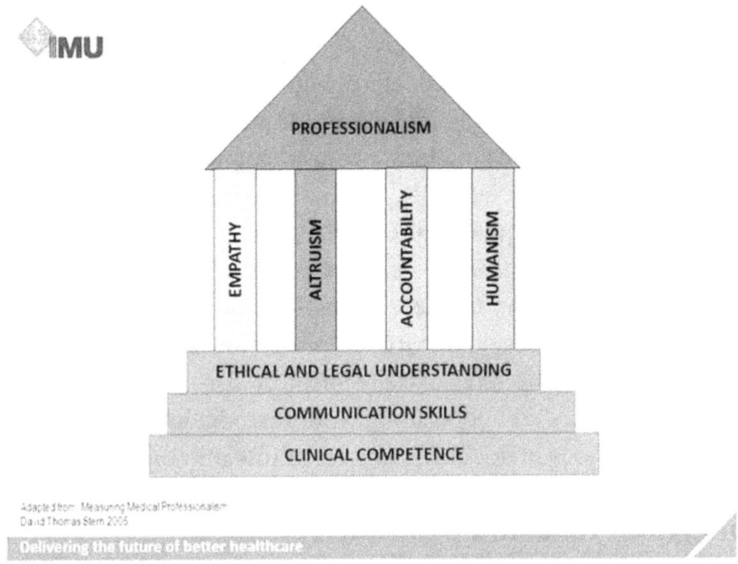

behaviors and attitudes in the graduating medical student must lead to a lifelong pursuit of continued professional development. These attributes can serve as a basis for developing curriculum for UME. Learning and assessment of these subcomponents of professionalism must be modified for the level of learner in each year of the undergraduate curriculum. Utilizing the model of EPAs, it is important to also address lifelong learning, empathy, teamwork, advocacy, wellness, trustworthiness, confidentiality, and integrity.

Technology that supports the continual development and evaluation of Professionalism includes:

1. Portfolios for submitting assignments and keeping up with deadlines and requirements,
2. 360 degree evaluations of Professional behaviors and attributes
3. Student online self-assessments,
4. Online clinical performance assessments of students on clinical rotations that capture the sub-competencies of professionalism,
5. Online peer assessments of professional attributes,
6. Online evaluation by staff and advisors

7. Online submissions of study plans and objectives.
8. Online record of timely use of teaching modalities can capture students responsibility in meeting deadlines

Technology and online evaluations can collate the results of multiple evaluations throughout the curriculum and can include 360 degree evaluations. The 360 degree evaluations are defined as evaluations obtained for learners from all that come into contact with them. For example, evaluations from faculty, residents, other students, administrators, health care professionals, and administrative coordinators that observe and can evaluate the learner is powerful feedback and can provide additional information for the learner. Technology provides opportunities for the assessment of longitudinal development of the professional attributes in the individual student. Annual reviews by advisors and mentors can also provide information about professional lapses and opportunities for remediation. This can be valuable to promotion committees in tracking progress of this important competency.

Technology for Teaching and Assessment in Practice-Based Learning and Improvement

The medical field is constantly evolving and with the advent of technology and the physician is exposed to new information daily. The physician needs to stay current on the practice of medicine by the continued recertification using a combination of continuing medical education (CME) activities and maintenance of certification within their specialty. Practice-based learning are activities discovered by physicians to keep their practice and knowledge current and constantly improving. Practice-based learning should be efficient to allow the busy physician to gain knowledge and be highly effective so the physician can apply that knowledge each day in practice (NEJM Knowledge+ Team, 2018).

The ACGME Core Competency of Practice-Based Learning and Improvement (PBLI) shows the both ability to comprehend relevant information and a practice of lifelong learning. Demonstration of competency in PBLI occurs when a resident displays the ability to:

- Investigate and evaluate patient care practices
- Appraise and assimilate scientific evidence, and
- Improve the practice of medicine.

Technology can provide online learning and assessment for continuing medical education, graduate medical education and undergraduate medical education. These systems will also allow for assessment of the activity to meet minimum requirements for meeting state standards for CME hours. Hospital credentialing bodies use online formats for annual required training and certification for compliance, Title IX and in certifying skills such as reading microscope slides.

For students in undergraduate medical education, it is important to develop lifelong learning and self-assessment skills. Students, residents and practicing professionals must be in charge of their learning and measuring the success of their learning. Ideally the use of technology in medical education will help develop the skills of lifelong learning so that after medical school, residents and practicing physicians will be responsible for their core learning and in preparing for certification examinations while keeping a busy clinical schedule in the balance. Technological systems that assist student learning, assessment and self-assessment of progress are most useful for this competency.

The development use of Portfolios in UME has increased to assist with this endeavor. Portfolios are offered by software vendors and schools have also developed homegrown systems. Portfolios should be reviewed by the learner and an advisor or mentor to verify progress and the quality of submissions and for reinforcement of PBLI. There should also be adequate time for reflection and review by the learner to modify learning objectives and progress on set goals to truly become a lifelong learner. The learner needs to be able to set objectives, find reliable teaching platforms, take assessments to show a level of performance and standard of competence.

The use of portfolios and online teaching formats in evidence-based medicine in patient care also teaches the PBLI elements. Students must have the opportunity to appraise the literature, answer a clinical question and apply current scientific evidence throughout their curriculum. Teaching students effective online literature searches and methods of application are essential. Online training in research methodology and preparing materials for an Institutional Review Board is also an effective method for teaching and assessing these competency objectives. The following EPA can be supported in this way:

Technology for Teaching and Assessment in Systems-Based Practice

The ACGME definition of Systems-Based Practice (SBP) "focuses on the underpinnings of health care in a good medical practice." The resident is required to engage in a healthcare system, patient safety and quality in healthcare, physician advocacy, health insurance, health care economics, transitions of care, different health care systems, pay for performance, patient centered medical home, and chronic care (NEJM Knowledge Team+, 2018). At the UME level, student clinical experiences occur in a system of care and it is important to identify these features of systems-based practice to make them practice ready to go into another system for residency and future clinical practice. The skills and attributes that a graduating medical student must have are:[62]

- Work effectively in various health care delivery settings and systems
- Coordinate patient care within the health care system
- Incorporate considerations of cost awareness and risk/benefit analysis in patient care
- Advocate for quality patient care and optimal patient care systems
- Work in interprofessional teams to enhance patient safety and improve patient care quality
- Participate in identifying systems errors and in implementing potential systems solutions

The EPAs also touch on these attributes with the following (Table 14).

SBP competency objectives should be developed for the medical student with year-specific behaviors that are measurable.

Technology to Teach and Model Systems-Based Practice

Telemedicine

Telemedicine is defined as using technology and electronic communications by clinicians and patients to educate, to deliver care, and to exchange information. E-visits where a patient speaks by telephone or using videoconferencing and secure messaging with a clinician where they then perform a remote evaluation, makes medical decisions, and prescribes medications or treatment plans. This form of

Table 14. EPAs

EPA 3: Recommend and interpret common diagnostic and screening tests
EPA 4: Enter and discuss patient orders/prescriptions
EPA 5: Provide documentation of a clinical encounter in written or electronic format
EPA 7: Form clinical questions and retrieve evidence to advance patient care
EPA 8: Give or receive a patient handover to transition care responsibility to another health care provider or team
EPA 9: Participate as a contributing and integrated member of an interprofessional team
EPA 10: Recognize a patient requiring urgent or emergent care, initiates evaluation and treatment, and seek help
EPA 11: Obtain informed consent for tests and/or procedures that the day 1 intern is expected to perform or order without supervision
EPA 13: Identify system failures and contribute to a culture of safety and improvement

providing care can reach more patients with the limited resources that the clinician and the healthcare system faces each day. This form of technology is a way for clinicians in practice to model how technology can improve patient care while working in a system of care (DeJong, Lucey & Dudley, 2017).

The ECHO Program or Project ECHO®

ECHO is Extension for Community Healthcare Outcome and is designed as an opportunity for specialists to bridge the gap with primary care to deliver evidence-based care to their patients without access to specialists. The ECHO model does not provide care to patients but provides increased specialty treatment in rural and underserved areas by providing front-line clinicians with the support to provide care to patients with complex medical conditions such as hepatitis C, HIV, tuberculosis, chronic pain, endocrinology, behavioral health disorders and more. It is a powerful opportunity for academic centers to provide evidence-based information and specialty input to primary care and their patients with complex medical problems. The University of New Mexico and the University of Missouri Kansas City have implemented this in their health system that engages their health professionals in this technological way.

Project ECHO® is a lifelong learning and guided practice model that revolutionizes medical education and exponentially increases workforce capacity to provide best-practice specialty care and reduce health disparities. The heart of the ECHO model™ is its hub-and-spoke knowledge-sharing networks, led by expert teams who use multi-point videoconferencing to conduct virtual clinics with community providers. In this way, primary care doctors, nurses, and other clinicians learn to provide excellent specialty care to patients in their own communities. (UNM, ProjectECHO www.echo.unmc.edu)

This system incorporates technology to address the healthcare system issues of inadequate or disparities in care related to cost, accessibility, system inefficiencies, and uses technology to improve opportunities to expand the workforce capacity to treat more patients using existing resources. This is a form of technology that can improve systems of care. If there is access to ECHO® at your institution this can be a powerful way for technology to provide teaching not only in the competency of Systems-based Practice but also in Interpersonal and Communication Skills, Practice-based Learning and Improvement, and Patient Care competency objectives.

Other afore mentioned technological tools that assist in teaching and assessment of the Systems-based Practice Competency are:

- **Simulation-Through Development of Simulation Cases:** Students can practice giving or receiving patient handover or transition of care, participate as the member of a team with other professionals, practice initiating care in a unique system, and practice patient safety and improvement.
- **Online Teaching and eLearning:** Modules can be developed to teach systems of care, patient safety and quality improvement. Students can be assessed through online examinations of their knowledge in these areas.
- **Online Assessment:** It can assess student SBP objectives during clinical rotations and the ability to obtain informed consent.
- **Virtual Humans:** It can be designed so that students incorporate cost considerations and the risk benefit analysis of certain procedures, tests, and therapies.
- **Electronic Health Record (EHR):** It allows the student to use the system to understand the impact on care, develop the skills to work with a specific EHR system, and develop a real understanding of the benefits and limitations of the EHR within a system. This allows them real-world experience on optimal and inefficient systems and how they impact the quality of patient care. Students can also practice reporting patient safety events using the EHR.
- **Gaming:** It can be developed to include working effectively with others in a realistic care delivery system, the coordination of care, and in working on interprofessional teams in an authentic system. Students can also practice on a team and serve as patient advocates
- **Reflective Writing:** Students can identify a system problem during a clinical rotation and propose a plan do study act method to make improvements in the quality of care in a system. Students can describe how they can contribute to a culture of safety and improvement.

Special Mention of Technology in Interprofessional Education

Interprofessional education (IPE) is the opportunity for professional students to learn with, from and about one another to provide safe patient care and to collaborate together on teams so professionals are practice ready to solve patient problems (World Health Organization, 2010). The IPE domains of practice as established by the Interprofessional Education Collaboration are Roles and Responsibilities, Values and Ethics, Interprofessional Communication, and Teams and Teamwork. Technology that support in-person IPE teams include interprofessional simulations designed to reinforce all 4 domains of Roles and Responsibilities, Values and Ethics, Interprofessional Communication, and Teams and Teamwork. Simulation is ideal for providing learning and assessment in all four domains. It provides students the

Table 15. A summary of technological tool useful for competency-based education

Technology	Patient Care and Procedures	Medical Knowledge	Interpersonal and Communication Skills	Practice-Based Learning and Improvement	Systems-Based Practice	Professionalism
Online Teaching, E-learning	X	X	X		X	X
Simulation	X	X	X	X	X	X
Online Assessment	X	X	X	X	X	X
Virtual Humans	X	X	X	X	X	X
EHR	X	X	X	X	X	X
Gaming	X	X	X	X	X	
Procedure Software	X	X		X		
Discussion Boards		X	X	X		X
Reflective Writing	X		X	X	X	X
Portfolios	X	X	X	X		X
Telemedicine/ ECHO Programs	X		X	X	X	

opportunity to interact together and develop skills in collaboration that hit all four domains. Simulation is important but requires development of cases and scheduling of multiple interprofessional teams while balancing the different schedules of professional program requirements including differing practice and education sites. This form of technological education is time consuming and expensive but is important and effective.

Another barrier and unique to IPE is the number of students that you need to educate with the engagement of more professional programs. The barriers of curriculum planning are the different schedules of live, in-class activities are difficult to find alignment and time for our learners to come together. Additionally, the numbers of learners increase exponentially as you add programs that value and want IPE for their students. Increasingly, programs have expended and include distance learning so students are not always physically present for leaning that is live and in the classroom. Technology can assist curriculum in IPE to deliver teaching and assessments in

IPE for large numbers of students, for distance learners, and for students located at a distance from one another. Students in interprofessional teams can use gaming to collaborate together without always needing to be together physically. They can develop skills to collaborate using technology such as online academic programs to share and disseminate online teaching and assessments including discussion boards and reflective writing; EHR-based teaching tools, portfolios using reflection and telemedicine tools.

University of Nebraska College of Medicine provides interprofessional clinical and nonclinical experiences with their nursing and allied health learners. Their goals is to extend IPE curricula into clinical learning environments, advance assessment of IPE competence, and improve teaching and learning strategies related to interprofessional education and practice. Their curriculum uses technology in shared resources with basic science teaching, in simulation and an EHR collaboration. Professional learners work together in blocks and interact with the EHR system. There is an infrastructure for tracking, monitoring and assessing interprofessional groups of learners. They also use this system as a repository for curricular materials and experiences. Education leaders at UNCOM have also developed the Interprofessional Experiential Center for Enduring Learning (iExcel, www.unmc.edu/iexcel) which is a building with highly interactive technology including an interactive digital wall. Interaction occurs between learners even from remote locations and classrooms. Writing on the digital wall is visible to the classroom and allows input from multiple professional learners. They are also using virtual reality/virtual humans in providing care on teams. Using virtual goggles students can work with a virtual nurse or pharmacist to solve problems and develop care plans. They are linking the needs of learners with the needs of the health care system to make them practice-ready to enter the system.[67]

The University of North Dakota School of Medicine and Health Sciences has developed a curriculum in telemedicine for IPE called Remotely Operated BiOmedical Telepresence Systems (ROBOTS). They have developed telemedicine teamwork interactions for students from five healthcare professions: medicine, nursing, occupational therapy, physical therapy, and social work. They have telemedicine consultants played by a medical student, faculty or a clinician. The simulations are real-life clinical scenarios that range from diagnosis, to intervention and treatment, and end-of-life care. Telemedicine is integrated as a natural part of the delivery of care for the learners and is designed to allow learners to rehearse and practice their roles and deliver care. The learners further develop their roles and relationships with one another, develop experience with the technology and how to use it in the patient care experience, and they teach reliance on one another in team-based care (Halaas, Van Eck, Allen, Johnson & Stauffenecker, 2018).

REFERENCES

Allen, M., Dirksen, J., Quinn, C., & Thalheimer, W. (2014). *The serious elearning manifesto.* Retrieved from http://elearningmanifesto.org

Arnold, L. (2002). Assessing professional behavior: Yesterday, today, and tomorrow. *Academic Medicine, 77*(6), 502–515. doi:10.1097/00001888-200206000-00006 PMID:12063194

Asch, D. A., Nicholson, S., Srinivas, S., Herrin, J., & Epstein, A. J. (2009). Evaluating obstetrical residency programs using patient outcomes. *Journal of the American Medical Association, 302*(12), 1277–1283. doi:10.1001/jama.2009.1356 PMID:19773562

Association of American Medical Colleges (AAMC). (2012). *Survey.* Retrieved from https://www.aamc.org/initiatives/cir/425112/14a.html

Beeson, M., Christopher, T., Heidt, J., Jones, J., Promes, S., Meyer, L., . . . Wagner, M. J. (2012). *American Board of Emergency Medicine. The Emergency Medicine Milestone Project.* Retrieved from https://www.abem.org/public/docs/default-source/migrated-documents-and-files/em-milestones.pdf?sfvrsn=6

Benson, B. J. (2014). Domain of competence: Interpersonal and communication skills. *Academic Pediatrics, 14*(2), S55–S65. PMID:24602649

Bergeron, B. P. (2006). *Developing Serious Games.* Charles River Media. Retrieved from www.designingdigitally.com

BreakAway. (n.d.). *Pulse!! Pulse!! Virtual clinical learning lab for health care training.* Retrieved from http://www.breakawaygames.com/serious-games/solutions/healthcare

Brookfield, S., & Peskill, S. (2005). *Discussion as A Way ofTeaching.* San Francisco, CA: Jossey-Bass. Retrieved from https://www.facultyfocus.com/articles/online-education/eight-tips-for-facilitating-effective-online-discussion-forums/

Brown, D. R., Warren, J. B., & Hyderi, A. (2017). AAMC Core Entrustable Professional Activities for Entering Residency Entrustment Concept Group. Finding a path to entrustment in undergraduate medical education: A progress report from the AAMC Core Entrustable Professional Activities for Entering Residency Entrustment Concept Group. *Acad Med, 92*, 774-779. Retrieved from https://members.aamc.org/eweb/upload/core%20EPA%20Curriculum%20Dev%20Guide.pdf

Carraccio, C., & Englander, R. (2004). Analyses/literature reviews: evaluating competence using a portfolio: a literature review and web-based application to the ACGME competencies. *Teaching and Learning in Medicine*, *16*(4), 381–387. doi:10.120715328015tlm1604_13 PMID:15582877

Carraccio, C., Englander, R., Gilhooly, J., Mink, R., Hofkosh, D., Barone, M. A., & Holmboe, E. S. (2017). Building a framework of entrustable professional activities, supported by competencies and milestones, to bridge the educational continuum. *Academic Medicine*, *92*(3), 324–330. doi:10.1097/ACM.0000000000001141 PMID:26959225

Carraccio, C., Englander, R., Van Melle, E., Ten Cate, O., Lockyer, J., Chan, M. K., ... Snell, L. S. (2016). Advancing competency-based medical education: A charter for clinician–educators. *Academic Medicine*, *91*(5), 645–649. doi:10.1097/ACM.0000000000001048 PMID:26675189

Carraccio, C., Wolfsthal, S. D., Englander, R., Ferentz, K., & Martin, C. (2002). Shifting paradigms: From Flexner to competencies. *Academic Medicine*, *77*(5), 361–367. doi:10.1097/00001888-200205000-00003 PMID:12010689

Carraccio, C. L., & Englander, R. (2013). From Flexner to competencies: Reflections on a decade and the journey ahead. *Academic Medicine*, *88*(8), 1067–1073. doi:10.1097/ACM.0b013e318299396f PMID:23807096

Charon, R. (2001). Narrative medicine: A model for empathy, reflection, profession, and trust. *Journal of the American Medical Association. Journal of the American Medical Association*, *286*(15), 1897–1902. doi:10.1001/jama.286.15.1897 PMID:11597295

Chen, C., Petterson, S., Phillips, R., Bazemore, A., & Mullan, F. (2014). Spending patterns in region of residency training and subsequent expenditures for care provided by practicing physicians for Medicare beneficiaries. *Journal of the American Medical Association*, *312*(22), 2385–2393. doi:10.1001/jama.2014.15973 PMID:25490329

Chen, H. C., van den Broek, W. S., & ten Cate, O. (2015). The case for use of entrustable professional activities in undergraduate medical education. *Academic Medicine*, *90*(4), 431–436. doi:10.1097/ACM.0000000000000586 PMID:25470310

Clark, D. B., Tanner-Smith, E. E., & Killingsworth, S. S. (2016). Digital games, design, and learning: A systematic review and meta-analysis. *Review of Educational Research*, *86*(1), 79–122. doi:10.3102/0034654315582065 PMID:26937054

Danoff, D., Corbett, E. C., Fortin, A. H., Novak, D. N., & McCurdy, F. (2005). *Recommendations for clinical skills curricula for undergraduate medical education*. Washington, DC: Task Force on the Clinical Skills Education of Medical Students. Association of American Medical Colleges, 40. Retrieved from https://members.aamc.org/eweb/upload/Recommendations%20for%20Clincial%20Skills%20Curricula%202005.pdf

DeJong, C., Lucey, C. R., & Dudley, R. A. (2015). Incorporating a new technology while doing no harm, virtually. *Journal of the American Medical Association, 314*(22), 2351–2352. doi:10.1001/jama.2015.13572 PMID:26647252

Epstein, R. M. (2007). Assessment in medical education. *The New England Journal of Medicine, 356*(4), 387–396. doi:10.1056/NEJMra054784 PMID:17251535

Evans, K. H., Daines, W., Tsui, J., Strehlow, M., Maggio, P., & Shieh, L. (2015). Septris: A novel, mobile, online, simulation game that improves sepsis recognition and management. *Academic Medicine, 90*(2), 180–184. doi:10.1097/ACM.0000000000000611 PMID:25517703

Frank, J. R., Snell, L. S., Cate, O. T., Holmboe, E. S., Carraccio, C., Swing, S. R., ... Harden, R. M. (2010). Competency-based medical education: Theory to practice. *Medical Teacher, 32*(8), 638–645. doi:10.3109/0142159X.2010.501190 PMID:20662574

Fremont, A. M., Cleary, P. D., Hargraves, J. L., Rowe, R. M., Jacobson, N. B., & Ayanian, J. Z. (2001). Patient-centered processes of care and long-term outcomes of myocardial infarction. *Journal of General Internal Medicine, 16*(12), 800–808. doi:10.1046/j.1525-1497.2001.10102.x PMID:11903758

George, D. R., & Dellasega, C. (2011). Use of social media in graduate-level medical humanities education: Two pilot studies from Penn State College of Medicine. *Medical Teacher, 33*(8), e429–e434. doi:10.3109/0142159X.2011.586749 PMID:21774639

Grace, S. (2017). *The Difference Between E-Learning and On-line Learning*. Retrieved from https://www.eztalks.com/elearning/difference-between-elearning-and-online-learning.html

Halaas, G. W., Van Eck, R. N., Allen, J., Johnson, E., & Stauffenecker, C. (2017). *Interprofessional Telemedicine Competency for Health Care Students With Remotely Operated BiOmedical Telepresence Systems (ROBOTS)*. Retrieved from https://www.ama-assn.org/sites/default/files/media-browser/public/medical-schools/ace-consortium-schools/consortium-images/spring-consortium-meeting-poster-university-of-north-dakota.pdf

Hammond, M., Skochelak, S., & Kirley, K. (2018). *Innovations in Medical Education Webinar: Interprofessional Education using Technology to Teach Team-based Care.* Retrieved from https://cme.ama-assn.org/Activity/6021873/Detail.aspx

Hammoud, M. M., Dalrymple, J. L., Christner, J. G., Stewart, R. A., Fisher, J., Margo, K., ... Pangaro, L. N. (2012). Medical student documentation in electronic health records: A collaborative statement from the Alliance for Clinical Education. *Teaching and Learning in Medicine*, *24*(3), 257–266. doi:10.1080/10401334.2012.692284 PMID:22775791

iExcel. (n.d.). Retrieved from https://www.unmc.edu/iexcel/about/index.html

Jakubek, K., & Welch, L. (2017). *AMA, Regenstrief Institute Heal Increase HER Training in Med Schools.* Retrieved from https://www.ama-assn.org/ama-regenstrief-institute-help-increase-ehr-training-med-schools

Johna, S., & Dehal, A. (2013). The power of reflective writing: Narrative medicine and medical education. *The Permanente Journal*, *17*(4), 84–85. doi:10.7812/TPP/13-043 PMID:24361026

Kapur, J., Han, T., Quek, S.T., Kanagasuntheram, R., Ng, Y.K., Lim, A., ... Samarasekera, D. (2016). The role of ultrasound teaching of clinical anatomy to first year medical students. *An International Association for Medical Education (AMEE) MedEdPublish* doi:10.15694/mep.2016.000029

Ludwig, S. (2014). Domain of competence: Professionalism. *Academic Pediatrics*, *14*(2), S66–S69. doi:10.1016/j.acap.2013.11.013 PMID:24602656

McDonnell, R., Breidt, M., & Bülthoff, H. H. (2012). Render me real?: Investigating the effect of render style on the perception of animated virtual humans. *ACM Transactions on Graphics*, *31*(4), 91. doi:10.1145/2185520.2185587

Nasca, T. J., Philibert, I., Brigham, T., & Flynn, T. C. (2012). The next GME accreditation system—rationale and benefits. *The New England Journal of Medicine*, *366*(11), 1051–1056. doi:10.1056/NEJMsr1200117 PMID:22356262

NEJM Knowledge+ Team. (n.d.a). *ACGME Core Competencies Interpersonal and Communication Skills.* Retrieved from https://knowledgeplus.nejm.org/blog/acgme-core-competencies-interpersonal-and-communication-skills/

NEJM Knowledge+ Team. (n.d.b). *ACGME Core Competencies Medical Knowledge.* Retrieved from https://knowledgeplus.nejm.org/blog/acgme-core-competencies-medical-knowledge/

NEJM Knowledge+ Team. (n.d.c). *ACGME Core Competencies Professionalism. Retrieved from* https://knowledgeplus.nejm.org/blog/acgme-core-competencies-professionalism/

NEJM Knowledge+ Team. (n.d.d). *ACGME Core Competencies Practice-based Learning and Improvement.* Retrieved from https://knowledgeplus.nejm.org/blog/practice-based-learning-and-improvement/

NEJM Knowledge+ Team. (n.d.e). *ACGME Core Competencies Systems-based Practice.* Retrieved from https://knowledgeplus.nejm.org/blog/acgme-core-competencies-systems-based-practice/

Parvati, D., Heinrichs, W. L., & Patricia, Y. (2011). CliniSpace: A multiperson 3D online immersive training environment accessible through a browser. Medicine Meets Virtual Reality 18. *NextMed, 163*, 173.

Patten, D. (2015). Using ultrasound to teach anatomy in the undergraduate medical curriculum: An evaluation of the experiences of tutors and medical students. *Ultrasound, 23*(1), 18–28. doi:10.1177/1742271X14542173 PMID:27433233

Pelletier, S. (2016). *Game On: Building the Case for Games in Medical Education.* Retrieved from https://news.aamc.org/medical-education/article/game-on-games-medical-education/

Qin, J., Chui, Y. P., Pang, W. M., Choi, K. S., & Heng, P. A. (2010). Learning blood management in orthopedic surgery through gameplay. *IEEE Computer Graphics and Applications, 30*(2), 45–57. doi:10.1109/MCG.2009.83 PMID:20650710

Ravindran, R., Kashyap, M., Lilis, L., Vivekanantham, S., & Phoenix, G. (2014). Evaluation of an online medical teaching forum. *The Clinical Teacher, 11*(4), 274–278. doi:10.1111/tct.12139 PMID:24917096

Richardson, W. C., Berwick, D. M., Bristow, L. R., Buck, C. R., Cassel, C. K., Chassin, M. R. … Warden, G.L. (2001). Committee on Quality of Health Care in America. Crossing the Quality Chasm: A New Health System for the 21st Century. Institute of Medicine. Washington, DC: National Academies Press.

Robbins, J. A., Bertakis, K. D., Helms, L. J., Azari, R., Callahan, E. J., & Creten, D. A. (1993). The influence of physician practice behaviors on patient satisfaction. *Family Medicine-Kansas City, 25*, 17–17. PMID:8454118

Rouf, E., Chumley, H. S., & Dobbie, A. E. (2008). Electronic health records in outpatient clinics: Perspectives of third year medical students. *BMC Medical Education, 8*(1), 13. doi:10.1186/1472-6920-8-13 PMID:18373880

SonoSim. (n.d.). Retrieved from www.sonosim.com

Stanford25. (n.d.). Retrieved from https://stanfordmedicine25.stanford.edu

Stern, D. T., & Papadakis, M. (2006). The developing physician—becoming a professional. *The New England Journal of Medicine*, *355*(17), 1794–1799. doi:10.1056/NEJMra054783 PMID:17065641

Stokes, B. G. (2005). Videogames have changed: Time to consider Serious Games'? *Development Education Journal*, *11*(3), 12.

Swing, S. R. (2007). The ACGME outcome project: Retrospective and prospective. *Medical Teacher*, *29*(7), 648–654. doi:10.1080/01421590701392903 PMID:18236251

Taekman, J. M., Segall, N., Hobbs, E., & Wright, M. (2007). 3DiTeams–Healthcare team training in a virtual environment. *Anesthesiology*, *107*(A2145), A2145.

ten Cate, O., & Billett, S. (2014). Competency-based medical education: Origins, perspectives and potentialities. *Medical Education*, *48*(3), 325–332. doi:10.1111/medu.12355 PMID:24528467

The Echo Project. (n.d.). Retrieved from https://echo.unm.edu

Thompson, L. R., Leung, C. G., Green, B., Lipps, J., Schaffernocker, T., Ledford, C., ... Kman, N. E. (2017). Development of an assessment for Entrustable Professional Activity (EPA) 10: Emergent patient management. *The Western Journal of Emergency Medicine*, *18*(1), 35–42. doi:10.5811/westjem.2016.10.31479 PMID:28116006

UNSW Sydney iLearn Resources. (n.d.). Retrieved from https://teaching.unsw.edu.au/assessment-blog-wiki-or-forum-which-should-you-use

Virtual Heroes 3diteams. (n.d.). Retrieved from http://www.virtualheroes.com/projects/3diteams

Von der Pütten, A., Krämer, N., & Gratch, J. (2010). How our Personality Shapes our Interactions with Virtual Characters-implications for Research and Development. In *Proceedings of the 10th International Conference on Intelligent Virtual Agents* (pp. 208-221). Springer.

Wald, H. S., Dube, C. E., & Anthony, D. C. (2007). Untangling the Web—The impact of Internet use on health care and the physician–patient relationship. *Patient Education and Counseling*, *68*(3), 218–224. doi:10.1016/j.pec.2007.05.016 PMID:17920226

Wald, H. S., George, P., Reis, S. P., & Taylor, J. S. (2014). Electronic health record training in undergraduate medical education: Bridging theory to practice with curricula for empowering patient-and relationship-centered care in the computerized setting. *Academic Medicine*, *89*(3), 380–386. doi:10.1097/ACM.0000000000000131 PMID:24448045

Walrod, B. J., Schroeder, A., Conroy, M. J., Boucher, L. C., Bockbrader, M., Way, D. P., ... Bahner, D. P. (2018). Does Ultrasound-Enhanced Instruction of Musculoskeletal Anatomy Improve Physical Examination Skills of First-Year Medical Students? *Journal of Ultrasound in Medicine*, *37*(1), 225–232. doi:10.1002/jum.14322 PMID:28795411

Weinberger, S. E., Pereira, A. G., Iobst, W. F., Mechaber, A. J., & Bronze, M. S. (2010). Competency-based education and training in internal medicine. *Annals of Internal Medicine*, *153*(11), 751–756. doi:10.7326/0003-4819-153-11-201012070-00009 PMID:21135298

World Health Organization (WHO). (2010). *Framework for action on Interprofessional education & collaborative practice*. Geneva: World Health Organization. Retrieved from http:/whqlibdoc.who.int/hq/2010/WHO.HRH.HPN 10.3.eng.pdf

Chapter 8
Are Electronic Medical Education and the EHR Helping or Hurting the Quality of Medical Education and Patient Care?
Taming Medicine's Leviathan

David Lee John
University of Missouri – Kansas City School of Medicine, USA

Deborah Kaercher
The Final Acts Project, USA

ABSTRACT

This chapter addresses some of the negative aspects of both electronic medical education and the electronic health record. This includes the dilution of the doctor/patient interface, the emphasis on documentation rather than on learning the healing arts, and the intellectual dishonesty that arises from the use of templates and automated fillers. The authors address concerns about the dehumanization of medicine, starting with the style of medical education carrying through to the style of function within the clinical environment.

DOI: 10.4018/978-1-5225-6289-4.ch008

INTRODUCTION

In recent decades, researchers have noted how the swift emergence and growth of digitized innovation, particularly in the healthcare and medical education sectors, has left little opportunity for end-users (medical students, residents and attending physicians) to reflect on how to best utilize these new technologies, or to question if they should be used in certain instances at all. Yet, our healthcare systems eagerly continue to employ these new innovations without much forethought. Right or wrong, technological innovations are now equated with greater efficiency, expediency and cost savings, though one can make a convincing argument that rather saving money with new educational technologies, we have actually shifted the costs – now hidden behind the electronic grid – with all the human support it actually entails. Technology is expensive – it just appears affordable when fewer people are standing in the room. While the bottom line will always be the bottom line, as a physician and educator, I can't help wondering at what cost?

It is important to bear in mind that technological innovations are not new, as noted by world renowned bioethicist and co-founder of the Hastings Center, Dr. Daniel Callahan. He reminds us how:

The culture of technological progress has a long history, going back to the Industrial Revolution, gathering more speed in the nineteenth and twentieth centuries, with Silicon Valley as a high point going into the twenty-first century. 'Innovative technology,' the marketing brand of Silicon Valley, is simply the older model of progress in new clothes, but moving faster and faster." Indeed, I would go a step further and argue that it is moving far more rapidly than we can possibly understand. (Callahan, 2017, pp. 169)

As a more senior physician, I acknowledge that I'm still working from an older model of healthcare education that was taught in the seventies, and that I'm also somewhat rebellious against the newer model of medical education for a variety reasons I consider valid. For instance, it is difficult to understand how the continuous streaming of medical education via digitized informational formats on a computer screen is an intelligent approach to medical education, particularly in a field that requires contextualization, understanding the complexities of team work and, most importantly, up-close and consistent engagement with the patient. Coordination of care is highly complex and requires a sophisticated 'human' infrastructure for the most efficient communication between team members. These communications are often highly nuanced. Important cues and clues can be easily missed or misinterpreted if the medical student, resident or attending physician is not in the room with the patient or has his/her back to the patient, typing . However, some researchers are now arguing for radical change in medical education to meet the needs of healthcare's growing demands. One researcher states that:

Changes in sites of health care delivery, from acute care institutions to community-based settings for chronic care, have required adaptations in educational venues. (Nair and Finucane, 2003)

Additionally, PO Ozuah suggests that:

Finding time to teach "new" fields such as genomics, palliative care, geriatrics, and complementary medicine is difficult when medical school curricula are already challenged to cover conventional materials. (Ozuah, 2002)

Indeed, it is true that medical staff and students are stretched, over-burdened and expected to do more with less, but does that imply technology is the golden egg? Technology is another slippery slope for the physicians who teach medical students. Physicians are not only concerned about technology superseding the trust in the physician/patient relationship – physicians can no longer afford to cling to the formal rigidity of ritualized exams that ultimately consume unreasonable amounts of time. Nor can physicians and medical students lean on the highly symbolic white coat that helped define medicine's power structure for many years. Today's physicians and medical students are now far more interested in relationship building that is constructed in partnership with their patients.

While most physicians do accept and value the benefits of new and emerging technologies that support patient care and blended learning – including technologies that support distance observation and surveillance of the medically fragile and chronically ill patient, as well as medical devices that allow self-care – many physicians remain concerned about the power of the 'ghost' in the room. The omnipresent ghost stands somewhere between the physician, the medical student and their patients – a ghost that was originally designed to facilitate learning, not lead, guide and instruct. It has little interest in the art of humanistic medical education. (Callahan, 2017)

On a more practical note, students must learn the importance of gowning the new and complex patient. If the patient isn't gowned, how can students learn to detect that hidden cutaneous malignancy, the oozing breast lesion or the testicular mass? Is cardiac auscultation or abdominal palpation through layers of clothing adequate? What have our students and young doctors become afraid of… or is it more an issue of expediency? Almost daily, I observe a hesitancy to touch, something that is basic to the art of medicine, the art of healing. In sum, asking our medical students and residents to sit in front of a computer screen, cutting and pasting patient information, will count for very little if the goal is to create good physicians and better patient outcomes. Returning significant value to the human touch will "require us to change entrenched values about progress and technological innovation."(Callahan, 2009) No small task.

In truth, technology provides us with a dual-edged sword – offering both benefits and risks. Unfortunately, we too often fail to do the evaluation and analysis first. Healthcare systems and educational institutions too frequently default into the position of thinking – IF IT CAN BE DONE… THEN WE MUST DO IT! Have we allowed ourselves to be hoodwinked into believing we must have the latest and 'best' to provide good patient care? Many factors are driving the hunger and near religious zeal in the United States to insert technology whenever possible, starting with competition between systems of care, economic incentives for providers, efficient time management of physicians and, lastly, the belief that the newest technologies are considered the new sexy (Callahan, 2009). In Callahan's book, *Taming the Beloved Beast*, he "likens medical technologies to a beloved dog, one that chews up the furniture, urinates on the floor, and is un-trainable – but for all that is a beloved, adored pet." Perhaps the most fitting response to this brilliant analogy is that the pet needs a stronger collar, shorter leash and wiser master!

In our postmodern world of health information construction and Internet technology, information and knowledge have become 'less linear' and less unidirectional (Loader, 1998), and this may ultimately be a great advantage for the patient interested in managing their health. (Kaercher, 2007, pp. 7) I also agree that, "unlike traditional bio-medical models of centralized knowledge construction, technology-based information construction holds a non-teleological posture, capturing ideas of diversity, negotiation, complexity and tension" (Loader, 1998). It is not a capitulation of human-centered healthcare to embrace the new complexities of technology but, while exploring ways to harness technology to meet the more humanistic needs in medical education, the unconditional acceptance of new and emerging technologies as the end-all to enhanced patient outcomes is unacceptable and dangerous, particularly with regard to medical education. In sum, this article is not a rallying cry for more technology but, rather, a cautionary stance surrounding the tale of the diminishing physician-patient relationship.

After 40-plus years of devotion to healing what is broken, I have experienced both private practice and, now, clinical academic medicine. As an internist/rheumatologist, I value the bedside, hands-on medical education I received in the seventies – one that demanded an in-depth knowledge of all aspects of each patient under my care. It was an education that taught me the value of intuition, even Gestalt, in my practice. I learned to look behind – and under – the box.

My medical education consisted of learning to take a multifaceted history, do an observant, thorough physical exam, make a diagnosis or, at the very least, identify the problem at hand and then treat/"work up" what was presented to me. I had a chart in my hands as I talked with my patient. Sometimes, I even browsed through it. This was usually AFTER my initial interaction with the patient. To this day, I still review outside records AFTER my own evaluation.

In today's world, when a medical student, resident and/or attending physician walks into a patient's room having already reviewed the patient's medical history beforehand, the health provider's intellectual trajectory has been set into motion, allowing assumptions to be often solidified, prior to the first word of introduction. It then becomes more difficult to hear what the patient is actually saying (and NOT saying) and/or SEE the body language, rich in clues. A diverted gaze, an awkward silence… all can deliver a powerful message.

With no exaggeration, because of the placement of the electronic health record (EHR) over patient needs, students and physicians are now working at a disadvantage. Yes, they might have saved a little time cutting and pasting on the computer before the exam, but once again, at what cost? Why should we expect our medical student's eyes and ears be open to anything in the room when they have already been informed by a series of previous documentations what to expect, what needs to be addressed? Often my students have almost completed 'their' notes before ever interacting with the patient. Is this a model we should emulate? Whose narrative matters more – the patient's narrative in the present tense or the information 'pre-loaded' from the EHR?

Many more mature physicians can be heard speaking wistfully of the days before coding, bullets and charges were the most important clinic topics. There were no templates in those days. The notes were short (and, I admit, often illegible) but they were ours. Our assessments and plans emerged from the initial conversation with the patient, who hopefully was given the first few minutes of the interaction to tell his or her story, without interruption. Not everything about the good old days was good – but this was. Sadly, the prognosis for this impressive and intuitive approach to the practice of medicine is very poor. Indeed, the artful practice of medicine is becoming moribund. I fear there's little hope for recovery, unless physicians and medical educators can secure a consensus that a return to this form of teaching is important… indeed, vital… to maintain the essence of our profession. The art of healing is sacred, and not for its theology but, rather, for its humanism. If we as physicians don't retain this, will there even be any reason for physicians when the robots are on the frontline?

As a rheumatologist, I'm often sent patients whose problems multiple physicians have had trouble understanding. If I have those work-ups and their prior analyses in my head as I enter the patient's room, I might well follow the same deductive path of others. Sir William Osler would not have approved of this, nor would any one of my esteemed mentors in medicine. But, what concerns me most is that our students see truth as 'fluid', and that documentation doesn't require the truth. While an epistemologist might argue this point with far more eloquence, in medicine and science most consider "the sentences on our lips or in our brains are true when and only when they correspond appropriately with the facts or with the reality." (Isa, 1993) But while truth based on the facts are indeed not considered all that 'fluid', facts do change over time based on new evidence in research, which then provides us with a new truth. 'Fluidity of truth', as my students like to think of it, is nearly bottomless, and virtually without reference to facts and/or external realities. There is a pronounced casualness to their approach to the truth in medicine that appears a little too easy for my comfort. Most of my senior medical students have never gowned a patient, including new patients, until they met with my insistence. I still can't grasp how one can attest to the presence of dorsals pedis pulses, or the degree of vibratory sensation through shoes and socks. As a seasoned clinician, I find this approach to bedside exams to be lazy, dishonest and dangerous. To nonchalantly hitting template after template, without modification or fact-checking, is not okay.

This brings me to my final point and concern about the placement of EHR (translate: insurance) documentation requirements above the intellectual honesty of the physician and the 'truth'. While electronic communications – a great idea that has drifted far from the original intent and objectives – could and should be a superb tool for patient care, there exist far too many failed scenarios for every good scenario to recount in this article. The advent of the electronic health record and communications via email has "result[ed] in fewer and fewer face-to-face interactions, making communications [with patients] even more challenging."(Palmieri, J., M.D. and Stern, T. A., M.D., 2009. pp. 163) According to an observational study in 2016, physicians are now spending greater amounts of time with their patients' health records than with their patients. This study revealed the gaps between EHR expectations and outcomes:

"For example, one might hypothesize that the new EHR activities decrease the time physicians spend engaging with patients," the authors write. "Our data quantify previous survey data showing that physicians report spending substantial work time using the EHR. These previous studies have suggested that decreased time with patients and increased workload from EHR tasks are major contributors to career dissatisfaction among physicians." (Sinsky, C., MD, et al, 2016).

The scarcity of personal time because of the electronic health record is just one of the many challenges facing our physicians, medical students and residents in today's world. The real issue is that the EHR is forcing thousands of honest physicians to work dishonestly. Physicians are now incentivized to practice medicine 'non-creatively' with EHR templates and the lack of hours in a day to see patients only increases the probability of physicians succumbing to this compromised way of practicing medicine. Some physicians "save time by writing illegibly. Some abbreviate liberally. Some use forms that have check-off items that are easy to use – so easy that the physician may check the box even if they only did part of what is implied by the presence of the check mark." (Essin, D., 2012). Most physicians can identify with this challenge, many feel compromised while others have accepted there is no alternative but to comply or risk no reimbursement for services provided. The physician is between a rock and a wall as:

EHRs have automated charting in way that makes it easy to incorporate material in a progress note that is fictitious. Check-boxes have proliferated. Some EHRs will, with a single click, generate a complete and detailed note. Were all those things examined? Was every finding exactly as described? Most physicians would never intentionally lie about things like this, but the EHR can make it so easy. (Essin, D. 2012)

Unfortunately, this is the new reality for our physicians, and the very world our young medical students and residents are being groomed to function in. The concern is that they will face the temptation to rely less and less on their clinical skills, and more and more on technology. We might as well march in the robots if abdication of critical thinking in a clinical setting is going to be the new norm. According to Essin, "in order to get the work done, everyone is forced to make a little compromise – enter the most plausible thing that the computer will accept even if it is not strictly true or correct. Eventually the senses get dulled to the point that these compromises no longer evoke an emotional response" (Essin, 2012). And eventually, these small compromises will create a record that will serve the patient poorly, if not disastrously. Records cannot be approximations. Edits count. We now have "a system that offers incentives to compromise the truth, encourage[ing] dishonest behavior. Today's EHR's do just this by demanding more of the physician's time while simultaneously creating situations that force ethical compromise and by appearing to sanction the compromises by providing features such as copy/paste and one-click normal exams." (Essin, D., 2012) Coding is not a science. It is not precise, ethical or meaningful in any way. Those who enforce coding often have limited understanding of what the practice of medicine is about. It is nothing short of tragic that our physicians and students are being both seduced and betrayed by a system of accountability that was developed by those who understand the practice and art of medicine the least. Make no mistake, the challenges around EHR and electronic medical education must be addressed if medicine is to retain its dignity, ethics and soul.

REFERENCES

Callahan, D. (2009). *Taming the Beloved Beast.* Princeton University Press.

Callahan, D. (2017). *The Five Horsemen of the Modern World: Climate, Food, Water, Disease, and Obesity.*

Essin, D. M. A. (2012). The Ethical Dilemma Created by EHRs. In *Physicians Practice, in Blog*. HER, Healthcare Careers.

Kaercher, D. (2007). *The Development of a South Texas Health Information Gateway: Negotiating the Construction of Information* (Dissertation). Edith Cowan University Press, Perth, Australia.

Loader, B. (1998). *Cyberspace divide: Equality, agency, policy in the information society*. New York: Routledge. doi:10.4324/9780203169537_chapter_1

Nair, B. R., & Finucane, P. M. (2003). Reforming Medical Education to Enhance the Management of Chronic Disease. *The Medical Journal of Australia, 20013*(179), 257–259. PMID:12924974

Ozuah, P. O. (2002). Undergraduate Medical Education: Thoughts on Future Challenges. *BMC Medical Education, 2*(1), 8–10. doi:10.1186/1472-6920-2-8 PMID:12149136

Palmieri, J. M. D., & Stern, T. M. D. (2009). Lies in the Doctor-Patient Relationship. *Primary Care Companion to the Journal of Clinical Psychiatry, 11*(4), 163–168. doi:10.4088/PCC.09r00780 PMID:19750068

Ruiz, J. G., Mintzer, M., & Leipzig, R. (2006). The Impact of E-Learning in Medical Education. Academic Medicine, 81(3).

Sinsky, C., Colligan, L., Li, L., Prgomet, M., Reynolds, Goeders, L., … Blike, G. (2016). Allocation of Physician Time in Ambulatory Practice: A Time and Motion Study in 4 Specialities. *Annals of Internal Medicine*.

Sosa, E. (1993). Epistemology, Realism, and Truth: The First Philosophical Perspectives Lecture. In *Philosophical Perspectives* (Vol. 7, pp. 1–16). Ridgeview Publishing.

Chapter 9
Apps and Their Applications:
Novel Uses of Technology in the Clinical Setting

Imran Nizamuddin
University of Missouri – Kansas City School of Medicine, USA

Raveena Basra
University of Missouri – Kansas City School of Medicine, USA

Sai Vanam
University of Missouri – Kansas City School of Medicine, USA

Nurbanu Pirani
University of Missouri – Kansas City School of Medicine, USA

ABSTRACT

In a society dominated by the use of technology as a primary method of communication and education, it should come as no surprise that medical professionals rely heavily on its use as well. The new dominance of smartphones over cell phones and pagers in medicine is largely influenced by convenience and efficiency, and over 70% of healthcare professionals have reported using a mobile device in their workplaces. This chapter aims to highlight the transition to mobile devices in the medical realm and the benefits for both clinicians and patients. For clinicians, mobile devices and apps may serve as diagnostic aids, med calculators, and clinical references. They can also be used for medical education purposes and access of electronic medical records. For patients, mobile devices and apps are often utilized to find resources and information about diseases, to help with disease management, and to promote lifestyle modification and fitness. Nevertheless, despite the numerous benefits of mobile devices in practice, potential risks and drawbacks must also be considered.

DOI: 10.4018/978-1-5225-6289-4.ch009

INTRODUCTION

In a society dominated by the use of technology as one of the main and most accessible ways of communication and education, it should come as no surprise that medical professionals rely heavily on its use as well. The transition from textbooks to mobile devices and their applications (apps) has revolutionized the practice of clinical medicine.

The gradual infiltration of technology into medicine began with the general concept of smartphones alone. Many hospitals analyzed the use of smartphones for clinical communication in the internal medicine wards. These studies found improved communication, efficiency, and accountability among clinicians and nurses with the use of smartphones. Specific advantages included quicker communication between nurses and physicians and fewer interruptions for non-urgent issues throughout the day (Ozdalga, Ozdalga, & Ahuja, 2012). To take matters a step further, smartphones are also integrated with electronic medical records (EMR). For example, Epic, one of the most popular EMR systems, is accessible via mobile applications on the leading platforms (Ozdalga et al.).

The new dominance of smartphones over cell phones and pagers in medicine is largely influenced by convenience and efficiency. The applications that smartphones and tablets offer provide the most important resources used by medical professionals in the most accessible and time-friendly manner. Several studies indicate that usage of medical apps have a positive impact on communication among healthcare professionals, as well as on patient management (Ozdalga, et al., 2012; Ventola, 2014). In fact, 70% of medical school healthcare professionals and students reported using at least one medical app regularly, with 50% using their favorite app daily (Ventola, 2014).

This chapter will explore and explain different categories of apps used to aid clinicians as well as patients. It includes general education tools for healthcare providers, and apps for patient education, diagnosis, treatment, and preventative health. It is not meant to include an exhaustive list of mobile apps for use in the clinical setting, but as an exposure to the possible benefits of technology on patient outcomes, patient education, and diagnosis. Nevertheless, the use of more technology in the clinical setting does not come without its drawbacks and concerns, which this chapter will address as well.

HISTORY OF TECHNOLOGY IN MEDICINE

As healthcare facilities began to include a variety of unrelated locations, such as outpatient clinics, inpatient services, emergency departments, radiology departments, and laboratories, mobile devices were initially implemented due to the vital need to establish an efficient means of communication. Up until the 1990's, medical professionals' chief means of mobile communication was a pager (Mosa, Yoo, & Sheets, 2012). The first pager system was used in 1950 by New York City's Jewish Hospital. About four decades later, personal digital assistants (PDAs) entered the medical scene. PDAs allowed physicians and other healthcare workers to organize some of their personal information, such as appointments, contacts, and schedules (Mosa et al., 2012). Nevertheless, these handheld PCs added yet another device that physicians needed to carry, along with a pager. As a result, with smartphones combining the features of a PDA, pager, and cell phone into one device, more and more people started adopting them instead. In fact, research conducted by Manhattan Research, LLC found that the use of smartphones by medical professionals doubled from 2001 to 2009, increasing from 31% to 64% (Mosa et al., 2012). With smartphones becoming an increasingly stable means of communication in the medical field, the next technological innovation to sweep the healthcare system was the development of mobile applications.

Smartphones and tablets provide many advantages in a clinical setting compared to other devices. In a single device, the latest models not only allow for traditional uses for mobile devices, such as communication via voice and text message, but also incorporate many advanced features. Current smartphones typically include high-quality cameras, Global Positioning System (GPS) sensors, microphones (which can help with recording sound), high-resolution screens, and powerful processing abilities. Taking advantage of these features, many applications are able to provide valuable resources that can be used in the clinical setting. With the rapid development of mobile technology, the reliance on computers, once considered essential in medical care, has started to decrease in favor of mobile devices.

With phones being an epicenter of technology, and specifically for the medical field, it is no surprise that some medical residency programs provide residents with a smartphone rather than the traditional pager. Well-known institutions, such as Barnes Jewish Hospital in St. Louis, MO, or Kaiser Permanente in California, utilize iPhones® as their residents' main communication resource. An advantage this system is the ease of contacting an individual, as users are able to directly call the necessary party instead of waiting for a response to a page. In addition, the system provides the opportunity for medical residents to download apps that can improve care for their patients.

MOBILE DEVICES

A mobile device is defined as a handheld tablet or device that is designed for portability. As mentioned earlier, older mobile devices included PDAs, which had color screen interfaces and access to specialized programs (i.e. e-mail clients, calculator) and the Internet. In the modern era, mobile devices typically refer to smartphones or tablet devices. These devices have a touchscreen interface providing a virtual keyboard. They are able to connect to the Internet as well as interconnect with other devices via technology such as Bluetooth® and near-field communication (NFC). Typically, mobile devices run mobile operating systems that influence available features and allow for the installation of third-party applications (Collins & Ellis, 2015).

One of the first mobile devices that incorporated both communication and computing features was the Blackberry®, which was introduced in 2002. Nevertheless, mobile devices did not gain significant popularity until the launch of the iPhone® and the iOS operating system in 2007, which revolutionized the industry with its multi-touch capacitative touch screen (Woyke, 2014). This development was soon followed by the introduction of Google's Android™ operating system in the same year. Yet, the first commercial Android device was not available until 2008 (Krajci & Cummings, 2015). In July of 2008, Apple® released its App Store®, a digital distribution platform allowing users to browse and install hundreds of apps, billed by Steve Jobs as "the biggest launch of my career" (Woyke, 2014).

Applications on iOS and Android were initially limited to smartphones. However, in 2010, Apple unveiled the iPad®, the first tablet device to run on its operating system, providing greater processing power and a larger screen. Tablets running the Android operating system quickly followed (Woyke, 2014).

Currently, Apple's iOS and Google's Android operating systems dominate in terms of market share on mobile devices. As of 2018, over 99% of new mobile devices ran either the iOS or Android operating systems (Kitagawa et al., 2018). iOS is exclusive to Apple devices, while the Android operating system runs on devices made by dozens of manufacturers, such as Samsung®, LG Electronics®, HTC®, and Google itself. Globally, up to 85% of mobile devices run Google's Android operating system, with Apple's iOS coming in at a distant second with 14% of the market share. However, iOS has greater market share in developed countries such as the United States (Kitagawa et al.). As of January 2017, over 2.2 million applications are available on the iOS App Store, along with over a million applications for Apple tablet devices (Apple Inc., 2017). Google's counterpart, the Google Play™ Store, houses over 3.5 million applications as well (Miller, 2017). According to App Annie, an app market data and insights company, global app downloads surpassed 175 billion in 2017 and consumer spending exceeded $86 billion (Sydow & Cheney, 2018).

mHealth (mobile health) is a general term for the use of mobile phones and other wireless technology in medical care (Becker et al., 2014). As of 2016, over 250,000 mHealth applications were available globally. Over 70% of mHealth application publishers develop for both iOS and Android operating systems. With over 59,000 application publishers, the healthcare application development industry is considered one of the fastest growing in the development realm. The global market for mobile medical apps is projected to reach $102.4 billion by 2022 (Zion Market Research, 2017).

The growth of this industry is readily apparent based on increased usage of mobile health applications by both healthcare providers and patients. Numerous studies have attempted to estimate the percentage of doctors that use mobile devices in their workplace. While the results vary, use of mobile devices appears to be pervasive. The Manhattan Research/Physician Channel Adoption Study in June 2012 found that 87% of doctors used a smartphone or tablet device in their workplace. Tablet device use is also increasing among healthcare professionals. One study estimated that 66% of doctors own a tablet computer, and 54% of them use these devices in the workplace (Moja & Kwag, 2015).

FOR CLINICIANS

Diagnostic Aids

Perhaps the most revolutionary aspect of smartphone applications in medicine is the ability to use them for diagnosis. Information about labs, images, and other diagnostic tools normally required for disease workup can, to an extent, now be found in a single handheld device.

One of the first medical applications to be included in the iOS App Store was called Mobile MIM. To this day, it continues to serve as a useful diagnostic aid, as it is an application that is designed to share images from radiology, radiation oncology, nuclear medicine, nuclear imaging, and cardiac imaging (Andrus, Forrester, Germain, & Eiland, 2015). The application is intended to provide greater access to images to help in coordinating care between physicians or consulting peers on challenging cases.

While some of these applications are used for more general diagnostic assistance, others are more specific. For medical students and physicians alike, oftentimes coming up with a proper and all-inclusive differential diagnosis can be challenging. Taking this into account, a number of applications, such as Diagnosaurus on iOS, can be used to form a general differential diagnosis based on a list of symptoms and physical exam findings. While these apps in no way serve to substitute the clinical decision-making role of a physician, they do help broaden the differential diagnosis so that less-common conditions are considered as well. In addition to apps used to form a differential diagnosis based on patient signs and symptoms, other applications may be used for diagnosing specific conditions, including the relevant cardiac, neurological, and surgical applications described below.

Electrocardiograms (ECGs) are one of the most widely utilized diagnostic tests in modern medicine, helpful for diagnosing dozens of conditions, including arrhythmias, acute coronary syndrome, pericarditis, and a number of other diseases. They are essential for diagnosis not only when patients demonstrate symptoms in the acute setting, but also to monitor the rhythms of asymptomatic or episodically symptomatic patients as well. Over the past several decades, the technology behind ambulatory recorders has flourished. As a result, with the advent of mobile devices, the opportunity to record ECGs in a convenient manner continues to thrive. Several companies have developed apps that allow for ambulatory monitoring of heart rhythms. Mobile applications are connected to mobile heart rhythm monitors that can record single-lead ECGs from the fingers of both hands. This field is rapidly gaining traction, and several comparable apps, including but not limited to AliveCor's KardiaMobile and Eko DUO, are currently available on multiple platforms. These companies are even branching out to incorporate wearable technology into their line of products. AliveCor's KardiaBand provides a replacement strap for the Apple Watch® including the company's single-channel electrocardiogram sensors (AliveCor Inc., 2017). Even Apple itself has entered this market, as they published a patent for a wrist-based ECG monitor that would compete with AliveCor's product. In September 2018, Apple unveiled the Apple Watch Series 4, adding heart health monitoring features to its traditional smartwatch. Electrodes and an electric heart sensor are found in different locations, allowing for the monitoring of arrhythmias, such as atrial fibrillation (Apple Inc., 2018).

The most popular mobile app that provides a single-lead ECG is KardiaMobile. KardiaMobile is a clinically-validated ECG monitor, cleared by the Food and Drug Administration (FDA), that allows physicians and patients alike to capture a medical-grade ECG in 30 seconds. The monitor is connected to a mobile app that allows for storage of heart activity data and sharing of the information with other physicians. This application may be utilized to detect arrhythmias "on the go" and is popularly used for improved detection and management of atrial fibrillation. Several studies continue to be conducted on the app, such as combining an embodied conversational agent with Kardia in the hopes of improving health-related quality of life and adherence to anticoagulation medication (Guhl et al., 2017). Other trials are investigating the effectiveness of the mobile app to detect atrial fibrillation in TIA and cryptogenic stroke patients (Treskes et al., 2017).

With cardiovascular disease being the most prevalent cause of morbidity in this country, the significance of listening to heart sounds on physical exam cannot be underestimated. Therefore, perhaps the most innovative and impactful mobile app to reach the medical technology realm is the FDA-approved Eko Core. This HIPAA-compliant app is linked to the Eko Core stethoscope via Bluetooth. This medical instrument is the first to wirelessly stream heart sounds and incorporate them into a patient's EMR via its adjacent mobile app. Similar apps are currently in progress and have the potential to aid with physical exam findings without requiring physical presence at all times.

In addition, tremors are another essential finding on physical exam that may help with the detection of underlying neurologic conditions and nutritional deficiencies. However, tremors and other movement disorders can be difficult to detect with the naked eye. Fortunately, new mobile apps relying on various sensors, including gyroscopes, may assist with diagnosis. One example is iSeisometer, available on iOS. This smartphone application is especially useful for detecting tremors, specifically orthostatic tremors (Joundi, Brittain, Jenkinson, Green, & Aziz, 2011).

Aside from applications that can be downloaded, multiple plug-in devices are now on the market that may help with diagnosis. For instance, mobile technology is taken to another level with mobile endoscopy applications. One application, endoscope-i, can be used take high definition pictures of the ear, nose, and throat (Mosa et al., 2012). In addition, portable ultrasound scanners are now available as well, such as Philips Lumify, which allow imaging via smartphones. Transducers simply need to be connected to a smartphone, which serve as the screen, allowing for convenient diagnostic capabilities. Other relevant apps include: eRoentgen (identifies which radiology exams to order), biomeme (smartphone kit to diagnose GC infections), Cupris Health/TYM otoscope (clips on phone that act as an otoscope), iGoniometer (measure angles for orthopedic diagnoses), EarTrumpet (audiometry), and Triton OR (assesses postsurgical blood loss).

There is an exhaustive list of well-known and developing apps that are now being used in the medical realm, such as the ones listed above. Nevertheless, their most important contributions are not their uses, but what they represent. The use of mobile apps reflects a more cost-efficient and time-efficient approach to clinical practice. For instance, the drawbacks of long-term heart rate monitoring systems that are currently being used, such as an implantable cardiac monitor (ICM) or loop recorder, is that they are expensive and must be worn on the body constantly. Therefore, in terms of accessibility, apps like Kardia are much more beneficial for long-term patient care and can improve quality of life (Treskes et al., 2017). In addition, mobile apps to assist with endoscopy can provide an easier alternative to the usual bulkier endoscopic instruments (Mosa et al., 2012). In addition, apps optimize the use of evidence-based resources at the bedside. As a result, not only do providers enhance their own efficiency in regards to patient care, but they are also able to educate patients in a quicker manner.

Med Calculators

One of the more tedious and error-prone aspects of medicine involves formulas and calculations. Even seasoned providers may forget how to calculate the fractional excretion of sodium (FeNa) or the components of the Wells Score. In this setting, mobile applications are especially useful. Medical calculators were first introduced onto personal computers for physician access and then progressed to availability on the Internet. However, many doctors encountered difficulties relying on computers to provide immediate access to medical calculators due to availability issues (Mosa et al., 2012). Therefore, providing these calculators via a mobile application is extremely helpful.

The advantages of these calculators range from providing standard formulas in order to make calculations and define risk scores to determining accurate drug dosing. Typically, calculation apps incorporate calculators for diverse fields. For example, MDCalc, the most popular online medical calculator, released a mobile application in 2016 that covers 200+ patient conditions across 35 specialties. These applications are helpful in both the adult and pediatric realms. One of the more difficult calculations in medicine is determining pediatric patients' drug doses based on their weight or age in years. Several drug-dosing calculators, such as Paeds ED, have options to account for pediatric populations. Many also provide instantaneous information regarding drug dosing for patients with renal failure, a topic that is often overlooked. (Mosa, et al., 2012). Newer apps, such as uBurn, may assist surgeons with determining the percentage of total body surface area affected in adult burn victims (Mosa et al.). Instead of manually calculating burn percentages using the Parkland formula, the information is now available immediately using these apps. Overall, the efficiency and stress relief that these mobile calculators provide cannot be underappreciated. Instead of memorizing every formula and computing calculations, physicians are able to devote more time to focus on patient communication and management, rather than tedious tasks.

Clinical References

To be a competent physician requires staying on top of the latest developments, changes, and additions in medicine. This requires consistent and copious amounts of reading and reviewing of the latest articles and studies. In regards to medical apps for references, their uses for physicians can be grouped into two main categories: literature review and information gathering. Literature review refers to accessing published articles in various journals that cover a wide array of medical topics. This is essential for research projects, practicing up-to-date evidence-based medicine, and routine clinical practice. Articles from recognized medical journals, such as the New England Journal of Medicine, the British Medical Journal, and the Lancet, can be viewed via mobile apps. In addition, literature search sites and databases, such as PubMed, are also easily available on a smartphone (Ventola, 2014). PubSearch and PubMed on Tap are two applications available via iOS that allow for access to PubMed and MEDLINE database searches (Mosa et al., 2012). Several "journal club" apps are also available on all platforms and provide quick take-home points regarding recent literature.

Nevertheless, information gathering often demands a majority of a healthcare professional's time. In fact, the Manhattan Research/Physician Channel Adoption Study discovered that physicians spend 64% of their time online to search for information to make or support clinical decisions (Ventola, 2014). Fortunately, several applications are available to assist clinicians with patient workup and management. For evidence-based medicine, UpToDate is a well-known app that provides the most recent clinical evidence on various topics, from drugs and medical conditions to recent changes in practice guidelines (Mosa et al., 2012). In fact, a study done at a community hospital found UpToDate to be among the top five resources used by physicians to search for general medical information, patient management, and evidence-based medicine (León, Fontelo, Green, Ackerman, & Liu, 2007; Mosa et al.). In another cross-sectional study done at a teaching hospital, 93.4% of residents reported that they would recommend UpToDate to another colleague (Phua & Lim, 2008). Several medical schools offer their medical students and resident physicians a free subscription to this application, which can be accessed via a desktop computer, tablet, or smartphone. Among medical students, UpToDate remains the most frequently used and trustworthy smartphone resource, with the perception that it improves patient care and diagnostic accuracy (Quant, Altieri, Torres, & Craft, 2016). Supporting this perception, a study was done among hospitals with access to UpToDate versus those without access. It revealed better outcomes in the hospitals with UpToDate in regards to patient safety and complications, along with a shorter length of stay among Medicare beneficiaries (Phua & Lim, 2008).

Similar to UpToDate, DynaMed is another evidence-based medical application that reviews literature and provides summaries on a given topic. DynaMed's greatest strength is that it is the most frequently updated point-of-care resource with a very low risk of conflict of interest (Andrews, et al., 2017). Moreover, unlike UpToDate, when the app is fully downloaded, it can be used offline without requiring an active Internet connection (Ozdalga et al., 2012).

Another frequently used education-focused medical application among medical professionals is Epocrates (Mosa et al., 2012). Although it has multiple features, this resource is most commonly used for pharmaceutical information. Epocrates extensively reviews medications regarding their uses, contraindications, drug interactions, dosing, and pharmacology (Bhanot & Sharma, 2017). Especially beneficial to patient outcomes and overall care is the app's ability to identify drug-to-drug interactions, a feature which can prevent treatment failure and adverse events. Other drug reference applications include Medscape, Skyscape's RxDrugs, SafeMed Pocket, and FDA drugs. Along with features similar to Epocrates, SafeMed Pocket is especially useful in nursing homes by warning against drug interactions, dosages, and therapies that are harmful to elderly patients (Mosa et al., 2012).

Having these references available via point-of-care access has truly improved the medical landscape. Diagnostic workup, management, and treatment are made easier and quicker, not only due to the availability of these apps, but also their user-friendly interfaces. For example, on UpToDate, medical topics are broken down into general headings and subheadings. This organization allows for the user to easily access exactly what he or she needs. Providing these features via smartphone apps further optimizes efficiency and accelerates the advantages that the resources already offer.

Electronic Medical Records (EMR)

Accessing patient information during hospital rounds and outpatient visits can be taxing if desktop computers are not nearby. Luckily, there are mobile applications on Android and iOS that allow for easy access to a patient's EMR. Two of the most popular EMR systems used nationwide are Epic and Cerner, both of which are accessible on smartphones via the Citrix Receiver app and Epic Haiku. Now, instead of having to spend extra time to find a computer to look up a simple lab result, providers have the freedom to safely and securely access patient information at any time. Moreover, these apps often provide unique features in addition to chart reviewing purposes. Some EMR apps provide communication servers that allow for HIPAA-compliant discussion of patients between providers. Several EMR apps even allow physicians to take pictures at bedside and upload them securely into the patient's EMR via the app. As of 2018, most of the leading EMR providers have mobile apps, which provide a majority of the information found on their PC counterparts, such as vital signs, lab results, patient notes, medication lists, and patient lists with room numbers and identifiers (Mosa et al., 2012). Furthermore, for obstetricians and gynecologists, EMR apps often have partnerships with other apps to provide access to fetal heart tracings remotely. One example, AirStrip, gives the provider immediate access to a patient's fetal strip in real time (Mosa et al.).

Medical Education/Training

Why haul around a dozen textbooks when most of the material can be found in a single handheld device? The convenience and resourcefulness of a smartphone and its applications has changed the landscape of medical students' training as well. Many of the classic textbooks of medical education, such as Netter's Atlas of Human Anatomy, now have mobile applications that present the information in a more interactive manner. These applications can be incredibly useful in the basic sciences portion of medical students' curriculum. Students can supplement anatomical knowledge using apps that serve as an interactive anatomy tool for dissection. One useful app is Cranial Nerves, which pictures and explains the role and location of cranial nerves while displaying them on high-resolution CT scans. Apps in this category can help medical students gain appreciation for the complexity of the human body, and also promote learning in a realistic manner (Mosa et al., 2012).

Most of the popular question banks that students use to prepare for clerkship and board exams, such as USMLE World and Kaplan, are available on mobile devices as well. Immediate access to these question banks via mobile devices allows students to study more frequently and wherever they please. Other applications can be used to share innovative images for learning purposes. For example, Figure 1 is a social media application where providers can share images of conditions that they encounter, much like an "Instagram for doctors." Additionally, applications exist that may assist students on the wards. For example, note-taking apps, such as I-Surgery, can be used to keep track of cases during surgery clerkships. From note-taking apps to question banks to apps with innovative images and visuospatial games, these apps provide a range of useful educational tools (Ventola, 2014).

One of the greatest advantages of these smartphone applications is the "on the go" accessibility. In a survey among medical students, residents, and faculty, well above half of the participants agreed that having an easily available mobile device with apps had a beneficial impact on their education (Ventola, 2014). Other benefits from mobile technology noted in this survey included rapid access to look up unfamiliar terms or pathology, ability to access various sources at the same time on one device, tools for time management, and easier communication among peers and faculty (Ventola, 2014).

A specific area of medical training where smartphone applications seem to be having an innovative impact is with simulated training. For instance, apps such as Touch Surgery or vCath provide simulated surgical training (Ventola, 2014). Moreover, in a study where physicians used a smartphone app during advanced life support training, researchers found an increase in cardiac arrest simulation testing scores (Ozdalga et al., 2012). Such apps include iCPR and iResus, both available for free on the iOS. iCPR aims to enhance proper chest compression rate by measuring the rate and giving audiovisual feedback. With iResus, the user can access both adult and pediatric resuscitation guideline algorithms in an interactive format (Mosa et al., 2012).

FOR PATIENTS

Patient Disease Management

Perhaps the best utilization of these smartphone apps is the ability to encourage patients to become more involved in their own care. Optimal management of chronic diseases requires a component of personal responsibility by the patient for his or her health. For patients with chronic conditions such as diabetes, cardiovascular disease, or COPD, many apps are available and can be helpful for monitoring at home and throughout their daily lives.

Several apps target patients with chronic cardiac conditions and can help control risk factors. For example, many apps include blood pressure logs, which allow patients to record their blood pressure readings and present them to their providers at clinic appointments. Other apps, such as QuitSTART, may assist those trying to quit smoking (Choi, Noh, & Park, 2014). These apps often provide tips and motivational messages that can encourage patients to avoid cigarettes. Taking cardiac disease management a step further, the National Heart Foundation introduced the My Heart, My Life app, which is designed to monitor an individual's medications and personal health statistics. It also features materials and videos on the warning signs of a heart attack for patient education (Choi et al.). For cardiac patients who struggle to reach a hospital for rehabilitation therapy, apps may help physicians monitor their clinical status. One app, Cardiomobile, is a programmed smartphone that tracks a patient's location, activity level, and heart rhythm, and subsequently sends that information to an expert for real-time monitoring (Mosa et al., 2012).

Another common disease gaining attention in the mobile health apps realm is diabetes. Patients often struggle with monitoring of blood sugars, and recent apps have made an effort to make monitoring easier. One app, known as Diabeo, gathers a patient's carbohydrate intake, pre-meal blood glucose levels, and presumed physical activity to help determine an individual's bolus insulin dose (Mosa et al., 2012). This information is then sent from a smartphone to a medical office computer via General Packet Radio Service (GPRS) connection (Mosa et al.). Implementation of this system is not only cost-efficient, but also holds patients accountable for their own care and improves communication with their providers.

For chronic respiratory conditions, self-monitoring apps can be helpful for optimal disease management. For example, a popular app on iOS is Pulmonary Rehabilitation, which can be used as an electronic peak flow meter and can also look at oxygen saturation through a pulse oximeter connected by Bluetooth technology. The electronic peak flow meter may be helpful for asthma patients and can securely send peak-flow readings to an online server via GPRS connections (Mosa et al., 2012).

Besides the more common chronic conditions, there are apps to help manage more specific, but also vital, health issues as well. Alzheimer's disease is progressive and can often lead to difficulties with activities of daily living. Recent technology has focused on avoiding preventable illnesses in this population. For example, an Android application known as iWander was developed to use GPS technology to monitor and track patients with early Alzheimer's disease who are prone to wandering (Ventola, 2014). Other apps useful for an elderly population are those addressing hearing loss and falls. Several apps are available that can assess for hearing loss. An iPhone app called Hearing Check provides users with a free hearing check by simply connecting them with a landline that conducts the test. Another app, uHear, also assesses hearing loss via tests that analyze hearing sensitivity and speech in noisy conditions (Mosa et al., 2012). One exciting concept is the ability to prevent falls through mobile apps. Some apps, such as iFall on Android, rely on the phone's accelerometer and gyroscope to detect a fall and automatically call for help. The Apple Watch Series 4, mentioned previously for its built-in features to act as an electrocardiogram, also can help in the case of a fall. Relying on its accelerometer and gyroscope, this watch can detect a fall based on immobility and automatically call emergency services and loved ones.

Fitness and Lifestyle Apps

Optimal and long-term patient management requires practicing holistic medical care. This consists of more than just treating the disease process itself, but also addressing the factors in an individual's life that influence his or her health. These factors include activity level, sleeping habits, diet, and much more. Counseling patients on healthy habits is one of healthcare providers' most essential responsibilities, and the patients assume responsibility to adhere to these recommendations. Maintaining a well-balanced lifestyle outside of a physician's office is now made easier with lifestyle modification apps addressing these concerns.

Some of the more popular topics of interest are fitness and nutrition. In fact, apps related to these categories were among the most frequently downloaded (Elavsky,

Smahel, & Machackova, 2017). In one study, 58% of smartphone owners were found to have at least one health-related app (Krebs & Duncan, 2015). As a result, hundreds of fitness and nutrition apps are available on all platforms. Some applications, including the popular MyFitnessPal and Lose It, serve as calorie counters and diet trackers with built-in barcode scanners. Therefore, by simply scanning a food item, consumers can measure caloric intake, as well as the carbohydrate, protein, or vitamin content of foods. MyFitnessPal also has a goal-setting feature in which users can set their ideal weight. The app then creates a personalized weight loss plan based on the individual's current weight, height, and activity level. Users can also track their weight loss progress and connect with other people using the app. The benefit of these nutrition apps for patients is not only accessibility, but also motivation. Being able to seamlessly track weight loss progress and connect with others going through the same struggles encourages people to make and maintain positive diet and fitness changes. Many studies have found that the benefits of these apps for patients are driven largely by autonomy, competence, and relatedness (Teixeira, Carraça, Markland, Silva, & Ryan, 2012). As such, the best mobile health apps give users the feeling of intrinsic motivation by putting them in control of how much they choose to use the app, as well as linking them with a community that shares the same struggles.

Patient Care/Resources

Moreover, apps may directly benefit patients by providing access to resources to assist with health management. Apps such as GoodRX compare prescription drug prices and find coupons at thousands of pharmacies, providing patients with affordable care.

In addition to helping with affording medications, other apps can assist with patient access to care. Several apps partner with surrounding doctors and clinics to encourage scheduling of appointments. For example, iTriage is an app that provides locations of nearby emergency rooms, doctors by specialty, and other practical information. The app even shows emergency room wait times and allows patients to schedule appointments at affiliated locations. Similarly, ZocDoc is an app that gives patients a chance to schedule appointments themselves with offices that utilize the system (Ozdalga et al., 2012). Applications such as these are excellent for time management and convenience.

Furthermore, apps can be utilized by both patients and clinicians to ensure proper preventative health practices. For patients, several apps can remind them of upcoming routine screenings, such as mammograms and colonoscopies. For providers, apps such as AHRQ ePSS can aid in identifying screening measures needed for a patient based on age, gender, sexual activity, and tobacco use (Ventola, 2014).

A frequent use of mobile apps, especially among youth populations, is for information regarding birth control measures. These apps are able to simplify options and provide visuals in an easy and discrete manner. One example is the Contraception application made by the Centers for Disease Control (CDC). This app details specific contraceptive methods that can be utilized by patients based on certain characteristics or medical comorbidities (Mangone, Lebrun, & Muessig, 2016). Other smartphone applications continue to be developed and utilized as patient educational assets, even in specialized fields such as plastic surgery, general surgery, and cardiology (Mosa et al., 2012).

Concerns

Despite the numerous benefits of incorporating smartphones and their applications into clinical training and practice, there are certainly concerns and drawbacks that should be addressed as well. Of course, with any new system, time is needed for smooth transitions. In the meantime, errors and poor follow-through are more likely to happen. For example, many of the more innovative applications are new, and, therefore, less reliable and prone to have bugs. On top of that, older physicians who are not as accustomed to newer technologies may be hesitant to adopt them.

In addition, opposition towards further incorporation of technology into the clinical setting focus on the impact on bedside manner and the patient-doctor relationship. More studies are needed regarding the impact of having a tablet or phone present during a clinical encounter. Questions, including how technology affects patient perception of provider attentiveness, should be addressed.

With the rapid increase of smartphone applications, there are inherent risks to the accuracy and safety of patient information. In 2016, the FDA released the 21st Century Cures Act, which outlines the regulatory requirements concerning medical smartphone applications (Ronquillo & Zuckerman, 2017). Still, with so many applications and a growing user base, safety concerns loom.

Moreover, there is concern that healthcare workers' mobile phones are a potential source for nosocomial infections. Researchers worry that phones are rarely cleaned and may transmit microorganisms after contact with patients (Ulger et al., 2009). Nevertheless, there are also studies to suggest that mobile phone applications prevent health-care associated infection by providing easy access to guidelines, hand hygiene monitoring support, or step-by-step procedures aimed at reducing infections at the point of clinical care (Schnall & Iribarren, 2015).

CONCLUSION

As the field of medicine progresses, technology is becoming more and more incorporated into practice and training. Driven by convenience and efficiency, the use of smartphones in particular is widely prevalent in the medical setting. Various smartphone applications have been developed to aid in different aspects of patient care. Some of these applications directly aid in the diagnosis of disease, while others provide reference materials or calculators for clinicians, medical personnel, and students. These applications provide efficient means to look up and gather information versus having to use a textbook. In addition, applications designed for patients are increasingly popular as well. These applications have allowed patients to educate themselves regarding various diseases and to have an active role in disease management. As smartphones have advanced in terms of functionality and ease of use over the years, they have become essential to the care of patients in the medical setting.

Aside from smartphones, other areas of technology have also shown great promise in the medical setting. Augmented reality, which is a type of technology that superimposes a computer into an individual's perception of the real world, has great potential in the future. For example, the Google Contact Lens aims to change diabetes management by measuring glucose levels from tears (Otis & Parvis, 2014). Also, Microsoft has designed the "hololens", which is a holographic computer allowing users to see three-dimensional images in real time (Case Western Reserve, 2015). This concept has very relevant applications for medical education. For example, the hololens has the potential to be a future replacement of cadavers that are used to learn anatomy in medical school.

Today, there are thousands of health and wellness applications that are available to download on the app store. The number of health and wellness applications projects to climb every year. Moving forward, technology will continue to play a greater role in medicine. As a result, medicine as a whole would benefit from continuing studies of its effects and embracing its revolutionary benefits.

REFERENCES

AliveCor, Inc. (2017). *FDA Clears First Medical Device Accessory for Apple Watch®* [Press release]. Retrieved from https://www.alivecor.com/press/press_release/fda-clears-first-medical-device-for-apple-watch/

Andrews, R., Mehta, N., Maypole, J., & Martin, S. A. (2017). Staying afloat in a sea of information: Point-of-care resources. *Cleveland Clinic Journal of Medicine*, *84*(3), 225–235. doi:10.3949/ccjm.84a.15087 PMID:28322678

Andrus, M. R., Forrester, J. B., Germain, K. E., & Eiland, L. S. (2015). Accuracy of pharmacy benefit manager medication formularies in an electronic health record system and the Epocrates mobile application. *Journal of Managed Care & Specialty Pharmacy*, *21*(4), 281–286. doi:10.18553/jmcp.2015.21.4.281 PMID:25803761

Apple Inc. (2017). *App Store shatters records on New Year's Day* [Press release]. Retrieved from https://www.apple.com/newsroom/2017/01/app-store-shatters-records-on-new-years-day/

Apple Inc. (2018). *Apple Watch Series 4: Beautifully redesigned with breakthrough communication, fitness and health capabilities* [Press release]. Retrieved from https://www.apple.com/newsroom/2018/09/redesigned-apple-watch-series-4-revolutionizes-communication-fitness-and-health/

Becker, S., Miron-Shatz, T., Schumacher, N., Krocza, J., Diamantidis, C., & Albrecht, U. V. (2014). mHealth 2.0: Experiences, possibilities, and perspectives. *JMIR mHealth and uHealth*, *2*(2), e24. doi:10.2196/mhealth.3328 PMID:25099752

Bhanot, S., & Sharma, A. (2017). App review series: Epocrates. *Journal of Digital Imaging*, *30*(5), 534–536. doi:10.100710278-017-9977-2 PMID:28523622

Bonis, P. A., Pickens, G. T., Rind, D. M., & Foster, D. A. (2008). Association of a clinical knowledge support system with improved patient safety, reduced complications and shorter length of stay among Medicare beneficiaries in acute care hospitals in the United States. *International Journal of Medical Informatics*, *77*(11), 745–753. doi:10.1016/j.ijmedinf.2008.04.002 PMID:18565788

Case Western Reserve University. (2015). *Case Western Reserve, Cleveland Clinic collaborate with Microsoft on earth-shattering mixed-reality technology for education.* Retrieved from http://case.edu/hololens/

Choi, J., Noh, G., & Park, D. (2014). Smoking cessation apps for smartphones: Content analysis with the self-determination theory. *Journal of Medical Internet Research*, *16*(2), e44. doi:10.2196/jmir.3061 PMID:24521881

Collins, L., & Ellis, S. R. (2015). *Mobile devices: Tools and technologies* (1st ed.). Boca Raton, FL: Chapman and Hall/CRC Press. doi:10.1201/b18165

Elavsky, S., Smahel, D., & Machackova, H. (2017). Who are mobile app users from healthy lifestyle websites? Analysis of patterns of app use and user characteristics. *Translational Behavioral Research*, *7*(4), 891–901. doi:10.100713142-017-0525-x PMID:28929368

Guhl, E. N., Schlusser, C. L., Henault, L. E., Bickmore, T. W., Kimani, E., Paasche-Orlow, M. K., & Magnani, J. W. (2017). Rationale and design of the atrial fibrillation health literacy information technology trial: (AF-LITT). *Contemporary Clinical Trials*, *62*, 153–158. doi:10.1016/j.cct.2017.09.005 PMID:28923492

Joundi, R. A., Brittain, J. S., Jenkinson, N., Green, A. L., & Aziz, T. (2011). Rapid tremor frequency assessment with the iPhone accelerometer. *Parkinsonism & Related Disorders*, *17*(4), 288–290. doi:10.1016/j.parkreldis.2011.01.001 PMID:21300563

Kheshti, R., Aalipour, M., & Namazi, S. (2016). A comparison of five common drug–drug interaction software programs regarding accuracy and comprehensiveness. *Journal of Research in Pharmacy Practice*, *5*(4), 257–263. doi:10.4103/2279-042X.192461 PMID:27843962

Kitagawa, M., Gupta, A., Cozza, R., Glenn, D., Atwal, R., Maita, K., … Wang, A. (2018). *Market share: Final PCs, ultramobiles and mobile phones, all countries, 4Q17* (ID: G00350384). Retrieved from Gartner database.

Krajci, I., & Cummings, D. (2013). *Android on x86: An introduction to optimizing for Intel® architecture* (1st ed.). New York, NY: Apress Media, LLC. doi:10.1007/978-1-4302-6131-5

Krebs, P., & Duncan, D. T. (2015). Health app use among US mobile phone owners: A national survey. *JMIR mHealth and uHealth*, *3*(4), e101. doi:10.2196/mhealth.4924 PMID:26537656

León, S. A., Fontelo, P., Green, L., Ackerman, M., & Liu, F. (2007). Evidence-based medicine among internal medicine residents in a community hospital program using smart phones. *BMC Medical Informatics and Decision Making*, *7*(5), 1–11. doi:10.1186/1472-6947-7-5 PMID:17313680

Mangone, E. R., Lebrun, V., & Muessig, K. E. (2016). Mobile phone apps for the prevention of unintended pregnancy: A systematic review and content analysis. *JMIR mHealth and uHealth*, *4*(1), e6. doi:10.2196/mhealth.4846 PMID:26787311

Miller, M. (2017). Top predictions for the app economy in 2018 [Blog post]. Retrieved from https://www.appannie.com/en/insights/market-data/predictions-app-economy-2018/

Moja, L., & Kwag, K. H. (2015). Point of care information services: A platform for self-directed continuing medical education for front line decision makers. *Postgraduate Medical Journal*, *91*(1072), 83–91. doi:10.1136/postgradmedj-2014-132965 PMID:25655251

Mosa, A. S., Yoo, I., & Sheets, L. (2012). A systemic review of healthcare applications for smartphones. *BMC Medical Informatics and Decision Making*, *12*(67), 1–31. doi:10.1186/1472-6947-12-67 PMID:22781312

Otis, B., & Parvis, B. (2014). Introducing our smart contact lens project [Blog post]. Retrieved from https://googleblog.blogspot.com/2014/01/introducing-our-smart-contact-lens.html

Ozdalga, E., Ozdalga, A., & Ahuja, N. (2012). The smartphone in medicine: A review of current and potential use among physicians and students. *Journal of Medical Internet Research*, *14*(5), e128. doi:10.2196/jmir.1994 PMID:23017375

Phua, J., & Lim, T. K. (2008). How residents and interns utilise and perceive the personal digital assistant and UpToDate. *BMC Medical Education*, *8*(1), 39. doi:10.1186/1472-6920-8-39 PMID:18625038

Quant, C., Altieri, L., Torres, J., & Craft, N. (2016). The self-perception and usage of medical apps amongst medical students in the United States: A cross-sectional survey. *International Journal of Telemedicine and Applications*, *1-5*. doi:10.1155/2016/3929741 PMID:27688752

Ronquillo, J. G., & Zuckerman, D. M. (2017). Software-related recalls of health information technology and other medical devices: Implications for FDA regulation of digital health. *The Milbank Quarterly*, *95*(3), 535–553. doi:10.1111/1468-0009.12278 PMID:28895231

Sanna, T., Diener, H. C., Passman, R. S., Di Lazzaro, V., Bernstein, R. A., Morillo, C. A., ... Brachmann, M. D. (2014). Cryptogenic stroke and underlying atrial fibrillation. *The New England Journal of Medicine*, *370*(26), 2478–2486. doi:10.1056/NEJMoa1313600 PMID:24963567

Schnall, R., & Iribarren, S. J. (2015). Review and analysis of existing mobile phone applications for health care-associated infection prevention. *American Journal of Infection Control*, *43*(6), 572–576. doi:10.1016/j.ajic.2015.01.021 PMID:25748924

Sydow, L., & Cheney, S. (2018). 2017 retrospective: A monumental year for the app economy [Blog post]. Retrieved from https://www.appannie.com/en/insights/market-data/app-annie-2017-retrospective/

Teixeira, P. J., Carraça, E. V., Markland, D., Silva, M. N., & Ryan, R. M. (2012). Exercise, physical activity, and self-determination theory: A systematic review. *The International Journal of Behavioral Nutrition and Physical Activity*, *9*(1), 78. doi:10.1186/1479-5868-9-78 PMID:22726453

Treskes, R. W., Gielen, W., Wermer, M. J., Grauss, R. W., Alem, A. P., Dehnavi, R. A., ... Trines, S. A. (2017). Mobile phones in cryptogenic stroke patients bringing single lead ECGs for atrial fibrillation detection (MOBILE-AF): Study protocol for a randomized controlled trial. *Trials*, *18*(1), 402. doi:10.118613063-017-2131-0 PMID:28851409

Ulger, F., Esen, S., Dilek, A., Yanik, K., Gunaydin, M., & Leblebicioglu, H. (2009). Are we aware how contaminated our mobile phones with nosocomial pathogens? *Annals of Clinical Microbiology and Antimicrobials*, *8*(1), 7. doi:10.1186/1476-0711-8-7 PMID:19267892

Ventola, C. L. (2014). Mobile devices and apps for health care professionals: uses and benefits. *Pharmacy and Therapeutics, 39*(5), 356-364. Retrieved from https://www.ncbi.nlm.nih.gov/pmc/articles/PMC4029126/pdf/ptj3905356.pdf

Woyke, E. (2014). *The smartphone: Anatomy of an industry* (1st ed.). New York, NY: The New Press.

Zion Market Research. (2017). *mHealth market by devices, by stakeholder, by service, by therapeutics, and by applications: Global industry perspective, comprehensive analysis, and forecast, 2014 - 2022*. Retrieved from https://www.zionmarketresearch.com/report/mhealth-market

KEY TERMS AND DEFINITIONS

Electronic Medical Record (EMR): Collection of patient health records protected under HIPAA that are electronically stored and can be shared among various healthcare facilities.

Health Insurance Portability and Accountability Act (HIPAA): Enacted in 1996 to establish national standards to protect individuals' medical records and other personal health information.

Healthcare Professional: An individual who is dedicated to diagnosing, treating and preventing disease. He or she is also a provider offering a variety of services in an effort to promote the health of an individual.

Medical Calculator: An application that allows users to input values into pre-stored formulas.

mHealth Apps: Use of mobile phones and other wireless technology in medical care.

Mobile Application: A program that is designed to run on a mobile platform. Applications can have various uses, such as setting reminders, making calculations, etc.

Mobile Device: Handheld tablet or device that is designed for portability.

Personal Digital Assistant (PDA): A personal device capable of organizing personal information, such as contacts, tasks, and appointments.

Smartphone: A personal device that uses a mobile network to make phone calls, send text messages, and connect to the internet. It is also capable of running software applications.

Chapter 10
Collaborative Learning for Histopathology Education

James L. Fishback
University of Kansas Medical Center, USA

Robert M. Klein
University of Kansas Medical Center, USA

ABSTRACT

The authors have developed a pedagogical approach to the teaching of histology and histopathology using a team-based, collaborative learning model. To accomplish this, students are assigned to small groups of "microdissection" teams, mirroring the approach used in gross anatomy dissection. These collaborative groups present the case, including history, relative labs, imaging, gross pathology, and microanatomy, to their classmates. Each clinical case contains normal and abnormal virtual microscopy slides with links to key areas of interest, as well as hyperlinked references to the medical literature (the electronic pathology text or an article from a general medical journal, e.g., The New England Journal of Medicine®). In order to facilitate this collaborative process, they use Microsoft Office 365® and the included OneNote® program. The approach has facilitated integration of histopathology into the curriculum with more interactive laboratories stimulating active learning to build improved diagnostic skills for the learners.

INTRODUCTION

Over the course of our combined 70+ years of teaching histology and histopathology in the pre-clinical phase of medical school, we have recognized that histology, and closely-related histopathology, are among the difficult subjects for medical students to master. Indeed, at the end of two years of coursework, the majority still seem to

DOI: 10.4018/978-1-5225-6289-4.ch010

see only blobs of pink and blue! Most students seem to focus on color or artifacts on their slides, rather than identifying the relevant diagnostic or pathognomonic morphological features. In retrospect, that should not be a surprise to those of us who are long-term medical educators. We often select medical students for admission to American medical schools based (largely) upon the standardized Medical College Admission Test (MCAT®) test, which consists of multiple choice questions. That standardized test tends to provide an advantage to those students who happen to possess the necessary learning skills to memorize and process large amounts of data (Pelley & Dalley, 2008; Pelley, 2018). Introverted, intuitive students (as determined by the Myers-Briggs Type Indicator®) (Pelley & Dalley, 2008; Pelley, 2018) may be at a disadvantage, as can be seen in Table 1 (Pelley & Dalley, 2008). Other types of learning inventory instruments, such as the Kolb Learning Style Inventory® classifies learners as "accommodators, assimilators, convergers, or divergers" (Kolb & Kolb, 2013). The Kolb Learning Inventory has shown that most of first-year medical students are "assimilators" and "convergers," although their learning style may change over the course of the undergraduate medical school curriculum (Engels & de Gara, 2010; Gurpinar, Bati, & Tetik, 2011). The study by Gurpinar et al. (2011) showed that the type of curriculum was not the driving force in the change in learning style. In contrast to medical students, medical residents and faculty are predominantly convergent and accommodative, with no statistically significant difference between residents and faculty members (Engels & de Gara, 2010).

Table 1. Well-developed type skills and underdeveloped type skills

Well-Developed Type Skills		Underdeveloped Type Skills	
Extraversion	**Introversion**	**Extraversion**	**Introversion**
Active approach	Reflective approach	Hyperactive	Withdrawn & secretive
Bring breadth	Bring depth	Superficial	Overly serious
Sensing	Intuition	Sensing	Intuition
Practical	Imaginative	Slow & dull	Careless
Brings data	Brings perspective	Narrow focus	Impractical & dreamy
Thinking	Feeling	Thinking	Feeling
Analyzes situations	Affiliate people	Cold & uncaring	Easily hurt
Brings consistency	Bring harmony	Overly competitive	Overly sentimental
Judging	Perceiving	Judging	Perceiving
Decisive	Inquisitive	Overly opinionated	Indecisive
Bring a plan	Bring options	Controlling	Procrastinating

Source: Adapted from Success types in medical education: A program for improving academic performance. Retrieved from https://www.ttuhsc.edu/medicine/medical-education/success-types/documents/stsinmeded.pdf

Given that the United States Medical Licensing Examination (USMLE) Step 1 Exam® consists largely of multiple choice questions, some may be tempted to ask, "Why attempt to teach histopathology at all?" Our answer to that question is that histology and histopathology can provide the learner with unique insight into the pathogenesis of disease, which may someday suggest alternative treatments to difficult clinical problems. A good example would be glioblastoma, a relatively common, but deadly, brain tumor. If the tissue is examined, one can see obviously malignant cells far from the main tumor mass seen on a CT Scan (see example case in the Appendix). This should suggest to the student that surgical resection alone will be ultimately ineffective, and that systemic or central nervous system chemotherapy, radiation, and/or immunologic therapies might provide better outcomes than surgery alone. An added advantage of teaching histopathology is that we may find that some students have the necessary aptitude for examining microscopic slides, and, therefore, may have sufficient aptitude to seek further training in anatomic pathology. At the very least, all students should realize diagnosing diseases from microscopic tissue slides is a difficult art, and gain some appreciation for how a pathologic diagnosis is made by an experienced pathologist. We should also seek to expand the students' medical vocabulary in the first two years, so that they can reasonably interpret pathology biopsy reports and communicate more precisely with their future patients and medical colleagues.

COLLABORATIVE LEARNING WITH MICRODISSECTION TEAMS

Our initial teaching concept, upon selecting the Aperio Scanscope® (now Leica®) system to digitize our respective histology and histopathology slide sets into "virtual microscopy" slides, was that each individual student would examine the assigned slide or slides, take selective photomicrographs, and generate their own histology and pathology atlas. What we found, however, over several years, was that many students were taking photomicrographs of histologic artifacts, or extremely high magnification views of pathologic specimens from patients with diseases that should be easily recognizable at low magnification (*e.g.*, liver cirrhosis). So, we created "talk-on" videos to help learners find the pathognomonic area of interest, only to have most of our students pause the videos and take a screenshot of the relevant area! Many students complained of how difficult it was for them to find these "diagnostic" areas of the slide, which would enable them to classify the slide as particular type of injury or disorder, based on etiology (see VINDICATE discussion in Pedagogy section, below).

To us, of course, our original concept of the lab exercise was to enable students to learn to direct their attention to the pathologic area of interest. As educators, we initially became extremely frustrated and confused, as we imagined we had developed a 21st century approach by eliminating microscopes and integrating histology and pathology (Karr, Fishback, & Klein, 2007).

We ultimately decided to assign the students to small groups of "microdissection" teams, modeling an approach we had previously learned about from Dana K. Townsend, Ph.D., at Kansas State University, who used it in her honors anatomy course (2009), and has also been used successfully by others (Marshak, Oakes, Hsieh, Chuang, & Cleary, 2015). These collaborative groups of 3 or 4 students would then present the case, including the history, relevant laboratory results, imaging, gross pathology, and microanatomy to their classmates. The exercise mimicked clinical students on rounds with the facilitator serving as attending physician. Each clinical case contained hyperlinked references to the medical literature (typically a pathology textbook or a general medical journal, *e.g.*, The *New England Journal of Medicine*®). To facilitate this collaborative process, we decided to use Microsoft Office 365® and the included OneNote® program.

The use of collaborative groups also offered an opportunity to leverage the diversity of learning skills seen in most medical school classes (Engels & de Gara, 2010; Gurpinar et al., 2011), and use that diversity in styles to enable deeper learning. Pelley and Dalley (2018) discuss this strategy in their book, a summary of which is reproduced in Table 2.

ONENOTE® AND NOTEBOOK CREATOR

Microsoft Office 365® (O-365) is the web version of the native Microsoft Office® program, available for both the PC and Mac platforms. Since O-365 is implemented through an internet browser, such as Internet Explorer® or Safari®, it is somewhat slower than the native (compiled) program, and has fewer features. However, O-365 does have the key advantage of being able to run on almost any type of personal computer, even if it does not have Microsoft Office® installed. We have a "bring your own device (BYOD)" program at our medical school, but we (strongly) recommend Microsoft Windows computers, which most students seem to choose. Apple MacIntosh® users also participate in the shared notebooks, with minimal technical problems.

Microsoft Education has developed a plugin for OneNote® called *Notebook Creator* for OneNote® that allows teachers to create collaborative notebooks. The process is relatively simple, although some input from information technology professionals may be necessary. The OneNote® notebooks are organized as follows:

Table 2. What the types can offer each other

Extraverts	Introverts
■ Provide the outwardly directed energy needed to move into action. ■ Offer responsiveness to what is going on in the environment. ■ Have a natural inclination to converse and to network.	■ Provide the inwardly directed energy needed for focused reflection. ■ Offer stability from attending to enduring ideas. ■ Have a natural tendency to think and work alone.
Sensing Types	**Intuitive Types**
■ Have a mastery of the facts. ■ Bring a knowledge of what materials and resources are available. ■ Appreciate knowing and doing what works.	■ Know by way of insight and attention to meanings. ■ Bring a grasp of what is possible and what the trends are. ■ Appreciate doing what hasn't been tried before.
Thinking Types	**Feeling Types**
■ Take a hard look at the pros and cons of situations, even when they have a personal stake. ■ Have an ability to analyze and solve problems. ■ Want to discover the "truth" and they naturally notice logical inconsistencies.	■ Know what is important to and for people, and adhere to that in the face of opposition. ■ Have an ability to build relationships and to be persuasive. ■ Want to uncover the greatest "good" in a situation and they notice when people may be harmed.
Judging Types	**Perceiving Types**
■ Can organize, plan, and follow through on projects. ■ Push to get things settled and decided. ■ Appreciate the well-oiled efficiency at work.	■ Can respond quickly and flexibly to the needs of the moment. ■ Strive to keep things open so new information may be gathered. ■ Appreciate the need for spontaneity and exploration at work.

Source: Adapted from Looking at type: The fundamentals. (p. 52)., by Charles R. Martin, 1997, Gainesville, FL: Center for Applications of Psychological Type.

- **Student Notebooks:** A space for individual student notes. Students do not see each other's notebook, unless they want to share with others. However, this space is shared with faculty, for collaboration with the student, when needed. Students can set up (an entirely separate) private notebooks or sections, and manage access as desired. Faculty will not be able to see these private notebook sections, unless granted access by the student.
- **Content Library:** A read-only notebook where faculty can share the histopathology case protocols and any other content with students. Students can then copy content from the Content Library and paste it into the collaboration space for a group mashup, or copy it to their private notebooks. The *read-only* nature of this section means that students cannot alter anything in the Content Library.

Figure 1. OneNote class notebook
Source: Microsoft 365 (2014)

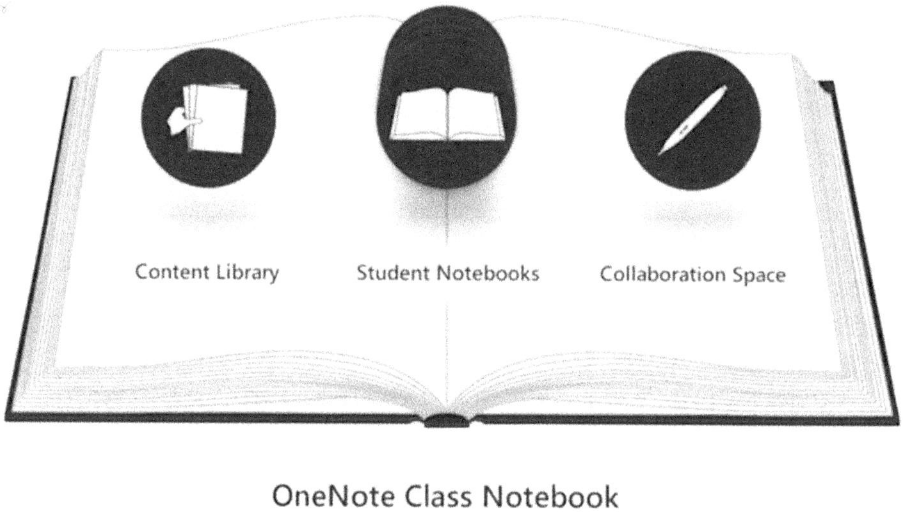

- **Collaboration Space:** A section for everyone in the lab group to share, organize, and collaborate. This is a good space to analyze cases as a group and prepare for clinical presentations. Both students and faculty can read and write into this space. This can be dangerous, as someone can accidently cut the collaborative content out of the space, and paste it to their individual notebook, thus leaving the community Collaboration Space blank. At first, students often need to be reminded to copy shared content (instead of cutting), so that they leave a copy of the collaborative content in its designated electronic space.

PEDAGOGY

We believe the main advantage to our pedagogical approach is that it promotes active and collaborative learning, through a strategy of *facilitated discovery* (Enosis Group, 2012; Pramas, Berres, Bjorklund, & Ellison, 2014), utilizing, for each case, what have been called Essential Questions (Wiggins, 2007; Wilson, 2014). We have further designated these essential questions into factual "What Must Be Known (WMBK)" questions, and conceptual "What Must Be Understood (WMBU)" questions. Thus, these essential questions help us to define the core Medical Knowledge Domain Competencies (Englander & Carraccio, 2014) for each case.

- Instructor/facilitator presence in OneNote shared notebooks provides an "over-the-shoulder" look for evidence of an individual student's critical thinking and reasoning processes. Ideally, to facilitate clinical reasoning, the facilitator would be a physician, although a "coached" basic scientist seems to work well for us.

The VINDICATE (Department of Radiology, University of Washington, n.d.) acronym is used as an organizing differential diagnosis framework for case collaboration, and to enhance differential diagnostic and clinical reasoning skills:

- Vascular
- Infectious, Inflammatory
- Neoplastic
- Degenerative
- Idiopathic
- Congenital
- Autoimmune
- Trauma / toxins
- Endocrine (metabolic)

Peer teaching, with oral presentation and discussion of findings to student groups and faculty facilitators, is essential. Students should be encouraged to follow the clinical model of oral case presentations, *i.e.*, Chief Complaint, History of the Present Illness, *etc.*, as they present the cases to their peers. The histology or histopathology is important only to demonstrate underlying pathophysiology, as we realize that most of our students will never look at a histologic slide again.

VIRTUAL MICROSCOPY

We have utilized servers from Aperio®, now Leica®, to serve up our virtual images. A web-based interphase, using Adobe Flash®, works best for most students. A more advanced native application, ImageScope®, provides some nicer features, such as the ability to make relative size comparisons with a micrometer, place images side by side, etc., but the differences are not material enough to prefer one over the other. Our Apple® users tend to prefer the web-based images. Both types of images are easily copied and pasted into OneNote® pages.

Despite the huge size of the images (typically >4 Gb), the server seems to have no trouble pre-fetching the desired part of the image, working similarly to what one sees in Google Maps®.

Since we heard loud and clear that students found it quite difficult to locate areas of diagnostic interest, we have now taken the relevant photomicrographs for them, and linked the images to the appropriate site in the virtual slide, which is trivial to do. An explanation of the pathognomonic feature of that area of interest is given beneath the photomicrograph, and any necessary arrows or text is added to the image to enhance understanding (see example lab protocol in the Appendix). In other words, we have created an electronic atlas, that student collaborative groups then supplement with any information they find relevant, from textbook, primary literature, or the web.

SUMMARY

Our approach has been well-received by students and faculty members in Pathology and Anatomy. Through peer preview sessions and "faculty notes," it has also served as a faculty development activity, enabling better instruction in our integrated curriculum. The University of Kansas School of Medicine is building on our initial collaborative team efforts in histopathology, as the curriculum undergoes a further transition to flipped classrooms and case-based collaborative learning. Histopathology lab exercises, such as these, can form the foundation for current and future curricular designs, leveraging technology to integrate content and enhance collaborative learning by our students. A recent metastudy showed students had a slight preference for virtual microscopy, compared to optical microscopy, but the difference was slight (Wilson, Taylor, Klein, Sugrue, Whipple, & Brokaw, 2016).

TECHNICAL REQUIREMENTS

Initially, we purchased the ScanScope® scanner, nearly a dozen years ago, from amongst a very limited number of competitors, to digitize our glass slide collection(s). We then purchased two servers, one for public use, and one for restricted use in hospital surgical pathology, which contained private patient data. The latter server was placed behind a firewall, so that access occurs through a virtual private network

Figure 2. Index page and resources for a typical weekly laboratory exercise

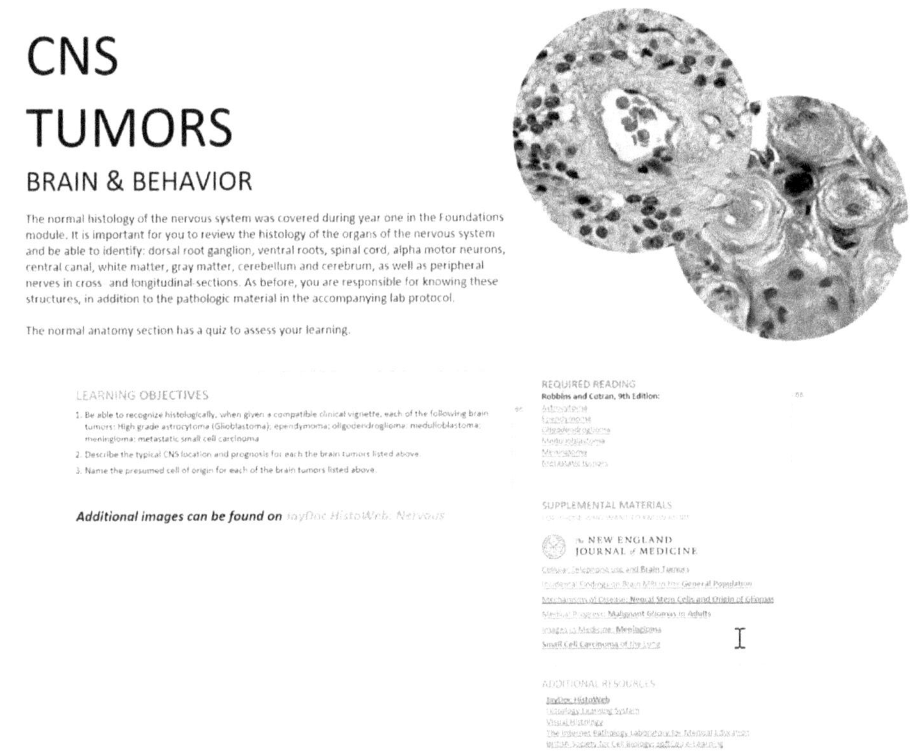
CNS
TUMORS
BRAIN & BEHAVIOR
The normal histology of the nervous system was covered during year one in the Foundations module. It is important for you to review the histology of the organs of the nervous system and be able to identify: dorsal root ganglion, ventral roots, spinal cord, alpha motor neurons, central canal, white matter, gray matter, cerebellum and cerebrum, as well as peripheral nerves in cross- and longitudinal-sections. As before, you are responsible for knowing these structures, in addition to the pathologic material in the accompanying lab protocol.
The normal anatomy section has a quiz to assess your learning.
LEARNING OBJECTIVES
1. Be able to recognize histologically, when given a compatible clinical vignette, each of the following brain tumors: High grade astrocytoma (Glioblastoma); ependymoma; oligodendroglioma; medulloblastoma; meningioma; metastatic small cell carcinoma
2. Describe the typical CNS location and prognosis for each the brain tumors listed above.
3. Name the presumed cell of origin for each of the brain tumors listed above.
Additional images can be found on
REQUIRED READING
Robbins and Cotran, 9th Edition:
SUPPLEMENTAL MATERIALS
The NEW ENGLAND JOURNAL of MEDICINE
ADDITIONAL RESOURCES

(VPN). We estimate, in the first few years, that we probably spent close to $500,000 on equipment, plus hundreds of faculty hours scanning slides, compiling patient histories, writing slide descriptions, and writing case study questions.

A school's investment (now, over a decade later) would require much less capital. Scanners have dropped in price, plus, there is an abundance of already scanned material available, either for free, or for purchase, from many vendors (including us). With a fast internet connection, serving up the virtual slides from the cloud is relatively simple, although with a slow connection (<10 Mb/Sec), having a locally mirrored version of the virtual slides probably makes more sense. Our current collect comprises about 500 slides, both normal and pathologic, and consumes almost 2 Terabytes of disk space. Our collaborative notebooks run on Office 365®, hosted in the cloud by Microsoft, on their cloud drive product called Microsoft OneDrive®. Local, private clouds could be constructed for schools with poor internet access, in countries outside the United States.

REFERENCES

Department of Radiology, University of Washington. (n.d.). *General principles: The universal differential diagnosis*. Retrieved from http://www.rad.washington.edu/academics/academic-sections/msk/teaching-materials/online-musculoskeletal-radiology-book/general-principles

Digital Pathology. (n.d.). Leica Biosystems. Aperio, ePathology Solutions. Available at: http://www.leicabiosystems.com/digital-pathology/

Engels, P. T., & de Gara, C. (2010). Learning styles of medical students, general surgery residents, and general surgeons: Implications for surgical education. *BMC Medical Education*, *10*(51). doi:10.1186/1472-6920-10-51 PMID:20591159

Englander, R., & Carraccio, C. (2014). Domain of competence: Medical knowledge. *Academic Pediatrics*, *14*(Suppl. 2), 536–537. doi:10.1016/j.acap.2013.10.006 PMID:24602633

Enosis Group. (2012). *Facilitated discovery. Eliciting and amplifying team brilliance*. Retrieved from http://www.facilitateddiscovery.com/

Gurpinar, E., Bati, H., & Tetik, C. (2011). Learning styles of medical students change in relation to time. *Advances in Physiology Education*, *35*(3), 307–311. doi:10.1152/advan.00047.2011 PMID:21908841

Karr, M., Fishback, J. L., & Klein, R. M. (2007). *Where did I put my microscope? Virtual microscopy*. Workshop presented at Slice of Life Conference, New Orleans, LA. Abstract retrieved from http://slice.utah.edu/2007/schedule/documents/07MichaelKarr1.pdf

Kolb, A. Y., & Kolb, D. A. (2013). *The Kolb learning style inventory 4.0: A comprehensive guide to the theory, psychometrics, research and validity and educational applications*. Retrieved from https://learningfromexperience.com/downloads/research-library/the-kolb-learning-style-inventory-4-0.pdf

Marshak, D. W., Oakes, J., Hsieh, P. H., Chuang, A. Z., & Cleary, L. J. (2015). Outcomes of a rotational dissection system in gross anatomy. *Anatomical Sciences Education*, *8*(5), 438–444. doi:10.1002/ase.1497 PMID:25358463

Martin, C. R. (1997). *Looking at type: The fundamentals*. Gainesville, FL: Center for Applications of Psychological Type.

Microsoft 365. (2014, October 12). *One Class Notebook*. Retrieved from https://www.microsoft.com/en-us/microsoft-365/blog/2014/10/07/introducing-onenote-class-notebooks-flexible-digital-framework-teaching-learning/

Microsoft Class Notebook Add-In. (n.d.). Available at: https://download.microsoft.com/download/5/0/0/500EF2CA-5192-49F2-8E0C-BDEB2D530788/ClassNotebook.Setup.exe

Microsoft Office 365. (n.d.). Available at: https://go.microsoft.com/fwlink/p/?LinkID=787538

Pelley, J. (2018). *The success types style type indicator*. John W. Pelley. Retrieved from https://www.ttuhsc.edu/medicine/medical-education/success-types/lsti.aspx

Pelley, J. W., & Dalley, B. K. (2008). *Success types in medical education: A program for improving academic performance version 1.1*. Retrieved from https://www.ttuhsc.edu/medicine/medical-education/success-types/documents/stsinmeded.pdf

Pramas, T. J., Berres, A., Bjorklund, S. L., & Ellison, S. J. (2014). Using technology to facilitate production of e-discovery. *William Mitchell Law Review*, *40*, 2–8. Retrieved from http://open.mitchellhamline.edu/wmlr/vol40/iss2/8

Townsend, D. (2009). *Cadaver dissection teams at Kansas State University*. Retrieved from https://www.k-state.edu/ksuhonors/courses/BIOL340-Sp10.htm

Wiggins, G. (2007, November 15). What is an essential question? *Big Ideas*. Retrieved from http://www.authenticeducation.org/ae_bigideas/article.lasso?artid=53

Wilson, A. B., Taylor, M. A., Klein, B. A., Sugrue, M. K., Whipple, E. C., & Brokaw, J. J. (2016). Meta-analysis and review of learner performance and preference: Virtual versus optical microscopy. *Medical Education*, *50*(4), 428–440. doi:10.1111/medu.12944 PMID:26995482

Wilson, L. O. (2014). *What are essential questions?* Retrieved from https://thesecondprinciple.com/teaching-essentials/essential-questions/

APPENDIX A

Example Histopathology Laboratory Protocol, With Hyperlinks

Glioblastoma

Astrocytoma, Grade IV

History of the Present Illness

This 58-year-old woman with a past medical history only of systemic hypertension presented with a 6-week history of worsening confusion, difficulty walking, and increased frequency of falls. In the 2 weeks preceding admission to the hospital, she was noted to have hallucinations, paranoia, and socially inappropriate behavior. She also was experiencing headache, nausea, and vomiting.

Physical Examination

On examination, she is alert, but confused. Her gait is wide based, and she requires assistance to walk. Otherwise, she has grossly intact cranial nerves, motor, and sensory neurologic examinations.

Hospital Course

The patient had a stereotactic needle biopsy, but died suddenly 3 days post-operatively. A post-mortem examination was performed, upon request of the family.

Imaging Studies

MRI images of the brain demonstrated an extensive enhancing area of tissue within the splenium of the corpus callosum, crossing the midline, and extending into the bilateral lateral ventricles to the frontal horns, right posterior horn, and third ventricle. The enhancing tissue extends through the septum pellucidum to the supracellar cistern and involves the genu of the corpus callosum. An additional lesion was noted in the right thalamus, and several others are scattered throughout the white matter adjacent to the lateral ventricles.

Figure 3. MRI images of the brain

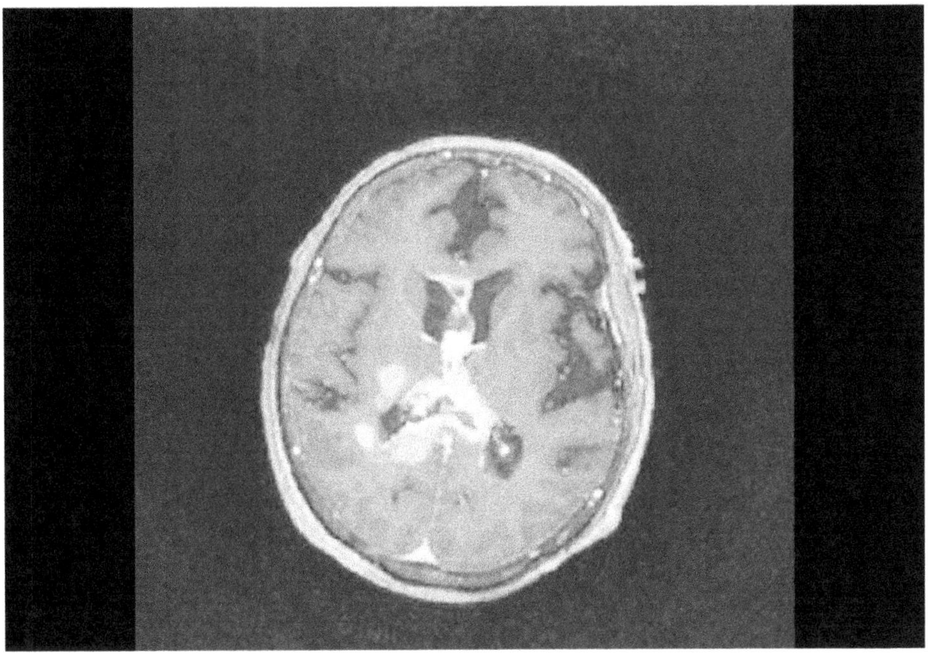

Histopathology

Brain, H&E, Glioblastoma, 1x. Glioblastomas are synonymous with high grade astrocytomas (Grade IV of IV astrocytomas). They are often quite large at discovery, and may cross the midline (so-called "Butterfly" glioblastomas). They are very fast-growing tumors, with striking cellularity. The histologic hallmark of glioblastoma, therefore, is *marked cellular pleomorphism* (often with *abundant mitotic figures* and *prominent necrosis* [black arrows]), and *microvascular proliferation*.

Brain, H&E, Glioblastoma, 20x. Cells on the left side of the photomicrograph still have distinct nuclei and cytoplasm, whereas on the right side the nuclei are gone, and only amorphous, necrotic debris remain.

Brain, H&E, Glioblastoma, 40x. Large atypical cells are common, with abundant pink cytoplasm (so-called "gemistocytic" astrocytes, black arrows). Glioblastomas are derived from astrocytes, and as such, are usually positive for the glial cell marker GFAP (glial fibrillary acidic protein).

Figure 4. Brain, H&E, glioblastoma, 1x

Virtual Slide: ***Glioblastoma.svs***	Watch Slide Tour

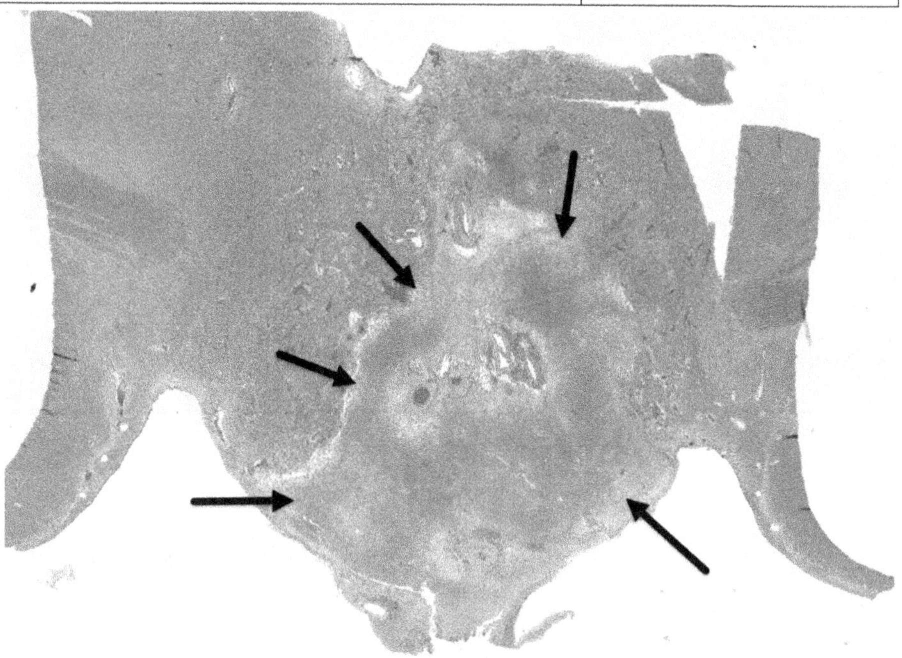

Figure 5. Brain, H&E, glioblastoma, 20x

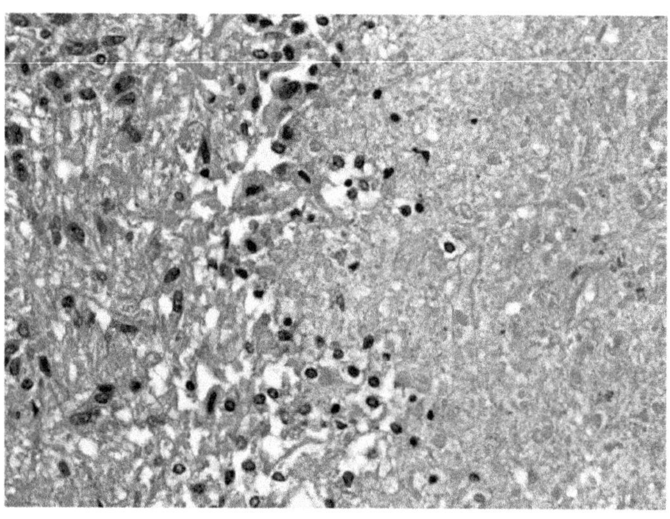

Figure 6. Brain, H&E, glioblastoma, 40x

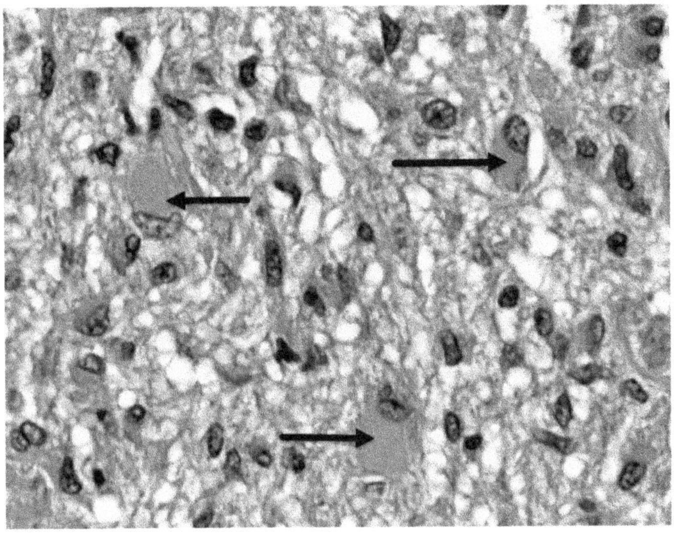

Table 3.

ESSENTIAL QUESTIONS WHAT MUST BE KNOWN (WMBK) 1.**What is the current treatment(s) for glioblastoma?** 2.**What is the clinical prognosis (5-year disease-free survival) for glioblastoma?** 3.**What are the molecular genetic alterations associated with low grade and high grade astrocytomas?**
ESSENTIAL CONCEPTS WHAT MUST BE UNDERSTOOD (WMBU) **4.The slide tour shows you some areas that quite far away from the main necrotic mass, yet still have atypical cells. What does this histologic feature tell you about the surgical resectability and ultimate prognosis of the tumor?**

APPENDIX B

Myers-Briggs. Information available at:
https://www.myersbriggs.org/my-mbti-personality-type/mbti-basics/home.htm?bhcp=1

APPENDIX C

Vendor Contacts

Digital Pathology: Leica Biosystems. Aperio, ePathology Solutions. Information available at: http://www.leicabiosystems.com/digital-pathology/

Microsoft Office 365, available download at: https://go.microsoft.com/fwlink/p/?LinkID=787538

Microsoft Class Notebook add-in. Available for download at: https://download.microsoft.com/download/5/0/0/500EF2CA-5192-49F2-8E0C-BDEB2D530788/ClassNotebook.Setup.exe

Chapter 11
Technological and Ethical Challenges of Online Education:
Adapting Medical Education to Digital Platforms

Lauren Haar
Loyola University Chicago, USA

Simon Kaja
Loyola University Chicago, USA

ABSTRACT

The impact of technology can be felt throughout the medical education continuum. From online learning environments in blended learning approaches to exclusively providing the preclinical curriculum online, there is a growing need to optimize the way that technology supports self-directed learning in the next generation of medical professionals. In this chapter, the authors address issues of best practice surrounding the development of virtual content for medical education. The information presented will be integral for medical education professionals, basic science/clinical faculty, and educational assessment specialists with an interest in the use of technology for contemporary medical education. The goal is to offer an overview of the theory and ethics behind adopting an online strategy for medical education. An emphasis is placed on developing best practices for presenting content, a comparison of blended and online-only approaches, and the ethical considerations necessary for the successful training of medical professionals online.

DOI: 10.4018/978-1-5225-6289-4.ch011

INTRODUCTION

In recent years, we have seen an explosion of technological advances that have transformed the way we teach, study and learn. The worldwide web now provides virtually instant and universal access to specialized information that used to be available only in university and public libraries. Modern communication tools furthermore provide global access to expert content and led to the implementation of distance and online learning in specialties that used to entirely rely on classroom teaching, such as medical and biomedical education. At the same time, the student body engaging in higher education has diversified, partly due to efforts in decreasing socioeconomic barriers to higher education and partly due to the opportunities of online learning.

Contemporary medical education has endorsed the use of online learning environments (OLE; also referred to as virtual learning environments, VLE) that provide an ever-expanding volume of curated educational content. Together with a trend toward instructional strategies that foster active learning to both tackle the exponential increase in medical knowledge and adapt to learners that have been described as "digital natives", educators face unprecedented challenges. These include implementation of curricula that combine traditional pedagogic approaches and learning microenvironments with OLEs, online content, and flipped classroom approaches.

In this chapter, we will address the opportunities and challenges associated with online education and learning, discuss the obstacles of transitioning from a traditional didactic model to online education, and offer an analysis of the ethical implications of digital learning and education.

DEFINING BEST PRACTICES IN MEDICAL EDUCATION

The increase in OLEs and online education has emphasized a need for devising novel metrics for learning outcomes and assessing whether the inclusion of OLEs and online classes, in fact, increases student achievements. Existing efforts have often been strongly biased by individuals' preconceptions on the effectiveness of OLEs. For example, in a study surveying the opinions of almost 3,000 chief academic officers of colleges, there was a strong positive association between the belief that students learn more in online classes and the extent of which the college was committed to online learning (Allen & Seaman, 2013).

Some of the earliest research on the topic of distance learning pointed out the challenges of accurately assessing educational outcomes. While most studies utilize three metrics to assess effectiveness, i.e. student grades, attitudes and overall student satisfaction, it is important to be aware of the inherent shortcomings of such research (Phipps & Merisotis, 1999; Moore & Thompson, 1990; Ni, 2013). Weak experimental designs, inappropriate statistics, lack of randomization, and an ensuing inability to distinguish cause and effect remain flaws of many studies that have been published on the assessment of online learning effectiveness (Phipps and Merisotis, 1999; McWilliam & Lee, 2006; Ni, 2013).

Classroom delivery has been directly compared to online delivery in the health professions and life sciences literature, specifically for pharmacy, nursing, paramedic, dental hygiene students, and for learners enrolled in a continuing medical education course (Rochester et al., 2008; Levett-Jones 2005; Buckley, 2003; Gallagher et al., 2005; Ryan et al., 2007; Alsharif et al. 2005; Faulkner et al 2005; Moazami et al., 2014; Porter et al., 2014). For example, in one recent study, no difference in student performance between traditional classroom learning and an online course was identified for an elective course on immunization in the University of Wisconsin School of Pharmacy Pharm.D. curriculum (Porter, Pitterle & Hayney, 2014). Notably, there is a paucity of studies making an effort to employ rigorous and unbiased experimental design to quantify the effectiveness of OLEs, active learning strategies, and flipped classrooms for the medical school curriculum. We speculate that the reason for such paucity is the evolving yet regulated nature of the medical school curriculum in the US. Over the past 30 years, we have seen a transition from traditional classroom learning, to "problem-based learning" (PBL), the incorporation of vertically integrated curricula, and the integration of a "blended learning" pedagogical approach (Brauer & Ferguson, 2015; Hartling et al., 2010). Blended learning refers to a combination of traditional and online learning approaches. In their pioneering article on the blended educational model, Garrison & Kanuka (2004) presented their case that integration of "asynchronous Internet communication technology" into live teaching serves to "facilitate a simultaneous independent and collaborative learning experience". A 2010 meta-analysis and review of online learning studies carefully conducted by the United States Department of Education provided support for blended learning strategies for a wide range of learners and learning environments.

Specifically, the study concluded, "despite what appears to be strong support for blended learning applications, the studies in this meta-analysis do not demonstrate that online learning is superior as a *medium*. [...] It was the *combination* of elements in the treatment conditions [...] that produced the observed learning advantages. At the same time, one should note that online learning is much more conducive to the expansion of learning time than is face-to-face instruction." (p. xviii)

Based on these findings, we have to identify the current best practices in medical education before making recommendations for educators. "Best practices" are defined as "procedures that have been shown by research and experience to produce optimal results and that are established or proposed as a standard suitable for widespread adoption".

Current best practice in medical education is based partly on the concept of andragogy as described by Knowles (1980). The term andragogy (*andra* – meaning "man"; agogos – meaning "learning") was initially used by Alexander Kapp in the 1830s to describe the educational theory of the Greek philosopher Plato. Theories of andragogy, albeit pursued in the 20th century by various individuals, remained outside of the mainstream of education research and philosophy until Malcolm Knowles further elaborated the concept (Knowles, 1980). His theory assumes that adults and adult learners (a) are independent and self-directing, (b) have experience, (c) integrate learning to the demand of their everyday life, (d) are more interested in immediate problem-centered approaches, and (e) are self-motivated.

In his review of learning theories, Abela (2009) raised two important criticisms on the concept of andragogy. Specifically, he noted the absence of "reflection" in Knowles' definition of adult learning. Reflection is not only an important difference between pedagogy and andragogy, but should also be considered an important contributing factor to the trait of self-motivation, which Knowles ascribes to adult learners. The importance of reflection is evident from David Kolb's learning theory in which he divided learning into four categories that can be described as diverging and assimilating (reflective observation) and converging and accommodating (active experimentation) (Kolb, 1984). The second omission is acknowledging the contribution of extrinsic motivation (Abela, 2009). Knowles assumes that all learners are equally intrinsically motivated. However, as educators we all are well aware that this is not the case: not only are there different learner styles, but motivation of learners is significantly affected by the learning environment (Sogunro, 2015), the mutual respect between teacher and learner (Brookfield, 2006), as well as exogenous factors, such as the learners' socioeconomic status or personal environment. This necessitates the "matching" of teaching styles to learner preferences (Grow, 1991; Newman & Peile, 2002).

How does this affect best practices and the role of the educator and the incorporation of OLEs into the medical curriculum? In the words of Gerald Grow (1991), "the teacher's purpose is to match the learner's stage of self-direction and prepare the learner to advance to higher stages". Grow defines these learner stages as "dependent", "interested", "involved", and "self-directed", each requiring a different pedagogical or andragogical approach. As such, it is critical that we identify our role as educators as one that is guided by our learners, in order to help them achieve greater degrees of self-directed learning. One useful tool for educators to guide learners is Bloom's taxonomy of learning (Bloom et al., 1956; Krathwohl, 2002). Bloom classified educational learning objectives into levels of complexity and specificity in three separate domains: cognitive, affective, and sensory. In the cognitive domain, these domains were categorized into six levels of objectives, i.e. Remember, Understand, Apply, Analyze, Evaluate, and Create. Bloom's taxonomy provides a basis for many teaching philosophies, including PBL (Krathwohl, 2002). In a blended classroom, application of Bloom's taxonomy can help motivate learners to utilize online resources, especially information searching (Jansen, Booth, & Smith, 2009).

In most medical school curricula, a blended approach that incorporates traditional classroom teaching, self-directed learning in small-group sessions and OLEs, and open discussions has been implemented to foster self-directed learning and, thereby, educate our future physicians. While this model certainly is not a "one size fits all", it does accommodate for learners in different stages. In conclusion, current best practices in medical education rely substantially on the principles of andragogy and blended learning approaches to enhance self-directed learning.

TRANSITIONING TO "ONLINE ONLY" EDUCATION

In the previous section, we have discussed how current best practices in medical education employ a blended learning approach that relies both on a physical face-to –face interaction in classrooms as small group sessions, and an OLE. Both approaches have been supported by learning philosophies and provide a rationale for use of both platforms as 'best practice'. However, as programs transition away from traditional classroom environments, and aim to exclusively provide preclinical basic science education through OLEs that enable self-directed learning, educators are now facing new challenges in preparing high-quality content suitable to meet that goal. The biggest difference between blended learning approaches and online-only learning is the lack of any physical interaction between educators and learners. Yet, blended learning, combining traditional strategies with online learning have been found to be the most effective approach to self-directed education. This requires educators to carefully devise novel strategies for online learning that can expand the learning microenvironments usually associated with OLEs to include those that closely mimic the unique aspects of face-to-face interaction.

Such strategies often rely on the concept of self-efficacy, as introduced by Professor Albert Bandura (1997). Self-efficacy refers to the personal judgment or perception of "how well one can execute courses of action required to deal with prospective situations" (Bandura, 1982, p. 122). In the context of learning, greater degrees of self-efficiency are positively associated with better learning outcomes and learner satisfaction (Tsai, Alqurashi). According to Bandura's theory, a learner's self-efficacy depends on four sources of information, i.e. (a) enactive attainment, (b) vicarious experience, (c) social persuasion, and (d) psychological states. Enactive attainment refers to an individual's experience of mastery and accomplishment, which is considered the primary factor in determining self-efficacy. The idea is that an individual's success can increase self-efficacy, and failure can attribute to decreasing it. This appears to be particularly effective in learners with low confidence in self or educational subject. Social (or verbal) persuasion generally contributes to increases or decreases in self-efficacy by encouragement or discouragement (respectively). While positive encouragement appears to have a lesser effect on self-efficacy than discouragement, it is this component of the learner-educator interaction that often significantly contributes to learner success in a traditional or blended classroom setting that requires an alternative approach in online-only courses. Lastly, physiological factors are considered factors critical for self-efficacy. However, rather than directly altering self-efficacy, it is the individual's perception and interpretation of physiological factors, such as stress, anxiety or nervousness, that will increase or decrease self-efficacy.

How do we utilize these theoretical concepts to increase self-efficacy in online-only learning? The first step is the acknowledgement that OLEs require an alternative andragogical approach than traditional face-to-face approaches, i.e. one that creates the positive reinforcement necessary to support self-efficacy. Fostering self-efficacy in an OLE structure can be accomplished through the generation of specific educational microenvironments that mimic the four sources of information that Bandura defined. For example, testimonials from previous students, video clips of interviews with recent graduates, statistics on USMLE Step I/II scores or the rate of successful placement into competitive residencies all can be utilized to model vicarious experience, which is typically achieved by informal discussions among peers in traditional learning settings or from information outside the OLEs. Implementation of a social persuasion component can be achieved by integration of instant messaging and social media components, or even live discussion sessions among learners in the OLE (Figure 1). Ultimately, we have to realize that a transition from blended learning to online-only approaches results in a transformed role of the educator away from being a motivator and provider of content to designer of learning microenvironments that appeal to digital natives and foster self-efficacy of learning.

A variety of tools exist that enable the construction of unique microenvironments that enhance self-efficacy in online learning and encourage interaction with teachers and educators. These tools can range from asynchronous discussion, which fosters conversation through logged posts on a forum, with educator feedback on ideas and

Figure 1.

Source of information	Traditional learning	Online-only learning
Attainment	Tests Exams Class participation	Online quizzes Simulations within and outside OLE
Modeling	Interaction with peers inside and outside the classroom	Testimonials Online chat rooms Example answers
Persuasion	Interaction with teachers and educators	Asynchronous discussion Digital conferencing Broadcast lectures
Physiological factors	Test and exam anxiety	Perceived anonymity in OLEs Anxiety due to lack of modeling

topics to broadcasting lectures to a fixed audience. Digital medium allow for a broad range of interactions on these mediums, and often digital preservation of complex idea formation can inform students and help them to moderate their own learning progression relative to those of their peers. Interaction between educators and learners in the arena of online only learning is not limited to a geographical location, and therefore may encompass a more flexible timetable for interaction. It also means that interactions can be paced at learner-determined intervals. To gauge this interaction a host of online tools are being developed to quantify learning and education in online settings. Adaptive Exams can offer new ways to challenge learners to rely on new knowledge and not a series of previously released exam content. Online problem sets offer a way to reward critical thinking and reasoning processes as well as final consolidation of knowledge. These can be released in a digital platform to compare or inspire self-directed learning in individuals who may be disengaging in an educational setting. The genesis of new tools for this medium is ongoing. With an increase in understanding of how online only learners interact with new digital platforms, and more consolidated research on effective microenvironments that foster learning in medical education, a more cohesive OLE can be maintained. It is then the goal of the instructor to observe the interaction of students in these new environments, and ensure that their progression is continuous.

ETHICAL CONSIDERATIONS FOR THE TRANSITION TO OLES

As the OLEs we build into our medical education continue to expand, so too do the ethical considerations for how we implement this technology. As the medical classroom shifts to digital content, it must maintain the same integrity and value based learning that exist in current classroom models. Specifically, for medical education, the implementation of content must serve to support the training obligations of the medical workforce. Though medical training has consistently shifted focus through history, the current system is viewed as a professional education, the goals of which are to master both theory and knowledge in the practice of medicine (Cooke, Irby, Sulivan & Ludmerer, 2006). The final goal of the instructor is not only to pass on the knowledge of the profession but also the skills and values of the medical community so that trainees can better prepare for practicing in their discipline (Collins, Brown & Neuman 1989; Cooke, Irby, Sulivan & Ludmerer, 2006; Maudsley & Strivens, 2000) The culmination of this learning is tested in board examinations, which are the foundation for residency and practice. The ethics of online course design are largely the same across many educational disciplines. The additional burden in medical education comes with the understanding that the foundational principles taught through most preclinical coursework will be the basis for medical practice. The topics of accountability, rigor and intellectual integrity are increasingly important ethical considerations for online course design that places a premium on not only transferring knowledge, but also values and skills to the learner (Figure 2).

Figure 2.

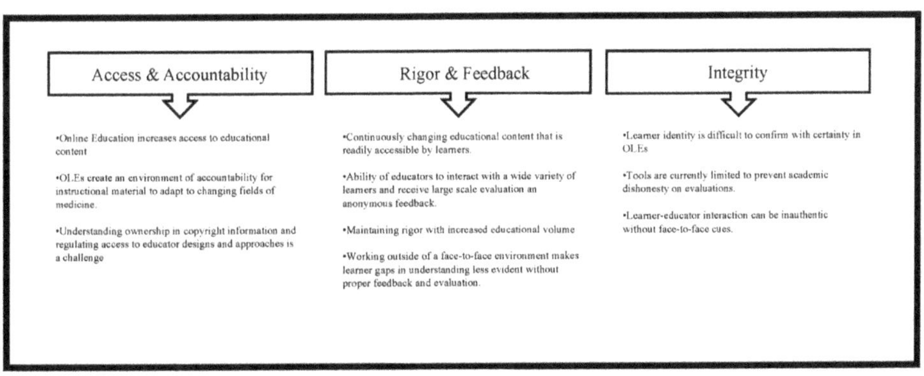

ACCESS AND ACCOUNTABILITY

The key difference between online and in person learning is physical presence. This makes the main challenge in transitioning to online learning, recapitulating the presence in a meaningful way through a digital medium. The clearest advantage to online learning is the increase in educational access that it offers. Eliminating physical boundaries of a classroom, constraints such as schedule, pace and timing also lessen. OLEs are customizable to each individual experience, and the use of learning microenvironments allows for learners to support their individual learning experience. It has been suggested that improvement in medical education could be possible by embracing a learning strategy that is self-paced and mastery based (Prober & Heath, 2012), both of which are supported in the OLE. There also exists it creates the possibility of expanding enrollment to match demand for physicians in areas without a local medical center. It is important that with this enrollment expansion there is also an increase in accountability for both the learning environment, and to the student who is doing the learning.

By nature, medical education is an immersive experience. It carries with it several conditions that may limit the ability of individuals to achieve a medical education. A few of these constraints include the volume of information, the time commitment to practice learned skills, and the pacing of course material by instructors. Designing online courses has great potential for expanding the student population that can complete medical training. Students who may have previously been unable to manage a classroom and transit would now be able to access course curriculum and examinations. Students for whom financing an education would have been preventative to achieving a medical degree, or who may have alternate family commitments that prevent them from traveling to a medical education center may also achieve work life balance. Furthermore, medical education would become attainable in parts of the world where no major medical center exists. At later stages of matriculation, the challenge of on site education may again be relevant, but early stages that require lecture based learning and traditional didactic education may be more able to reach a broad audience.

Another advantage of a broad audience is broad feedback. Online learning offers an easy way to ensure that coursework is communicated. In medical education, this is a distinct advantage. It offers a great benefit in adapting educational standards to board skills, or to advancing new and more adaptive forms of learning. Examples of this can be seen as new fields of medicine are beginning to take shape in a digital age. The advent of genomics and personalized medicines, and all of the rules and requirements that they carry will be a challenge for medical education in the coming decades. Online education also offers students the ability to interact on an online platform effectively. They must communicate with each other and with instructors during their education, and in doing so they develop skills that may assist them in specialties that may also require this type of communication. The expanse of online education can carry with it an ability to adapt and change outside an institutional level. Each of these advances should motivate medical educators to invest in building course curriculum online. Though, there are some considerations that should be taken to maintain accountability in education when in person content is not being presented, and when the audience for this content is expanded.

The challenges of facing a broad audience exist in understanding how course content is disseminated and what claim the author of that content may have to its use. Educational environments face a particular challenge in the application of copyright to course design. Instructors create content based on their practice and experience, as such it is unique to their experience as well as their discipline. As the online community changes the range of reach from a classroom to the Internet, there is more of a risk of this information being co-opted for other use. This presents several issues in medical education. First, because of the nature of change in medical education, disseminating information that is not up to date may impact a student's ability to matriculate or to function in a clinical capacity. Second, the ownership of information in the student/instructor relationship becomes unclear with broad distribution. Institutional structures that balance these two factors are critical for the ethical implementation of medical education. Without safeguards in place both sides are at risk.

RIGOR AND FEEDBACK

Rigor and Feedback are two closely related sides of the learning spectrum. Rigor addresses the quality and accuracy of the course content, as well as the application of the learning environment to the students enrolled in the course. These factors create an educational standard that must be met in order to say a student has learned enough to matriculate. Feedback largely refers to the reporting of obtained information for the purpose of learning or refining a course. This could encompass the student opinion of a particular course section and it's learning objectives or it could be viewed more as instructor commentary on student learning in the online platform. Feedback is useful in interpreting the level of rigor of the coursework. Each of these concepts raises specific challenges in the online education world.

Online learning makes continuous education a reality. It allows students to access information in real time as they need it or as it fits into their learning plan. A drawback of this is that the content of this medical information must be monitored, and the identity of the students accessing it must be confirmed. Many critics have cautioned of the decline in rigor of online education (Cole, Shelley & Swartz, 2014).

They offer that without direct feedback from an in person-learning environment, it may be difficult to gage learning. The digital environment offers several advantages in providing feedback for instructors. First, the anonymity of each student and the lack of a direct contact on a physical campus can make criticism and feedback of teaching more quantitative. Instructors can gage the efficacy of responses through digital learning, or log conversation in asynchronous forum environments that better describe a student's interaction with literature or content material, for example. Without the physical restraint of a classroom, a larger audience can be reached for feedback on learning materials. With more voices in the conversation, better design can be executed to support learning, and a clearer picture of areas of strength or improvement can be built around course material. They can also contribute content to online microenvironments that could be used by learners to improve self-efficacy.

The key drawback to a complete change to a digital medium is the learning curve required to make it an effective tool. Because of this it is imperative that instructors work to modify their online instruction so they foster communication in their course and incentivize students to engage with online course platforms. Until recently, in person education was the format for most primary education. While increasingly, medical education will be pursued by 'digital natives', it is important to understand the bias that accompanies those who may not fit into this distinction. Adopting an online curriculum means some students will be interacting online for the first time in an educational setting. Because of this, it may be difficult to use traditional methods of understanding how much retention of course content a student is capable of. As the online classroom takes independent learning to a new level, it may be difficult to understand how much understanding a student has, even if they complete the required milestones of a course.

The same can be true of in person education. But, the model for online learning more drastically divides instructor and student for problem solving activities by placing them in different physical locations. Where before an instructor could easily modify instruction to address a student who is clearly losing attention or struggling visibly with material, online instruction may create more of a vacuum for student experience, or a curated experience that the student self selects. Course design strategies that implement feedback between the student and the instructor are imperative for understanding these weaknesses. In medical education, where the primary goals are to gain broad knowledge of physiological systems as well as the skills necessary to practice medicine, this feedback could be organized in a number of course dependent ways. Studies have indicated that online learning is only useful when it is paired with interactive learning (Castaño-Muñoz, Duart, & Sancho-Vinuesa, 2014). Tools like asynchronous conversation and digital communication platforms are decreasing the burden of this style of learning, and should be considered by instructors for the promotion of educational goals. Instructors moving to this format have a duty to students to modify their teaching so that student learning is accurately quantified. The goal of online education remains the same as the in person classroom, and as such instructors should work to overcome any barriers that their online platform presents to students, so they can more adequately determine the medical knowledge and course objectives that their students have met.

INTEGRITY

Perhaps the most concerning element of expanding medical education to online platforms is the issue of integrity. More specifically, it is imperative to make sure that each student is completing their own educational training. The competitive nature of medical education, and the emphasis on rank for matriculation and matching makes the ability to measure outcomes of specific individuals a particularly important task. Without a physical presence it is difficult to determine if outside sources (such as the internet, textbooks, or other individuals) are being used to complete assessments and evaluations. Traditionally, examinations for medical training have been organized as a multiple-choice answer system. These can be difficult to administer in an online setting, and some restructuring may be required until more adequate tools are built for identifying individuals as they complete their work.

With decreasing presence-based learning, comes many advantages in influencing a broader audience and allowing students to more appropriately moderate their own learning environment and information intake. Distance also increases the challenge of accountability and isolation. In a changing landscape it is important to consider the implications of both sides of the coin and to continue to develop feedback based assessment that enhances the professional development both of instructors seeking to present course material and students seeking to obtain and utilize this information. Ultimately, it is impossible to ensure that all participants in academic training uphold academic integrity. A study conducted on health science education students indicated that simply defining academic integrity in an online environment and emphasizing professional behavior expectations greatly improved conduct in a blended learning environment (Azulay, Chertok, Barnes & Gilleland, 2014). Online education will develop and grow it's capacity to regulate this over time, much as in person education has shown itself how to. As that development takes place, it is important for instructors to consider the purpose of the content, and be innovative in their approach to evaluating student knowledge as they design online courses, as well as stating their expectations for professional conduct and integrity clearly.

CONCLUSION

In recent years, an explosion of technological advances has transformed the way we teach, study and learn. Notably, they have created the ability to access education completely independent of person-to-person instruction or the need for local expertise. As part of this development, we have seen a rise in OLEs and an associated growing need for new ways to quantify and assess the quality of education delivered via such platforms.

Contemporary medical education has encouraged the use of OLEs that provide an ever-expanding volume of curated educational content. However, we believe that the current environment is lacking in evidence-based best practice, and would benefit from the expansion of data-driven studies of online medical education. Current education approaches medical training through the principles of andragogy, assuming that learners are self-directed and not only able to adequately access digital learning platforms, but also to effectively utilize them for self-directed learning. The goal of an instructor, then, is to generate beneficial microenvironments in OLEs that enable learners to support their progress through the medical online curriculum. Successful utilization of these microenvironments will create quantifiable outcomes in student learning.

During the development of curriculum, educators must also consider the ethical implications of digital environments. For educators in the health sciences and medical disciplines, the implementation of content still serves the purpose of supporting the training obligations of a medical workforce. While OLEs provide expanded access to medical education, they must maintain the same accountability for precision and educational quality as is maintained in face-to-face classroom environments. Instructors must ensure that the content they provide adequately reflects a vastly changing field, and must be aware of the way in which the content they generate is disseminated. Through a system of feedback between learners and instructors, the classroom should continue to evolve microenvironments that support student efficacy as well as challenge the learners to expand their medical understanding. Finally, the problem of academic integrity must be managed through the development of novel platforms of learning that confirm identity and ensure individual work from each learner participating in the course.

The digital age of education brings with it a great opportunity to transform the way in which we approach medical education. It is important to continue to consider these topics as we progress further from the genesis of distance education, and form new quantitative means to understand how to best interact with new OLEs that make available an ever-expanding volume of curated educational content. The burden for instruction is now to create instructional strategies that foster active and self-directed learning to both tackle the exponential increase in medical knowledge and adapt to learners that have been described as "digital natives". By better defining the relationship between learning and educating, and endorsing the opportunities technology provides, we can continue to tackle these challenges head on.

REFERENCES

Abela, J. (2009). Adult learning theories and medical education: A review. *Malta Medical Journal*, *21*(1), 11–18.

Albarrak, A. I. (2011). E-learning in Medical Education and Blended Learning Approach. In A. Méndez-Vilas (Ed.), Education in a technological world: communicating current and emerging research and technological efforts. Academic Press.

Allen, I. E., & Seaman, J. (2013). *Changing course: Ten years of tracking online education in the United States*. Babson Survey Research Group. Pearson Publishers and Sloan Foundation.

Alqurashi, E. (2016). Self-Efficacy In Online Learning Environments: A Literature Review. *Contemporary Issues in Education Research*, *9*(1), 45–52. doi:10.19030/cier.v9i1.9549

Alsharif, N. Z., Roche, V. F., Ogunbadeniyi, A. M., Chapman, R., & Bramble, J. D. (2005). Evaluation of performance and learning parity between campus-based and web-based medicinal chemistry courses. *American Journal of Pharmaceutical Education*, *69*(2), 33. doi:10.5688/aj690233

Azulay Chertok, I. R., Barnes, E. R., & Gilleland, D. (2014, October). Academic integrity in the online learning environment for health sciences students. *Nurse Education Today*, *34*(10), 1324–1329. doi:10.1016/j.nedt.2013.06.002 PMID:23870688

Bandura, A. (1982). Self-Efficacy Mechanism in Human Agency. *The American Psychologist*, *37*(2), 122–147. doi:10.1037/0003-066X.37.2.122

Bandura, A. (1997). *Self-efficacy: The exercise of control*. New York: W.H. Freeman.

Bloom, B. S., Engelhart, M. D., Furst, E. J., Hill, W. H., & Krathwohl, D. R. (1956). *Taxonomy of educational objectives: The classification of educational goals. Handbook I: Cognitive domain*. New York: David McKay Company.

Brauer, D. G., & Ferguson, K. J. (2015). The integrated curriculum in medical education: AMEE Guide No. 96. *Medical Teacher*, *37*(4), 312–322. doi:10.3109/0142159X.2014.970998 PMID:25319403

Brookfield, S. D. (1986). *Understanding and Facilitating Adult Learning*. Milton Keynes, UK: Open University Press.

Buckley, K. M. (2003). Evaluation of classroom-based, web-enhanced, and web-based distance learning nutrition courses for undergraduate nursing. *The Journal of Nursing Education*, *42*(8), 367–370. PMID:12938900

Castaño-Muñoz, J., Duart, J. M., & Sancho-Vinuesa, T. (2014). The Internet in face-to-face higher education: Can interactive learning improve academic achievement? *British Journal of Educational Technology*, *45*(1), 149–159. doi:10.1111/bjet.12007

Cole, M., Shelley, D., & Swartz, L. (2014). Online instruction, e-learning, and student satisfaction: A three year study. International Review of Research in Open and Distance Learning., 15(6). *International Review of Research in Open and Distance Learning*, *15*(6). doi:10.19173/irrodl.v15i6.1748

Collins, A., Brown, J. S., & Newman, S. E. (1989). Cognitive Apprenticeship: Teaching the Craft of Reading, Writing, and Mathematics. In L. B. Resnick (Ed.), *Knowing, learning and Instruction:Essays in honor of Robert Glaser* (pp. 453–494). Hillsdale, NJ: Lawrence Erlbaum Associates.

Cooke, M., Irby, D., Sullivan, W., & Ludmerer, K. (2006). American Medical Education 100 Years after the Flexner Report. *The New England Journal of Medicine*, *355*(13), 1339–1344. doi:10.1056/NEJMra055445 PMID:17005951

Faulkner, T. P., Christoff, J. J., Sweeney, M. A., & Oliver, N. (2005). Pilot study of a distance-learning methodology used on campus for first professional degree pharmacy students in an integrated therapeutics module. *American Journal of Pharmaceutical Education*, *69*(1), 7. doi:10.5688/aj690107

Gallagher, J. E., Dobrosielski-Vergona, K. A., Wingard, R. G., & Williams, T. M. (2005). Web-based vs. traditional classroom instruction in gerontology: A pilot study. *Journal of Dental Hygiene*, *79*(3). PMID:16197772

Garrison, D. R. & Kanuka, H. (2004). Blended learning: Uncovering its transformative potential in higher education. *Internet and Higher Education, 7*, 95–105.

Grow, G. O. (1991). Teaching learners to be self-directed. *Adult Education Quarterly*, *41*(3), 125–149. doi:10.1177/0001848191041003001

Hartling, L., Spooner, C., Tjosvold, L., & Oswald, A. (2010). Problem-based learning in pre-clinical medical education: 22 years of outcome research. *Medical Teacher*, *32*(1), 28–35. doi:10.3109/01421590903200789 PMID:20095771

Jansen, B. J., Booth, D., & Smith, B. (2009). Using the taxonomy of cognitive learning to model online searching. *Information Processing & Management*, *45*(6), 643–663. doi:10.1016/j.ipm.2009.05.004

Knowles, M. S. (1980). *The modern practice of adult education: From pedagogy to andragogy*. Chicago: Follett.

Kolb, D. A. (1984). *Experiential learning: experience as the source of learning and development*. Englewood Cliffs, NJ: Prentice Hall.

Krathwohl, D. (2002). A revision of Bloom's taxonomy: An overview. *Theory into Practice*, *41*(4), 212–218. doi:10.120715430421tip4104_2

Levett-Jones, T. L. (2005). Self-directed learning: Implications and limitations for undergraduate nursing education. *Nurse Education Today*, *25*(5), 363–368. doi:10.1016/j.nedt.2005.03.003 PMID:15894411

Maudsley G. & Strivens J. (2000) Promoting professional knowledge, experiential learning and critical thinking for medical students. *Med Edu, 34*(7), 535-44

McWilliam, E., & Lee, A. (2006). The problem of 'the problem with educational research'. *Australian Educational Researcher*, *33*(2), 43–60. doi:10.1007/BF03216833

Moazami, F., Bahrampour, E., Azar, M. R., Jahedi, F., & Moattari, M. (2014). Comparing two methods of education (virtual versus traditional) on learning of Iranian dental students: A post-test only design study. *BMC Medical Education*, *14*(1), 1. doi:10.1186/1472-6920-14-45 PMID:24597923

Moore, M. G., & Thompson, M. M. (1990). *The effects of distance learning: A summary of literature*. ERIC Document Reproduction Service No. ED 330 321.

Newman, P., & Peile, E. (2002). Valuing Learners' experience and supporting further growth: Educational models to help experienced adult learners in medicine. *British Medical Journal*, *325*(7357), 200–202. doi:10.1136/bmj.325.7357.200 PMID:12142310

Ni, A. Y. (2013). Comparing the Effectiveness of Classroom and Online Learning: Teaching Research Methods. *Journal of Public Affairs Education*, *19*(2), 199–215. doi:10.1080/15236803.2013.12001730

Phipps, R. A., & Merisotis, J. P. (1999). *What's the difference: A review of contemporary research on the effectiveness of distance learning in higher education*. Washington, DC: The Institute for Higher Education Policy.

Porter, A. L., Pitterle, M. E., & Hayney, M. S. (2014). Comparison of Online Versus Classroom Delivery of an Immunization Elective Course. *American Journal of Pharmaceutical Education*, *78*(5), 96. doi:10.5688/ajpe78596 PMID:24954936

Prober, C. G., & Heath, C. (2012, May 3). Lecture halls without lectures--a proposal for medical education. *The New England Journal of Medicine*, *366*(18), 1657–1659. doi:10.1056/NEJMp1202451 PMID:22551125

Rochester, C. D., & Pradel, F. (2008). Students' perceptions and satisfaction with a web-based human nutrition course. *American Journal of Pharmaceutical Education*, *72*(4), 91. doi:10.5688/aj720491 PMID:19002289

Ryan, G., Lyon, P., Kuma, K., Bell, J., Barnet, S., & Shaw, T. (2007). Online CME: An effective alternative to face-to-face delivery. *Medical Teacher*, *29*(8), e251–e257. doi:10.1080/01421590701551698 PMID:18236269

Sogunro, O. A. (2015). Motivating factors for adult learners in higher education. *International Journal of Higher Education*, *4*(1), 22–37.

Summers, J. J., Waigandt, A., & Whittaker, T. A. (2005). A comparison of student achievement and satisfaction in an online versusa traditional face-to-face statistics class. *Innovations in Higher Education.*, *29*(3), 233–250. doi:10.100710755-005-1938-x

Tsai, C.-C., Chuang, S.-C., Liang, J.-C., & Tsai, M.-J. (2011). Self-efficacy in Internet-based Learning Environments: A Literature Review. *Journal of Educational Technology & Society*, *14*(4), 222–240.

U.S. Department of Education, Office of Planning, Evaluation, and Policy Development. (2010). *Evaluation of Evidence-Based Practices in Online Learning: A Meta-Analysis and Review of Online Learning Studies*. Washington, DC: Author.

KEY TERMS AND DEFINITIONS

Andragogy: The method and practice of teaching adult learners.

Best Practices: Procedures that have been shown by research and experience to produce optimal results and that are established or proposed as a standard suitable for widespread adoption.

Blended Learning: A pedagogical/andragogical approach that refers to the combination of traditional and online learning approaches.

Online Microenvironments: The unique assembly of interactions that take place between course participants, or with course resources and tools, built in the virtual learning environment.

Problem-Based Learning: A learner-centered approach in which learners study a subject by working in groups to solve an open-ended problem.

Self-Directed Learning: Self-directed learning is an instructional strategy that places the responsibility for the learning progress on the learner.

Virtual Learning Environment (VLE)/Online Learning Environment (OLE): A digital platform for online learning often used in blended-learning approaches.

Compilation of References

Abela, J. (2009). Adult learning theories and medical education: A review. *Malta Medical Journal, 21*(1), 11–18.

Abrahamson, S., Denson, J. S., & Wolf, R. M. (1969). Effectiveness of a simulator in training anesthesiology residents. *Journal of Medical Education, 44*, 515–519. doi:10.1136/qhc.13.5.395 PMID:5789592

Agency for Healthcare Research and Quality. (2016). *The Six Domains of Health Care Quality*. Retrieved from https://www.ahrq.gov/professionals/quality-patient-safety/talkingquality/create/sixdomains.html

Al Habeeb, A., Evans, A., & Ghazarian, D. (2012). Virtual microscopy using whole-slide imaging as an enabler for teledermatopathology: A paired consultant validation study. *Journal of Pathology Informatics, 3*(1), 2. doi:10.4103/2153-3539.93399 PMID:22439122

Albarrak, A. I. (2011). E-learning in Medical Education and Blended Learning Approach. In A. Méndez-Vilas (Ed.), Education in a technological world: communicating current and emerging research and technological efforts. Academic Press.

AliveCor, Inc. (2017). *FDA Clears First Medical Device Accessory for Apple Watch®* [Press release]. Retrieved from https://www.alivecor.com/press/press_release/fda-clears-first-medical-device-for-apple-watch/

AliveCor® KardiaMobile EKG Monitor. (2018). *AliveCor*. Retrieved Sept. 12 2018 from www.alivecor.com/getkardiamobile/

Al-Janabi, S., Huisman, A., & Van Diest, P. J. (2012). Digital pathology: Current status and future perspectives. *Histopathology, 61*(1), 1–9. doi:10.1111/j.1365-2559.2011.03814.x PMID:21477260

Allen Interactions. (2017). *Agile eLearning Development with SAM*. Retrieved from http://www.alleninteractions.com/sam-process

Allen, M., Dirksen, J., Quinn, C., & Thalheimer, W. (2014). *The serious elearning manifesto*. Retrieved from http://elearningmanifesto.org

Allen, I. E., & Seaman, J. (2013). *Changing course: Ten years of tracking online education in the United States*. Babson Survey Research Group. Pearson Publishers and Sloan Foundation.

Alotaibi, O., & ALQahtani, D. (2016). Measuring dental students' preference: A comparison of light microscopy and virtual microscopy as teaching tools in oral histology and pathology. *The Saudi Dental Journal*, *28*(4), 169–173. doi:10.1016/j.sdentj.2015.11.002 PMID:27872547

Alqurashi, E. (2016). Self-Efficacy In Online Learning Environments: A Literature Review. *Contemporary Issues in Education Research*, *9*(1), 45–52. doi:10.19030/cier.v9i1.9549

Alsharif, N. Z., Roche, V. F., Ogunbadeniyi, A. M., Chapman, R., & Bramble, J. D. (2005). Evaluation of performance and learning parity between campus-based and web-based medicinal chemistry courses. *American Journal of Pharmaceutical Education*, *69*(2), 33. doi:10.5688/aj690233

American Board of Dermatology. (2017). *Certification examination details*. Retrieved from https://www.abderm.org/residents-and-fellows/primary-certification-examination/certification-examination-details.aspx

Andrews, R., Mehta, N., Maypole, J., & Martin, S. A. (2017). Staying afloat in a sea of information: Point-of-care resources. *Cleveland Clinic Journal of Medicine*, *84*(3), 225–235. doi:10.3949/ccjm.84a.15087 PMID:28322678

Andrus, M. R., Forrester, J. B., Germain, K. E., & Eiland, L. S. (2015). Accuracy of pharmacy benefit manager medication formularies in an electronic health record system and the Epocrates mobile application. *Journal of Managed Care & Specialty Pharmacy*, *21*(4), 281–286. doi:10.18553/jmcp.2015.21.4.281 PMID:25803761

Apple Inc. (2017). *App Store shatters records on New Year's Day* [Press release]. Retrieved from https://www.apple.com/newsroom/2017/01/app-store-shatters-records-on-new-years-day/

Apple Inc. (2018). *Apple Watch Series 4: Beautifully redesigned with breakthrough communication, fitness and health capabilities* [Press release]. Retrieved from https://www.apple.com/newsroom/2018/09/redesigned-apple-watch-series-4-revolutionizes-communication-fitness-and-health/

Arnold, L. (2002). Assessing professional behavior: Yesterday, today, and tomorrow. *Academic Medicine, 77*(6), 502–515. doi:10.1097/00001888-200206000-00006 PMID:12063194

Asch, D. A., Nicholson, S., Srinivas, S., Herrin, J., & Epstein, A. J. (2009). Evaluating obstetrical residency programs using patient outcomes. *Journal of the American Medical Association, 302*(12), 1277–1283. doi:10.1001/jama.2009.1356 PMID:19773562

Association of American Medical Colleges (AAMC). (2012). *Survey*. Retrieved from https://www.aamc.org/initiatives/cir/425112/14a.html

Azulay Chertok, I. R., Barnes, E. R., & Gilleland, D. (2014, October). Academic integrity in the online learning environment for health sciences students. *Nurse Education Today, 34*(10), 1324–1329. doi:10.1016/j.nedt.2013.06.002 PMID:23870688

Balls-Berry, J. E. (2012). *Mayo Clinic Learners' Perceptions of Health Disparities*. Paper presented at the 13th RCMI International Symposium on Health Disparities, San Juan, Puerto Rico.

Balls-Berry, J. E., Billings, H., Ernste, L., Valdez Soto, M., Frimannsdottir, K., Weavers, K., ... Patten, C. A. (2017). Development of a self-directed, online-learning curriculum to increase community-engaged research in clinical and translational science. *J Clin Transl Sci, 1*(2), 135–139. doi:10.1017/cts.2016.19 PMID:28649456

Bandura, A. (1982). Self-Efficacy Mechanism in Human Agency. *The American Psychologist, 37*(2), 122–147. doi:10.1037/0003-066X.37.2.122

Bandura, A. (1997). *Self-efficacy: The exercise of control*. New York: W.H. Freeman.

Becker, S., Miron-Shatz, T., Schumacher, N., Krocza, J., Diamantidis, C., & Albrecht, U. V. (2014). mHealth 2.0: Experiences, possibilities, and perspectives. *JMIR mHealth and uHealth, 2*(2), e24. doi:10.2196/mhealth.3328 PMID:25099752

Beeson, M., Christopher, T., Heidt, J., Jones, J., Promes, S., Meyer, L., . . . Wagner, M. J. (2012). *American Board of Emergency Medicine. The Emergency Medicine Milestone Project*. Retrieved from https://www.abem.org/public/docs/default-source/migrated-documents-and-files/em-milestones.pdf?sfvrsn=6

Bellina, L., & Missoni, E. (2009). Mobile cell-phones (M-phones) in telemicroscopy: Increasing connectivity of isolated laboratories. *Diagnostic Pathology*, *4*(1), 19–22. doi:10.1186/1746-1596-4-19 PMID:19545373

Benson, B. J. (2014). Domain of competence: Interpersonal and communication skills. *Academic Pediatrics*, *14*(2), S55–S65. PMID:24602649

Bergeron, B. P. (2006). *Developing Serious Games*. Charles River Media. Retrieved from www.designingdigitally.com

Berger, W. A., Townsend-Kraft, M., Murphy, M. J., & Elaba, Z. (2017). Randomized comparison of virtual microscopy and glass microscopy among dermatology and pathology residents during a simulated in-training examination. *Journal of Cutaneous Pathology*, *44*(4), 409–410. doi:10.1111/cup.12896 PMID:28150326

Bhanot, S., & Sharma, A. (2017). App review series: Epocrates. *Journal of Digital Imaging*, *30*(5), 534–536. doi:10.100710278-017-9977-2 PMID:28523622

Blake, C. A., Lavoie, H. A., & Millette, C. F. (2003). Teaching medical histology at the University of South Carolina school of medicine: Transition to virtual slides and virtual microscopes. *Anatomical Record. Part B, New Anatomist*, *275*(1), 196–206. doi:10.1002/ar.b.10037 PMID:14628320

Bloom, B. S., Engelhart, M. D., Furst, E. J., Hill, W. H., & Krathwohl, D. R. (1956). *Taxonomy of educational objectives: The classification of educational goals. Handbook I: Cognitive domain*. New York: David McKay Company.

Bonis, P. A., Pickens, G. T., Rind, D. M., & Foster, D. A. (2008). Association of a clinical knowledge support system with improved patient safety, reduced complications and shorter length of stay among Medicare beneficiaries in acute care hospitals in the United States. *International Journal of Medical Informatics*, *77*(11), 745–753. doi:10.1016/j.ijmedinf.2008.04.002 PMID:18565788

Boutonnat, J., Paulin, C., Faure, C., Colle, P. E., Ronot, X., & Seigneurin, D. (2006). A pilot study in two French medical schools for teaching histology using virtual microscopy. *Morphologie*, *90*(288), 21–25. doi:10.1016/S1286-0115(06)74314-4 PMID:16929817

Boyce, B. F. (2015). Whole slide imaging: Uses and limitations for surgical pathology and teaching. *Biotechnic & Histochemistry*, *90*(5), 321–330. doi:10.3109/1052029 5.2015.1033463 PMID:25901738

Brauer, D. G., & Ferguson, K. J. (2015). The integrated curriculum in medical education: AMEE Guide No. 96. *Medical Teacher, 37*(4), 312–322. doi:10.3109/0142159X.2014.970998 PMID:25319403

Braveman, P. A., Egerter, S. A., Woolf, S. H., & Marks, J. S. (2011). When Do We Know Enough to Recommend Action on the Social Determinants of Health? *Strong Medicine for a Healthier America, 40*(1Supplement 1), S58–S66. doi:10.1016/j.amepre.2010.09.026 PMID:21146780

BreakAway. (n.d.). *Pulse!! Pulse!! Virtual clinical learning lab for health care training*. Retrieved from http://www.breakawaygames.com/serious-games/solutions/healthcare

Breen, D. P., Duncan, C. W., Pope, A. E., Gray, A. J., & Al-Shahi Salman, R. (2008). Emergency department evaluation of sudden, severe headache. *QJM: An International Journal of Medicine, 101*(6), 435–443. doi:10.1093/qjmed/hcn036 PMID:18443002

Brewer, A. C., Endly, D. C., Henley, J., Amir, M., Sampson, B. P., Moreau, J. F., & Dellavalle, R. P. (2013). Mobile applications in dermatology. *JAMA Dermatology, 149*(11), 1300–1304. doi:10.1001/jamadermatol.2013.5517 PMID:24067948

Brick, K. E., Sluzevich, J. C., Cappel, M. A., DiCaudo, D. J., Comfere, N. I., & Wieland, C. N. (2013). Comparison of virtual microscopy and glass slide microscopy among dermatology residents during a simulated in-training examination. *Journal of Cutaneous Pathology, 40*(9), 807–811. doi:10.1111/cup.12189 PMID:23808673

Bronfenbrener, R. (2014). Learning dermatopathology in the digital age. *Cutis, 94*(4), E22–E24. PMID:25372265

Brookfield, S., & Peskill, S. (2005). *Discussion as A Way of Teaching*. San Francisco, CA: Jossey-Bass. Retrieved from https://www.facultyfocus.com/articles/online-education/eight-tips-for-facilitating-effective-online-discussion-forums/

Brookfield, S. D. (1986). *Understanding and Facilitating Adult Learning*. Milton Keynes, UK: Open University Press.

Brown, D. R., Warren, J. B., & Hyderi, A. (2017). AAMC Core Entrustable Professional Activities for Entering Residency Entrustment Concept Group. Finding a path to entrustment in undergraduate medical education: A progress report from the AAMC Core Entrustable Professional Activities for Entering Residency Entrustment Concept Group. *Acad Med, 92*, 774-779. Retrieved from https://members.aamc.org/eweb/upload/core%20EPA%20Curriculum%20Dev%20Guide.pdf

Brown, B., Adhikari, S., Marx, J., Lander, L., & Todd, G. L. (2012). Introduction of ultrasound into gross anatomy curriculum: Perceptions of medical students. *The Journal of Emergency Medicine*, *43*(6), 1098–1102. doi:10.1016/j.jemermed.2012.01.041 PMID:22459597

Bruce, B. B., Lamirel, C., Wright, D. W., Ward, A., Heilpern, K., Biousse, V., & Newman, N. J. (2011). Nonmydriatic ocular fundus photography in the emergency department. *The New England Journal of Medicine*, *364*(4), 387–289. doi:10.1056/NEJMc1009733 PMID:21268749

Bruch, L. A., De Young, B. R., Kreiter, C. D., Haugen, T. H., Leaven, T. C., & Dee, F. R. (2009). Competency assessment of residents in surgical pathology using virtual microscopy. *Human Pathology*, *40*(8), 1122–1128. doi:10.1016/j.humpath.2009.04.009 PMID:19552936

Brunye, T.T., Carney, P.A., Allison, K.H., Shapiro, L.G., Weaver, D.L., & Elmore, J.G. (2014). Eye movements as an index of pathologist visual expertise: a pilot study. *PLoS One, 9*(8), 1-7.

Buckley, K. M. (2003). Evaluation of classroom-based, web-enhanced, and web-based distance learning nutrition courses for undergraduate nursing. *The Journal of Nursing Education*, *42*(8), 367–370. PMID:12938900

Callahan, D. (2009). *Taming the Beloved Beast.* Princeton University Press.

Callahan, D. (2017). *The Five Horsemen of the Modern World: Climate, Food, Water, Disease, and Obesity.*

Callard, A. (2011). *5 Points on Ultrasound for Pain Management.* Retrieved January 20, 2018, from https://www.beckersspine.com/pain/item/9956-5-points-on-ultrasound-for-pain-management

Carraccio, C. L., & Englander, R. (2013). From Flexner to competencies: Reflections on a decade and the journey ahead. *Academic Medicine*, *88*(8), 1067–1073. doi:10.1097/ACM.0b013e318299396f PMID:23807096

Carraccio, C., & Englander, R. (2004). Analyses/literature reviews: evaluating competence using a portfolio: a literature review and web-based application to the ACGME competencies. *Teaching and Learning in Medicine*, *16*(4), 381–387. doi:10.120715328015tlm1604_13 PMID:15582877

Carraccio, C., Englander, R., Gilhooly, J., Mink, R., Hofkosh, D., Barone, M. A., & Holmboe, E. S. (2017). Building a framework of entrustable professional activities, supported by competencies and milestones, to bridge the educational continuum. *Academic Medicine*, *92*(3), 324–330. doi:10.1097/ACM.0000000000001141 PMID:26959225

Carraccio, C., Englander, R., Van Melle, E., Ten Cate, O., Lockyer, J., Chan, M. K., ... Snell, L. S. (2016). Advancing competency-based medical education: A charter for clinician–educators. *Academic Medicine*, *91*(5), 645–649. doi:10.1097/ACM.0000000000001048 PMID:26675189

Carraccio, C., Wolfsthal, S. D., Englander, R., Ferentz, K., & Martin, C. (2002). Shifting paradigms: From Flexner to competencies. *Academic Medicine*, *77*(5), 361–367. doi:10.1097/00001888-200205000-00003 PMID:12010689

Case Western Reserve University. (2015). *Case Western Reserve, Cleveland Clinic collaborate with Microsoft on earth-shattering mixed-reality technology for education.* Retrieved from http://case.edu/hololens/

Castaño-Muñoz, J., Duart, J. M., & Sancho-Vinuesa, T. (2014). The Internet in face-to-face higher education: Can interactive learning improve academic achievement? *British Journal of Educational Technology*, *45*(1), 149–159. doi:10.1111/bjet.12007

Chan, I., Brown, A.R., Park, K., & Winfree, C.J. (2010). Ultrasound-guided, percutaneous peripheral nerve stimulation: Technical note. *Neurosurgery, 67*(3), 136-9. doi:10.1227/01.NEU.0000383137.33503.EB

Chang, C.-H. (2013). Medical simulation is needed in anesthesia training to achieve patient's safety. *Korean Journal of Anesthesiology*, *64*(3), 204–211. doi:10.4097/kjae.2013.64.3.204 PMID:23560184

Chang, D. R., Lin, R. P., Bowe, S., Bunegin, L., Weitzel, E. K., McMains, K. C., ... Chen, P. G. (2017). Fabrication and Validation of a Low-Cost, Medium-Fidelity Silicone Injection Molded Endoscopic Sinus Surgery Simulation Model. *Larygoscope*, *127*(4), 781–786. doi:10.1002/lary.26370 PMID:28000224

Charon, R. (2001). Narrative medicine: A model for empathy, reflection, profession, and trust. *Journal of the American Medical Association. Journal of the American Medical Association*, *286*(15), 1897–1902. doi:10.1001/jama.286.15.1897 PMID:11597295

Chen, C., Petterson, S., Phillips, R., Bazemore, A., & Mullan, F. (2014). Spending patterns in region of residency training and subsequent expenditures for care provided by practicing physicians for Medicare beneficiaries. *Journal of the American Medical Association, 312*(22), 2385–2393. doi:10.1001/jama.2014.15973 PMID:25490329

Chen, H. C., van den Broek, W. S., & ten Cate, O. (2015). The case for use of entrustable professional activities in undergraduate medical education. *Academic Medicine, 90*(4), 431–436. doi:10.1097/ACM.0000000000000586 PMID:25470310

Choi, J., Noh, G., & Park, D. (2014). Smoking cessation apps for smartphones: Content analysis with the self-determination theory. *Journal of Medical Internet Research, 16*(2), e44. doi:10.2196/jmir.3061 PMID:24521881

Chopra, V., Gesink, B. J., de Jong, J., Bovill, J. G., Spierdijk, J., & Brand, R. (1994). Does training on an anesthesia simulator lead to improvement in performance? *British Journal of Anaesthesia, 73*(3), 293–297. doi:10.1093/bja/73.3.293 PMID:7946851

Clark, D. B., Tanner-Smith, E. E., & Killingsworth, S. S. (2016). Digital games, design, and learning: A systematic review and meta-analysis. *Review of Educational Research, 86*(1), 79–122. doi:10.3102/0034654315582065 PMID:26937054

Cole, M., Shelley, D., & Swartz, L. (2014). Online instruction, e-learning, and student satisfaction: A three year study. International Review of Research in Open and Distance Learning., 15(6). *International Review of Research in Open and Distance Learning, 15*(6). doi:10.19173/irrodl.v15i6.1748

Collins, A., Brown, J. S., & Newman, S. E. (1989). Cognitive Apprenticeship: Teaching the Craft of Reading, Writing, and Mathematics. In L. B. Resnick (Ed.), *Knowing, learning and Instruction:Essays in honor of Robert Glaser* (pp. 453–494). Hillsdale, NJ: Lawrence Erlbaum Associates.

Collins, L., & Ellis, S. R. (2015). *Mobile devices: Tools and technologies* (1st ed.). Boca Raton, FL: Chapman and Hall/CRC Press. doi:10.1201/b18165

Cooke, M., Irby, D., Sullivan, W., & Ludmerer, K. (2006). American Medical Education 100 Years after the Flexner Report. *The New England Journal of Medicine, 355*(13), 1339–1344. doi:10.1056/NEJMra055445 PMID:17005951

Cooper, J. B., & Taqueti, V. R. (2008). A brief history of the development of mannequin simulators for clinical education and training. *Postgraduate Medical Journal, 84*(997), 563–570. doi:10.1136/qshc.2004.009886 PMID:19103813

Cotter, J. R. (2001). Laboratory instruction in histology at the University at Buffalo: Recent replacement of microscope exercises with computer applications. *The Anatomical Record*, *265*(5), 212–221. doi:10.1002/ar.10010 PMID:11745105

Crabtree, N. A., Chandra, D. B., Weiss, I. D., Joo, H. S., & Naik, V. N. (2008). Fibreoptic airway training: Correlation of simulator performance and clinical skill. *Canadian Journal of Anaesthesia*, *55*(2), 100–104. doi:10.1007/BF03016321 PMID:18245069

Crane, G. M., & Gardner, J. M. (2016). Pathology image-sharing on social media: Recommendations for protecting privacy while motivating education. *AMA Journal of Ethics*, *18*(8), 817–825. doi:10.1001/journalofethics.2016.18.8.stas1-1608 PMID:27550566

Crowley, R. S., Naus, G. J., Stewart, J., & Friedman, C. P. (2003). Development of visual diagnostic expertise in pathology: An information-processing study. *Journal of the American Medical Informatics Association*, *10*(1), 39–51. doi:10.1197/jamia.M1123 PMID:12509356

Dabbagh, N., & Bannan-Ritland, R. (2005). *Online Learning: Concepts, Strategies, and Application*. Upper Saddle River, NJ: Pearson/Merrill/Prentice Hall.

Danoff, D., Corbett, E. C., Fortin, A. H., Novak, D. N., & McCurdy, F. (2005). *Recommendations for clinical skills curricula for undergraduate medical education*. Washington, DC: Task Force on the Clinical Skills Education of Medical Students. Association of American Medical Colleges, 40. Retrieved from https://members.aamc.org/eweb/upload/Recommendations%20for%20Clincial%20Skills%20Curricula%202005.pdf

DeJong, C., Lucey, C. R., & Dudley, R. A. (2015). Incorporating a new technology while doing no harm, virtually. *Journal of the American Medical Association*, *314*(22), 2351–2352. doi:10.1001/jama.2015.13572 PMID:26647252

Demiroz, E. (2016). Principles of Instructional Design for E-Learning and Online Learning Practices: Implications for Medical Education. In V. Wang (Ed.), *Handbook of Research on Advancing Health Education through Technology* (pp. 419–451). Hershey, PA: IGI Global; doi:10.4018/978-1-4666-9494-1.ch018

Demiryürek, D., Bayramoğlu, A., & Ustaçelebi, S. (2002). Infective agents in fixed human cadavers: A brief review and suggested guidelines. *Anat Rec.*, *269*(4), 194-7.

Department of Radiology, University of Washington. (n.d.). *General principles: The universal differential diagnosis*. Retrieved from http://www.rad.washington.edu/academics/academic-sections/msk/teaching-materials/online-musculoskeletal-radiology-book/general-principles

Dickson, D., Fouzdar-Jain, S., MacDonald, C., Song, H., Agraz, D., Morgan, L., & Suh, D. (2017). Comparison study of funduscopic exam of pediatric patients using the D-EYE method and conventional indirect ophthalmoscopic methods. *Open Journal of Ophthalmology*, *145*(03), 145–152. doi:10.4236/ojoph.2017.73020

Digital Pathology. (n.d.). Leica Biosystems. Aperio, ePathology Solutions. Available at: http://www.leicabiosystems.com/digital-pathology/

Donohoe, C., Gratton, S., & Vallurupalli, V. R. (2018, April). *Implementation of Smartphone-Compatible Non-Mydriatic Ocular Fundoscopy in the Evaluation of Headaches in Clinical Settings*. Poster session presented at the 2018 UMKC Health Sciences Research Summit, Kansas City, MO.

Dorey, S. (2010). *Link Aviation, A History. Susan Dorey Designs*. Accessed from www.susandoreydesigns.com/genealogy/clirehugh/LinkAviationHistory.pdf

Drake, J. (1998). Commercial simulation market drives industry's future growth. *National Defense Magazine*. Accessed November 12, 2007 from http://www.nationaldefensemagazine.org

Drake, R. L., McBride, J. M., Lachman, N., & Pawlina, W. (2009). Medical education in the anatomical sciences: The winds of change continue to blow. *Anatomical Sciences Education*, *2*(6), 253–259. doi:10.1002/ase.117 PMID:19890982

Drobac, P., & Morse, M. (2016). Medical Education and Global Health Equity. *AMA Journal of Ethics*, *18*(7), 702–709. doi:10.1001/journalofethics.2016.18.7.medu1-1607 PMID:27437820

Dziegielewski, M., Velan, G. M., & Kumar, R. K. (2003). Teaching pathology using 'hotspotted' digital images. *Medical Education*, *37*(11), 1047–1048. doi:10.1046/j.1365-2923.2003.01646.x PMID:14629446

Elavsky, S., Smahel, D., & Machackova, H. (2017). Who are mobile app users from healthy lifestyle websites? Analysis of patterns of app use and user characteristics. *Translational Behavioral Research*, *7*(4), 891–901. doi:10.100713142-017-0525-x PMID:28929368

Engels, P. T., & de Gara, C. (2010). Learning styles of medical students, general surgery residents, and general surgeons: Implications for surgical education. *BMC Medical Education*, *10*(51). doi:10.1186/1472-6920-10-51 PMID:20591159

Englander, R., & Carraccio, C. (2014). Domain of competence: Medical knowledge. *Academic Pediatrics*, *14*(Suppl. 2), 536–537. doi:10.1016/j.acap.2013.10.006 PMID:24602633

Enosis Group. (2012). *Facilitated discovery. Eliciting and amplifying team brilliance*. Retrieved from http://www.facilitateddiscovery.com/

Epstein, R. M. (2007). Assessment in medical education. *The New England Journal of Medicine*, *356*(4), 387–396. doi:10.1056/NEJMra054784 PMID:17251535

Essin, D. M. A. (2012). The Ethical Dilemma Created by EHRs. In *Physicians Practice, in Blog*. HER, Healthcare Careers.

Evans, K. H., Daines, W., Tsui, J., Strehlow, M., Maggio, P., & Shieh, L. (2015). Septris: A novel, mobile, online, simulation game that improves sepsis recognition and management. *Academic Medicine*, *90*(2), 180–184. doi:10.1097/ACM.0000000000000611 PMID:25517703

Evans, L. V., Dodge, K. L., Shah, T. D., Kaplan, L. J., Siegel, M. D., Moore, C. L., ... D'Onofrio, G. (2010). Simulation training in central venous catheter insertion: Improved performance in clinical practice. *Academic Medicine*, *85*(9), 1462–1469. doi:10.1097/ACM.0b013e3181eac9a3 PMID:20736674

Fakoya, F.A. (2013). Integrating ultrasound technology into teaching gross anatomy: point of order! *Medical Education Online*. doi:. doi:10.3402/meo.v18i0.20888

Farahani, N., Parwani, A. V., & Pantanowitz, L. (2015). Whole slide imaging in pathology: Advantages, limitations, and emerging perspectives. *Pathology and Laboratory Medicine International: PLMI*, *7*, 23–33.

Farahani, N., Post, R., Duboy, J., Ahmed, I., Kolowitz, B. J., Krinchai, T., ... Pantanowitz, L. (2016). Exploring virtual reality technology and the Oculus Rift for the examination of digital pathology slides. *Journal of Pathology Informatics*, *7*(1), 22–26. doi:10.4103/2153-3539.181766 PMID:27217972

Faulkner, T. P., Christoff, J. J., Sweeney, M. A., & Oliver, N. (2005). Pilot study of a distance-learning methodology used on campus for first professional degree pharmacy students in an integrated therapeutics module. *American Journal of Pharmaceutical Education*, *69*(1), 7. doi:10.5688/aj690107

Fernandez, E., & Williams, D. G. (2009). Training and the European working time directive: A 7 year review of paediatric anesthetic trainee caseload data. *British Journal of Anaesthesia*, *103*(4), 566–569. doi:10.1093/bja/aep170 PMID:19556272

Filho, A. P., & Romano, M. M. D. (2007). Simulacao: Aspectos conceituais. *Rev Fac Med Ribeirao Preto*, *40*(2), 167–170.

Finlayson, R. J. (2017). Ultrasound Guidance for Trigger Point Injections: Gold Standard or Fool's Gold? *Regional Anesthesia and Pain Medicine*, *42*(3), 279–280. doi:10.1097/AAP.0000000000000599 PMID:28419045

Flin, R., & Maran, N. (2004). Identifying and training non-technical skills for teams in acute medicine. *Quality & Safety in Health Care*, *13*(Suppl. 1), i80–i84. doi:10.1136/qshc.2004.009993 PMID:15465960

Foster, K. (2010). Medical education in the digital age: Digital whole slide imaging as an e-learning tool. *Journal of Pathology Informatics*, *1*(1), 14–16. doi:10.4103/2153-3539.68331 PMID:20922031

Frank, J. R., Snell, L. S., Cate, O. T., Holmboe, E. S., Carraccio, C., Swing, S. R., ... Harden, R. M. (2010). Competency-based medical education: Theory to practice. *Medical Teacher*, *32*(8), 638–645. doi:10.3109/0142159X.2010.501190 PMID:20662574

Fremont, A. M., Cleary, P. D., Hargraves, J. L., Rowe, R. M., Jacobson, N. B., & Ayanian, J. Z. (2001). Patient-centered processes of care and long-term outcomes of myocardial infarction. *Journal of General Internal Medicine*, *16*(12), 800–808. doi:10.1046/j.1525-1497.2001.10102.x PMID:11903758

Fuller, M. Y., Mukhopadhyay, S., & Gardner, J. M. (2016). Using the periscope live video-streaming application for global pathology education: A brief introduction. *Archives of Pathology & Laboratory Medicine*, *140*(11), 1273–1280. doi:10.5858/arpa.2016-0268-SA PMID:27441785

Gallagher, J. E., Dobrosielski-Vergona, K. A., Wingard, R. G., & Williams, T. M. (2005). Web-based vs. traditional classroom instruction in gerontology: A pilot study. *Journal of Dental Hygiene*, *79*(3). PMID:16197772

Garrison, D. R. & Kanuka, H. (2004). Blended learning: Uncovering its transformative potential in higher education. *Internet and Higher Education, 7*, 95–105.

George, D. R., & Dellasega, C. (2011). Use of social media in graduate-level medical humanities education: Two pilot studies from Penn State College of Medicine. *Medical Teacher*, *33*(8), e429–e434. doi:10.3109/0142159X.2011.586749 PMID:21774639

Gerolemou, L., Fidellagra, A., Rose, K., Cooper, S., & Venturanza, M. (2014). Simulation-based training for nurses in sterile techniques during central vein catheterization. *American Journal of Critical Care*, *23*(1), 40–48. doi:10.4037/ajcc2014860 PMID:24382616

Gertz, R., Longley, B. J., Bennett, D., Ranheim, E., Rajamanickam, V., Kawahara, T., & Endo, J. (2015). Integrating virtual dermatopathology as part of formative and summative assessment of residents: A feasibility pilot study. *Journal of Cutaneous Pathology*, *42*(10), 779–781. doi:10.1111/cup.12503 PMID:25990466

Goldberg, H. R., & Dintzis, R. (2007). The positive impact of team-based virtual microscopy on student learning in physiology and histology. *Advances in Physiology Education*, *31*(3), 261–265. doi:10.1152/advan.00125.2006 PMID:17848592

Gonzalez, R. S., Amer, S. M., Yahia, N. B., D'Almeida Costa, F., Noatay, M., Qiao, J. H., ... Gardner, J. M. (2017). Facebook discussion groups provide a robust worldwide platform for free pathology education. *Archives of Pathology & Laboratory Medicine*, *141*(5), 690–695. doi:10.5858/arpa.2016-0369-OA PMID:27763789

Gonzalez, S. (2008). Clinical applications of reflectance confocal microscopy in the management of cutaneous tumors. *Actas Dermo-Sifiliograficas*, *99*(7), 528–531. doi:10.1016/S0001-7310(08)74737-9 PMID:18682165

Good, M. L. (2003). Patient simulation for training basic and advanced clinical skills. *Medical Education*, *37*(1), 14–21. doi:10.1046/j.1365-2923.37.s1.6.x PMID:14641634

Grace, S. (2017). *The Difference Between E-Learning and On-line Learning*. Retrieved from https://www.eztalks.com/elearning/difference-between-elearning-and-online-learning.html

Graff, B., Gąsecki, D., Rojek, A., Boutouyrie, P., Nyka, W., Laurent, S., & Narkiewicz, K. (2013). Heart rate variability and functional outcome in ischemic stroke. *Journal of Hypertension*, *31*(8), 1629–1636. doi:10.1097/HJH.0b013e328361e48b PMID:23751963

Gregoski, M. J., Mueller, M., Vertegel, A., Shaporev, A., Jackson, B. B., Frenzel, R. M., ... Treiber, F. A. (2012). Development and validation of a smartphone heart rate acquisition application for health promotion and wellness telehealth applications. *International Journal of Telemedicine and Applications*, *2012*, 1–7. doi:10.1155/2012/696324 PMID:22272197

Grow, G. O. (1991). Teaching learners to be self-directed. *Adult Education Quarterly*, *41*(3), 125–149. doi:10.1177/0001848191041003001

Guhl, E. N., Schlusser, C. L., Henault, L. E., Bickmore, T. W., Kimani, E., Paasche-Orlow, M. K., & Magnani, J. W. (2017). Rationale and design of the atrial fibrillation health literacy information technology trial: (AF-LITT). *Contemporary Clinical Trials*, *62*, 153–158. doi:10.1016/j.cct.2017.09.005 PMID:28923492

Guo, K., Liao, J., Bian, Z., Heng, X., & Zheng, G. (2015). InstantScope: A low-cost whole slide imaging system with instant focal plane detection. *Biomedical Optics Express*, *6*(9), 3210–3216. doi:10.1364/BOE.6.003210 PMID:26417493

Gurpinar, E., Bati, H., & Tetik, C. (2011). Learning styles of medical students change in relation to time. *Advances in Physiology Education*, *35*(3), 307–311. doi:10.1152/advan.00047.2011 PMID:21908841

Haddock, L. J., Kim, D. Y., & Mukai, S. (2013). Simple, inexpensive technique for high-quality smartphone fundus photography in human and animal eyes. *Journal of Ophthalmology*, 518479. PMID:24171108

Halaas, G. W., Van Eck, R. N., Allen, J., Johnson, E., & Stauffenecker, C. (2017). *Interprofessional Telemedicine Competency for Health Care Students With Remotely Operated BiOmedical Telepresence Systems (ROBOTS).* Retrieved from https://www.ama-assn.org/sites/default/files/media-browser/public/medical-schools/ace-consortium-schools/consortium-images/spring-consortium-meeting-poster-university-of-north-dakota.pdf

Halcox, J. P., Wareham, K., Cardew, A., Gilmore, M., Barry, J. P., Phillips, C., & Gravenor, M. B. (2017). Assessment of remote heart rhythm sampling using the AliveCor heart monitor to screen for atrial fibrillation: The REHEARSE-AF study. *Circulation*, *136*(19), 1784–1794. doi:10.1161/CIRCULATIONAHA.117.030583 PMID:28851729

Hamilton, P. W., Wang, Y., & McCullough, S. J. (2012). Virtual microscopy and digital pathology in training and education. *APMIS*, *120*(4), 305–315. doi:10.1111/j.1600-0463.2011.02869.x PMID:22429213

Hammond, M., Skochelak, S., & Kirley, K. (2018). *Innovations in Medical Education Webinar: Interprofessional Education using Technology to Teach Team-based Care.* Retrieved from https://cme.ama-assn.org/Activity/6021873/Detail.aspx

Hammoud, M. M., Dalrymple, J. L., Christner, J. G., Stewart, R. A., Fisher, J., Margo, K., ... Pangaro, L. N. (2012). Medical student documentation in electronic health records: A collaborative statement from the Alliance for Clinical Education. *Teaching and Learning in Medicine*, *24*(3), 257–266. doi:10.1080/10401334.2012.692284 PMID:22775791

Hanna, M. G., Parwani, A. V., Pantanowitz, L., Punjabi, V., & Singh, R. (2015). Smartphone applications: A contemporary resource for dermatopathology. *Journal of Pathology Informatics*, *6*(1), 44–48. doi:10.4103/2153-3539.161612 PMID:26284155

Hartling, L., Spooner, C., Tjosvold, L., & Oswald, A. (2010). Problem-based learning in pre-clinical medical education: 22 years of outcome research. *Medical Teacher*, *32*(1), 28–35. doi:10.3109/01421590903200789 PMID:20095771

Hartman, D. J. (2016). Mobile technology for the practice of pathology. *Advances in Anatomic Pathology*, *23*(2), 118–124. doi:10.1097/PAP.0000000000000093 PMID:26849818

Haskins, S. C., Boublik, J., & Wu, C. L. (2017). Point-of-Care Ultrasound for the Regional Anesthesiologist and Pain Specialist: A Series Introduction. *Regional Anesthesia and Pain Medicine*, *42*(3), 281–282. doi:10.1097/AAP.0000000000000570 PMID:28419046

Heckler, M. (1985). *Report of the Secretary's Task Force on Black & Minority Health*. Retrieved from https://minorityhealth.hhs.gov/assets/pdf/checked/1/ANDERSON.pdf

Helmreich, R. L. (2000). On error management: Lessons from aviation. *BMJ (Clinical Research Ed.)*, *320*(7237), 781–785. doi:10.1136/bmj.320.7237.781 PMID:10720367

Higgins, C. (2015). Applications and challenges of digital pathology and whole slide imaging. *Biotechnic & Histochemistry*, *90*(5), 341–347. doi:10.3109/10520295.2015.1044566 PMID:25978139

Hinshaw, M. A. (2012). Dermatopathology education: An update. *Dermatologic Clinics*, *30*(4), 815–826. doi:10.1016/j.det.2012.06.003 PMID:23021060

Hinshaw, M., Hsu, P., Lee, L. Y., & Stratman, E. (2009). The current state of dermatopathology education: A survey of the Association of Professors of Dermatology. *Journal of Cutaneous Pathology*, *36*(6), 620–628. doi:10.1111/j.1600-0560.2008.01128.x PMID:19515041

Horn, A. J., Czarnecki, D., & Lele, S. M. (2012). Interactive case vignettes utilizing simulated pathologist-clinician encounters with whole slide imaging and video tutorials of whole slide scans improve student understanding of disease processes. *Journal of Pathology Informatics*, *3*(1), 34–38. doi:10.4103/2153-3539.101786 PMID:23243552

Houghton, J. P., Smoller, B. R., Leonard, N., Stevenson, M. R., & Dornan, T. (2015). Diagnostic performance on briefly presented digital pathology images. *Journal of Pathology Informatics*, *6*(1), 56–61. doi:10.4103/2153-3539.168517 PMID:26605121

iExcel. (n.d.). Retrieved from https://www.unmc.edu/iexcel/about/index.html

Isom, J., Walsh, M., & Gardner, J. (2017). Social media and pathology: Where are we now and why does it matter? *Advances in Anatomic Pathology*, *24*(5), 294–303. doi:10.1097/PAP.0000000000000159 PMID:28719442

Izzard, L. C., & Bhalla, A. (2015). Post-stroke cardiac complications. *Management of Post-Stroke Complications,* 21-31. doi:4_3 doi:10.1007/978-3-319-17855

Jaarsma, T., Jarodzka, H., Nap, M., van Merrienboer, J. J., & Boshuizen, H. P. (2014). Expertise under the microscope: Processing histopathological slides. *Medical Education*, *48*(3), 292–300. doi:10.1111/medu.12385 PMID:24528464

Jaarsma, T., Jarodzka, H., Nap, M., van Merrienboer, J. J., & Boshuizen, H. P. (2015). Expertise in clinical pathology: Combining the visual and cognitive perspective. *Advances in Health Sciences Education: Theory and Practice*, *20*(4), 1089–1106. doi:10.100710459-015-9589-x PMID:25677013

Jackson, C. S., & Gracia, J. N. (2014). Addressing Health and Health-Care Disparities: The Role of a Diverse Workforce and the Social Determinants of Health. *Public Health Reports (Washington, D.C.)*, *129*(Suppl 2), 57–61. doi:10.1177/00333549141291S211 PMID:24385666

Jahan-Tigh, R. R., Chinn, G. M., & Rapini, R. P. (2016). A comparative study between smartphone-based microscopy and conventional light microscopy in 1021 dermatopathology specimens. *Archives of Pathology & Laboratory Medicine*, *140*(1), 86–90. doi:10.5858/arpa.2014-0593-OA PMID:26717060

Jakubek, K., & Welch, L. (2017). *AMA, Regenstrief Institute Heal Increase HER Training in Med Schools.* Retrieved from https://www.ama-assn.org/ama-regenstrief-institute-help-increase-ehr-training-med-schools

James, J. T. (2013). A new, evidence-based estimate of patient harms associated with hospital care. *Journal of Patient Safety*, *9*(3), 122–128. doi:10.1097/PTS.0b013e3182948a69 PMID:23860193

Jansen, B. J., Booth, D., & Smith, B. (2009). Using the taxonomy of cognitive learning to model online searching. *Information Processing & Management*, *45*(6), 643–663. doi:10.1016/j.ipm.2009.05.004

Johna, S., & Dehal, A. (2013). The power of reflective writing: Narrative medicine and medical education. *The Permanente Journal*, *17*(4), 84–85. doi:10.7812/TPP/13-043 PMID:24361026

Jones, F., Passos-Neto, C. E., & Braghiroli, O. F. M. (2015). Simulation in medical education: Brief history and methodology. *J PPCR*, *1*(2), 56–63.

Joundi, R. A., Brittain, J. S., Jenkinson, N., Green, A. L., & Aziz, T. (2011). Rapid tremor frequency assessment with the iPhone accelerometer. *Parkinsonism & Related Disorders*, *17*(4), 288–290. doi:10.1016/j.parkreldis.2011.01.001 PMID:21300563

Kaercher, D. (2007). *The Development of a South Texas Health Information Gateway: Negotiating the Construction of Information* (Dissertation). Edith Cowan University Press, Perth, Australia.

Kai, L., Zhang, X., Wang, Y., Suibiao, H., Ning, G., Wangyong, P., ... Chen, H. (2011). A system of portable ECG monitoring based on Bluetooth mobile phone. *2011 IEEE International Symposium on IT in Medicine and Education*. doi:10.1109/itime.2011.6132113

Kapur, J., Han, T., Quek, S.T., Kanagasuntheram, R., Ng, Y.K., Lim, A., ... Samarasekera, D. (2016). The role of ultrasound teaching of clinical anatomy to first year medical students. *An International Association for Medical Education (AMEE) MedEdPublish* doi:10.15694/mep.2016.000029

Karr, M., Fishback, J. L., & Klein, R. M. (2007). *Where did I put my microscope? Virtual microscopy*. Workshop presented at Slice of Life Conference, New Orleans, LA. Abstract retrieved from http://slice.utah.edu/2007/schedule/documents/07MichaelKarr1.pdf

Kelly, L. P., Garza, P. S., Bruce, B. B., Graubart, E. B., Newman, N. J., & Biousse, V. (2013). Teaching ophthalmoscopy to medical students (the TOTeMS study). *American Journal of Ophthalmology*, *156*(5), 1056–1061. doi:10.1016/j.ajo.2013.06.022 PMID:24041982

Kelly, R. (2015). *Kelly Report: Health Disparities in America*. Washington, DC: United States Congress. Retrieved from https://robinkelly.house.gov/sites/robinkelly.house.gov/files/2015%20Kelly%20Report.pdf

Kennedy, C. C., Cannon, E. K., Warner, D. O., & Cook, D. A. (2014). Advanced airway management simulation training in medical education: A systematic review and meta-analysis. *Critical Care Medicine*, *42*(1), 169–178. doi:10.1097/CCM.0b013e31829a721f PMID:24220691

Kennedy, C. C., Maldonado, F., & Cook, D. A. (2013). Simulation-based bronchoscopy training: Systemic review and meta-analysis. *Chest*, *144*(1), 183–192. doi:10.1378/chest.12-1786 PMID:23370487

Kent, M., Olsen, T., Feeser, T., Tesno, K. C., Moad, J. C., Conroy, M. P., ... Bottomley, M. A. (2017). Diagnostic accuracy of virtual pathology vs traditional microscopy in a large dermatopathology study. *JAMA Dermatology*, E1–E7. PMID:29049424

Kheshti, R., Aalipour, M., & Namazi, S. (2016). A comparison of five common drug–drug interaction software programs regarding accuracy and comprehensiveness. *Journal of Research in Pharmacy Practice*, *5*(4), 257–263. doi:10.4103/2279-042X.192461 PMID:27843962

Kitagawa, M., Gupta, A., Cozza, R., Glenn, D., Atwal, R., Maita, K., … Wang, A. (2018). *Market share: Final PCs, ultramobiles and mobile phones, all countries, 4Q17* (ID: G00350384). Retrieved from Gartner database.

Knowles, M. S., Holton, E. F., & Swanson, R. A. (2012). The Adult Learner: the Definitive Classics in Adult Education and Human Resource Development (7th ed.). New York, NY: Taylor & Francis.

Knowles, M. S. (1980). *The modern practice of adult education: From pedagogy to andragogy*. Chicago: Follett.

Knowles, M. S. (1990). *The Adult Learner: A Neglected Species*. Houston, TX: Gulf.

Koch, L. H., Lampros, J. N., Delong, L. K., Chen, S. C., Woosley, J. T., & Hood, A. F. (2009). Randomized comparison of virtual microscopy and traditional glass microscopy in diagnostic accuracy among dermatology and pathology residents. *Human Pathology*, *40*(5), 662–667. doi:10.1016/j.humpath.2008.10.009 PMID:19144382

Kohn, L. T., Corrigan, J. M., & Donaldson, M. S. (1999). *To err is human: Building a safer health system*. Washington, DC: National Academy Press.

Kolb, A. Y., & Kolb, D. A. (2013). *The Kolb learning style inventory 4.0: A comprehensive guide to the theory, psychometrics, research and validity and educational applications*. Retrieved from https://learningfromexperience.com/downloads/research-library/the-kolb-learning-style-inventory-4-0.pdf

Kolb, D. A. (1984). *Experiential learning: experience as the source of learning and development*. Englewood Cliffs, NJ: Prentice Hall.

Korbe, S., Udoji, E. N., Ness, T. J., & Udoji, M. A. (2015). Ultrasound-guided interventional procedures for chronic pain management. *Pain Management*, *5*(6), 465–482. doi:10.2217/pmt.15.46 PMID:26402316

Krajci, I., & Cummings, D. (2013). *Android on x86: An introduction to optimizing for Intel® architecture* (1st ed.). New York, NY: Apress Media, LLC. doi:10.1007/978-1-4302-6131-5

Krathwohl, D. (2002). A revision of Bloom's taxonomy: An overview. *Theory into Practice*, *41*(4), 212–218. doi:10.120715430421tip4104_2

Krebs, P., & Duncan, D. T. (2015). Health app use among US mobile phone owners: A national survey. *JMIR mHealth and uHealth*, *3*(4), e101. doi:10.2196/mhealth.4924 PMID:26537656

Krippendorf, B. B., & Lough, J. (2005). Complete and rapid switch from light microscopy to virtual microscopy for teaching medical histology. *Anatomical Record. Part B, New Anatomist*, *285*(1), 19–25. doi:10.1002/ar.b.20066 PMID:16032757

Krupinski, E. A., Graham, A. R., & Weinstein, R. S. (2013). Characterizing the development of visual search expertise in pathology residents viewing whole slide images. *Human Pathology*, *44*(3), 357–364. doi:10.1016/j.humpath.2012.05.024 PMID:22835956

Kumar, R. K., Velan, G. M., Korell, S. O., Kandara, M., Dee, F. R., & Wakefield, D. (2004). Virtual microscopy for learning and assessment in pathology. *The Journal of Pathology*, *204*(5), 613–618. doi:10.1002/path.1658 PMID:15470688

L3 Link. (2017). *Innovation heritage*. Accessed October 15, 2017 from http://www.link.com/about#our-innovation-heritage

Laerdal Medical. (2006). *The girl from the River Seine (History in brief)*. Accessed September 24, 2017 from http://www.laerdal.com/about/default.htm

LaVeist, T. A., & Pierre, G. (2014). Integrating the 3Ds--social determinants, health disparities, and health-care workforce diversity. *Public Health Reports (Washington, D.C.)*, *129* (Suppl 2), 9–14. doi:10.1177/00333549141291S204 PMID:24385659

Lee, J. J., Jedrych, J., Pantanowitz, L., & Ho, J. (2017). Validation of digital pathology for primary histopathological diagnosis of routine, inflammatory dermatopathology cases. *The American Journal of Dermatopathology*, *0*, 1–7. PMID:28763335

Lee, P., Chen, C. F., Wan, H. T., Jian, W. S., Hsu, M. H., Syed-Abdul, S., ... Li, Y. C. (2015). iSlide: A 'big picture' interactive teledermatopathology e-learning system. *British Journal of Dermatology*, *172*(3), 692–699. doi:10.1111/bjd.13274 PMID:25040884

Lehman, J. S., & Gibson, L. E. (2013). Smart teledermatopathology: A feasibility study of novel, high-value, portable, widely accessible and intuitive telepathology methods using handheld electronic devices. *Journal of Cutaneous Pathology*, *40*(5), 513–518. doi:10.1111/cup.12108 PMID:23472602

Leifer, Z. (2015). The use of virtual microscopy and a wiki in pathology education: Tracking student use, involvement, and response. *Journal of Pathology Informatics*, *6*(1), 30–36. doi:10.4103/2153-3539.158063 PMID:26110097

Leinweber, B., Massone, C., Kodama, K., Kaddu, S., Cerroni, L., Haas, J., ... Smolle, J. (2006). Teledermatopathology: A controlled study about diagnostic validity and technical requirements for digital transmission. *The American Journal of Dermatopathology*, *28*(5), 413–416. doi:10.1097/01.dad.0000211523.95552.86 PMID:17012916

León, S. A., Fontelo, P., Green, L., Ackerman, M., & Liu, F. (2007). Evidence-based medicine among internal medicine residents in a community hospital program using smart phones. *BMC Medical Informatics and Decision Making*, *7*(5), 1–11. doi:10.1186/1472-6947-7-5 PMID:17313680

Levett-Jones, T. L. (2005). Self-directed learning: Implications and limitations for undergraduate nursing education. *Nurse Education Today*, *25*(5), 363–368. doi:10.1016/j.nedt.2005.03.003 PMID:15894411

Lippa, L. M., Boker, J., Duke, A., & Amin, A. (2006). A novel 3-year longitudinal pilot study of medical students' acquisition and retention of screening eye examination skills. *Ophthalmology*, *113*(1), 133–139. doi:10.1016/j.ophtha.2005.09.003 PMID:16310854

Liu, Y., Glass, N. L., Glover, C. D., Power, R. W., & Watcha, M. F. (2013). Comparison of the development of performance skills in ultrasound-guided regional anesthesia simulations with different phantom models. *Simulation in Healthcare*, *8*(6), 368–375. doi:10.1097/SIH.0b013e318299dae2 PMID:24096912

Loader, B. (1998). *Cyberspace divide: Equality, agency, policy in the information society*. New York: Routledge. doi:10.4324/9780203169537_chapter_1

Loftin, B. (2002). Med school 1.0: Can computer simulation aid physician training. *Quest*, *5*(5), 16–19.

Lord, R. K., Shah, V. A., San-Filippo, A. N., & Krishna, R. (2010). Novel uses of smartphones in ophthalmology. *Ophthalmology*, *117*(6), 1274–1274. doi:10.1016/j.ophtha.2010.01.001 PMID:20522335

Ludwig, S. (2014). Domain of competence: Professionalism. *Academic Pediatrics*, *14*(2), S66–S69. doi:10.1016/j.acap.2013.11.013 PMID:24602656

Mackay, D. D., Garza, P. S., Bruce, B. B., Bidot, S., Graubart, E. B., Newman, N. J., ... Kelly, L. P. (2014). Teaching ophthalmology to medical students (TOTeMS) II: A one-year retention study. *American Journal of Ophthalmology*, *157*(3), 747–748. doi:10.1016/j.ajo.2013.12.013 PMID:24528937

Mackay, D. D., Garza, P. S., Bruce, B. B., Newman, N. J., & Biousse, V. (2015). The demise of direct ophthalmoscopy: A modern clinical challenge. *Neurology. Clinical Practice*, *5*(2), 150–157. doi:10.1212/CPJ.0000000000000115 PMID:26137422

Madke, B., & Gardner, J. (2017). Enhanced worldwide dermatology–pathology interaction via facebook, twitter, and other social media platforms. *The American Journal of Dermatopathology*, *0*, 1–5. PMID:28796693

Maizels, M. (2001). Headache evaluation and treatment by primary care physicians in an emergency department in the era of triptans. *Archives of Internal Medicine*, *161*(16), 1969–1973. doi:10.1001/archinte.161.16.1969 PMID:11525699

Maldonado, M. E., Fried, E. D., DuBose, T. D., Nelson, C., & Breida, M. (2014). The role that graduate medical education must play in ensuring health equity and eliminating health care disparities. *Annals of the American Thoracic Society*, *11*(4), 603–607. doi:10.1513/AnnalsATS.201402-068PS PMID:24708150

Mangone, E. R., Lebrun, V., & Muessig, K. E. (2016). Mobile phone apps for the prevention of unintended pregnancy: A systematic review and content analysis. *JMIR mHealth and uHealth*, *4*(1), e6. doi:10.2196/mhealth.4846 PMID:26787311

Marshak, D. W., Oakes, J., Hsieh, P. H., Chuang, A. Z., & Cleary, L. J. (2015). Outcomes of a rotational dissection system in gross anatomy. *Anatomical Sciences Education*, *8*(5), 438–444. doi:10.1002/ase.1497 PMID:25358463

Martin, C. R. (1997). *Looking at type: The fundamentals*. Gainesville, FL: Center for Applications of Psychological Type.

Massone, C., Soyer, P. H., Lozzi, G. P., Di Stefani, A., Leinweber, B., Gabler, G., ... Kerl, H. (2007). Feasibility and diagnostic agreement in teledermatopathology using a virtual slide system. *Human Pathology*, *38*(4), 546–554. doi:10.1016/j.humpath.2006.10.006 PMID:17270240

Maudsley G. & Strivens J. (2000) Promoting professional knowledge, experiential learning and critical thinking for medical students. *Med Edu, 34*(7), 535-44

McComiskie, J. E., Greer, R. M., & Gole, G. A. (2004). Panoptic vs conventional ophthalmoscope. *Clinical & Experimental Ophthalmology*, *32*(3), 238–242. doi:10.1111/j.1442-9071.2004.00810.x PMID:15180833

McDonnell, R., Breidt, M., & Bülthoff, H. H. (2012). Render me real?: Investigating the effect of render style on the perception of animated virtual humans. *ACM Transactions on Graphics*, *31*(4), 91. doi:10.1145/2185520.2185587

McLachlan, J. C., Bligh, J., Bradley, P., & Searle, J. (2004, April). Teaching anatomy without cadavers. *Medical Education*, *38*(4), 418–424. doi:10.1046/j.1365-2923.2004.01795.x PMID:15025643

McWilliam, E., & Lee, A. (2006). The problem of 'the problem with educational research'. *Australian Educational Researcher*, *33*(2), 43–60. doi:10.1007/BF03216833

Mello-Thoms, C., Mello, C. A., Medvedeva, O., Castine, M., Legowski, E., Gardner, G., ... Crowley, R. (2012). Perceptual analysis of the reading of dermatopathology virtual slides by pathology residents. *Archives of Pathology & Laboratory Medicine*, *136*(5), 551–562. doi:10.5858/arpa.2010-0697-OA PMID:22540304

Michael S. Gordon Center for Research in Medical Education. (2007). *History/ Overview*. Accessed September 24, 2017 from http://www.crme.med.miami.edu/history.html

Microsoft 365. (2014, October 12). *One Class Notebook*. Retrieved from https://www.microsoft.com/en-us/microsoft-365/blog/2014/10/07/introducing-onenote-class-notebooks-flexible-digital-framework-teaching-learning/

Microsoft Class Notebook Add-In. (n.d.). Available at: https://download.microsoft.com/download/5/0/0/500EF2CA-5192-49F2-8E0C-BDEB2D530788/ClassNotebook.Setup.exe

Microsoft Office 365. (n.d.). Available at: https://go.microsoft.com/fwlink/p/?LinkID=787538

Milani, B. Y., Majdi, M., Green, W., Mehralian, A., Moarefi, M., Oh, F. S., ... Djalilian, A. R. (2013). The use of peer optic nerve photographs for teaching direct ophthalmoscopy. *Ophthalmology*, *120*(4), 761–765. doi:10.1016/j.ophtha.2012.09.020 PMID:23246117

Miller, M. (2017). Top predictions for the app economy in 2018 [Blog post]. Retrieved from https://www.appannie.com/en/insights/market-data/predictions-app-economy-2018/

Mione, S., Valcke, M., & Cornelissen, M. (2013). Evaluation of virtual microscopy in medical histology teaching. *Anatomical Sciences Education*, *6*(5), 307–315. doi:10.1002/ase.1353 PMID:23463716

Mitchell, A. R., & Page, P. L. (2015). Living with the handheld ECG. *BMJ Innovations*, *1*(2), 46–48. doi:10.1136/bmjinnov-2014-000029

Moazami, F., Bahrampour, E., Azar, M. R., Jahedi, F., & Moattari, M. (2014). Comparing two methods of education (virtual versus traditional) on learning of Iranian dental students: A post-test only design study. *BMC Medical Education*, *14*(1), 1. doi:10.1186/1472-6920-14-45 PMID:24597923

Mobasheri, M. H., King, D., Johnston, M., Gautama, S., Purkayastha, S., & Darzi, A. (2015). The ownership and clinical use of smartphones by doctors and nurses in the UK: A multicentre survey study. *BMJ Innovations*, *1*(4), 174–181. doi:10.1136/bmjinnov-2015-000062

Moja, L., & Kwag, K. H. (2015). Point of care information services: A platform for self-directed continuing medical education for front line decision makers. *Postgraduate Medical Journal*, *91*(1072), 83–91. doi:10.1136/postgradmedj-2014-132965 PMID:25655251

Mooney, E., & Hedblad, M. A. (2012). Virtual dermatopathology: Current technology and use. *Forum for Nordic Dermato-Venerology*, *17*(2), 40–43.

Mooney, E., Hood, A. F., Lampros, J., Kempf, W., & Jemec, G. B. E. (2011). Comparative diagnostic accuracy in virtual dermatopathology. *Skin Research and Technology*, *17*(2), 251–255. doi:10.1111/j.1600-0846.2010.00493.x PMID:21251087

Moore, M. G., & Thompson, M. M. (1990). *The effects of distance learning: A summary of literature.* ERIC Document Reproduction Service No. ED 330 321.

Morillo, C. A., Banerjee, A., Perel, P., Wood, D., & Jouven, X. (2017). Atrial fibrillation: The current epidemic. *Journal of Geriatric Cardiology*, *14*(3), 195–203. 5411.2017.03.011 doi:10.11909/j.issn.1671

Morrison, A. O., & Gardner, J. M. (2015a). Microscopic image photography techniques of the past, present, and future. *Archives of Pathology & Laboratory Medicine*, *139*(12), 1558–1564. doi:10.5858/arpa.2014-0315-RA PMID:25989285

Morrison, A. O., & Gardner, J. M. (2015b). The Morrison technique: A free-hand method for capturing photomicrographs using a smartphone. *Journal of Cutaneous Pathology*, *43*(5), 472–474. doi:10.1111/cup.12650 PMID:26679477

Morrison, A. S., & Gardner, J. M. (2014). Smart phone microscopic photography: A novel tool for physicians and trainees. *Archives of Pathology & Laboratory Medicine*, *138*(8), 1002. doi:10.5858/arpa.2013-0425-ED PMID:24199830

Mosa, A. S., Yoo, I., & Sheets, L. (2012). A systemic review of healthcare applications for smartphones. *BMC Medical Informatics and Decision Making*, *12*(67), 1–31. doi:10.1186/1472-6947-12-67 PMID:22781312

Mottow-Lippa, L. (2009). Ophthalmology in the medical school curriculum: Reestablishing our value and effecting change. *Ophthalmology*, *116*(7), 1235–1236. doi:10.1016/j.ophtha.2009.01.012 PMID:19576494

Myers, B. A. (1998). A brief history of human computer interaction technology. *Interactions (New York, N.Y.)*, *5*(2), 44–54. doi:10.1145/274430.274436

Naik, V. N., & Brien, S. E. (2013). Review article: Simulation: A means to address and improve patient safety. *Canadian Journal of Anaesthesia*, *60*(2), 192–200. doi:10.100712630-012-9860-z PMID:23239487

Naik, V. N., Matsumoto, E. D., Houston, P. L., Hamstra, S. J., Yeung, R. Y.-M., Mallon, J. S., & Martire, T. M. (2001). Fiberoptic orotracheal intubation on anesthetized patients: Do manipulation skills learned on a simple model transfer into the operating room? *Anesthesiology*, *95*(2), 343–348. doi:10.1097/00000542-200108000-00014 PMID:11506104

Nair, B. R., & Finucane, P. M. (2003). Reforming Medical Education to Enhance the Management of Chronic Disease. *The Medical Journal of Australia*, *20013*(179), 257–259. PMID:12924974

Nasca, T. J., Philibert, I., Brigham, T., & Flynn, T. C. (2012). The next GME accreditation system—rationale and benefits. *The New England Journal of Medicine*, *366*(11), 1051–1056. doi:10.1056/NEJMsr1200117 PMID:22356262

NEJM Knowledge+ Team. (n.d.a). *ACGME Core Competencies Interpersonal and Communication Skills.* Retrieved from https://knowledgeplus.nejm.org/blog/acgme-core-competencies-interpersonal-and-communication-skills/

NEJM Knowledge+ Team. (n.d.b). *ACGME Core Competencies Medical Knowledge.* Retrieved from https://knowledgeplus.nejm.org/blog/acgme-core-competencies-medical-knowledge/

NEJM Knowledge+ Team. (n.d.c). *ACGME Core Competencies Professionalism. Retrieved from* https://knowledgeplus.nejm.org/blog/acgme-core-competencies-professionalism/

NEJM Knowledge+ Team. (n.d.d). *ACGME Core Competencies Practice-based Learning and Improvement.* Retrieved from https://knowledgeplus.nejm.org/blog/practice-based-learning-and-improvement/

NEJM Knowledge+ Team. (n.d.e). *ACGME Core Competencies Systems-based Practice.* Retrieved from https://knowledgeplus.nejm.org/blog/acgme-core-competencies-systems-based-practice/

Nelson, D., Ziv, A., & Bandali, K. S. (2012). Going glass to digital: Virtual microscopy as a simulation-based revolution in pathology and laboratory science. *Journal of Clinical Pathology*, *65*(10), 877–881. doi:10.1136/jclinpath-2012-200665 PMID:22791768

Newman, P., & Peile, E. (2002). Valuing Learners' experience and supporting further growth: Educational models to help experienced adult learners in medicine. *British Medical Journal*, *325*(7357), 200–202. doi:10.1136/bmj.325.7357.200 PMID:12142310

Ni, A. Y. (2013). Comparing the Effectiveness of Classroom and Online Learning: Teaching Research Methods. *Journal of Public Affairs Education*, *19*(2), 199–215. doi:10.1080/15236803.2013.12001730

Nickson, C. P., & Cadogan, M. D. (2014). Free Open Access Medical education (FOAM) for the emergency physician. *Emergency Medicine Australasia*, *26*(1), 76–83. doi:10.1111/1742-6723.12191 PMID:24495067

Nielsen, P. S., Lindebjerg, J., Rasmussen, J., Starklint, H., Waldstrom, M., & Nielsen, B. (2010). Virtual microscopy: An evaluation of its validity and diagnostic performance in routine histologic diagnosis of skin tumors. *Human Pathology*, *41*(12), 1770–1776. doi:10.1016/j.humpath.2010.05.015 PMID:20869750

Office of the Legislative Counsel. (2010). *Compilation of Patient Protection and Affordable Care Act*. Retrieved from http://housedocs.house.gov/energycommerce/ppacacon.pdf

Oluleye, T. S., Rotimi-Samuel, A., & Adenekan, A. (2016). Mobile phones for retinopathy of prematurity screening in Lagos, Nigeria, Sub-Saharan Africa. *European Journal of Ophthalmology*, *26*, 1–102. PMID:26044377

Ordi, O., Bombí, J. A., Martínez, A., Ramirez, J., Alos, L., Saco, A., ... Ordi, J. (2015). Virtual microscopy in the undergraduate teaching of pathology. *Journal of Pathology Informatics*, *6*(1), 1–6. doi:10.4103/2153-3539.150246 PMID:25722941

Otis, B., & Parvis, B. (2014). Introducing our smart contact lens project [Blog post]. Retrieved from https://googleblog.blogspot.com/2014/01/introducing-our-smart-contact-lens.html

Owen, H. (2012, April). Early use of simulation in medical education. *Simulation in Healthcare*, *7*(2), 102–116. doi:10.1097/SIH.0b013e3182415a91 PMID:22374231

Ozdalga, E., Ozdalga, A., & Ahuja, N. (2012). The smartphone in medicine: A review of current and potential use among physicians and students. *Journal of Medical Internet Research*, *14*(5), e128. doi:10.2196/jmir.1994 PMID:23017375

Ozuah, P. O. (2002). Undergraduate Medical Education: Thoughts on Future Challenges. *BMC Medical Education*, *2*(1), 8–10. doi:10.1186/1472-6920-2-8 PMID:12149136

Palmieri, J. M. D., & Stern, T. M. D. (2009). Lies in the Doctor-Patient Relationship. *Primary Care Companion to the Journal of Clinical Psychiatry*, *11*(4), 163–168. doi:10.4088/PCC.09r00780 PMID:19750068

Pantanowitz, L., Valenstein, P. N., Evans, A. J., Kaplan, K. J., Pfeifer, J. D., Wilbur, D. C., ... Colgan, T. J. (2011). Review of the current state of whole slide imaging in pathology. *Journal of Pathology Informatics*, *2*(1), 36–45. doi:10.4103/2153-3539.83746 PMID:21886892

Parvati, D., Heinrichs, W. L., & Patricia, Y. (2011). CliniSpace: A multiperson 3D online immersive training environment accessible through a browser. Medicine Meets Virtual Reality 18. *NextMed*, *163*, 173.

Pasquel, F. J., Hendrick, A. M., Ryan, M., Cason, E., Ali, M. K., & Narayan, K. M. (2016). Cost-effectiveness of different diabetic retinopathy screening modalities. *Journal of Diabetes Science and Technology*, *10*(2), 301–307. doi:10.1177/1932296815624109 PMID:26719134

Passiment, M., Sacks, H., & Huang, G. (2011, Sept.). *Medical simulation in medical education: Results of an AAMc survey*. Association of American Medical Colleges. Accessed from https://www.aamc.org/download/259760/data/

Patten, D. (2015). Using ultrasound to teach anatomy in the undergraduate medical curriculum: An evaluation of the experiences of tutors and medical students. *Ultrasound*, *23*(1), 18–28. doi:10.1177/1742271X14542173 PMID:27433233

Pelletier, S. (2016). *Game On: Building the Case for Games in Medical Education*. Retrieved from https://news.aamc.org/medical-education/article/game-on-games-medical-education/

Pelley, J. (2018). *The success types style type indicator*. John W. Pelley. Retrieved from https://www.ttuhsc.edu/medicine/medical-education/success-types/lsti.aspx

Pelley, J. W., & Dalley, B. K. (2008). *Success types in medical education: A program for improving academic performance version 1.1*. Retrieved from https://www.ttuhsc.edu/medicine/medical-education/success-types/documents/stsinmeded.pdf

Peltan, I. D., Shiga, T., Gordon, J. A., & Currier, P. F. (2015). Simulation improves procedural protocol adherence during central venous catheter placement: A randomized-controlled trial. *Simulation in Healthcare*, *10*(5), 270–276. doi:10.1097/SIH.0000000000000096 PMID:26154250

Phipps, R. A., & Merisotis, J. P. (1999). *What's the difference: A review of contemporary research on the effectiveness of distance learning in higher education*. Washington, DC: The Institute for Higher Education Policy.

Phua, J., & Lim, T. K. (2008). How residents and interns utilise and perceive the personal digital assistant and UpToDate. *BMC Medical Education*, *8*(1), 39. doi:10.1186/1472-6920-8-39 PMID:18625038

Piatkowska, A., Nowicka, A., Szymanowska, M., Kandziora, M., & Wierzchowiecki, M. (2005). *Evaluation of prognostic value of heart rate variability (HRV) and heart rate turbulence (HRT) in patients with congestive heart failure* EP. Europace Oxford Academic. Retrieved September 12, 2018 from https://academic.oup.com/europace/article/7/Supplement_1/137/696396

Porter, A. L., Pitterle, M. E., & Hayney, M. S. (2014). Comparison of Online Versus Classroom Delivery of an Immunization Elective Course. *American Journal of Pharmaceutical Education*, *78*(5), 96. doi:10.5688/ajpe78596 PMID:24954936

Pramas, T. J., Berres, A., Bjorklund, S. L., & Ellison, S. J. (2014). Using technology to facilitate production of e-discovery. *William Mitchell Law Review*, *40*, 2–8. Retrieved from http://open.mitchellhamline.edu/wmlr/vol40/iss2/8

Prober, C. G., & Heath, C. (2012, May 3). Lecture halls without lectures--a proposal for medical education. *The New England Journal of Medicine*, *366*(18), 1657–1659. doi:10.1056/NEJMp1202451 PMID:22551125

Qin, J., Chui, Y. P., Pang, W. M., Choi, K. S., & Heng, P. A. (2010). Learning blood management in orthopedic surgery through gameplay. *IEEE Computer Graphics and Applications*, *30*(2), 45–57. doi:10.1109/MCG.2009.83 PMID:20650710

Quant, C., Altieri, L., Torres, J., & Craft, N. (2016). The self-perception and usage of medical apps amongst medical students in the United States: A cross-sectional survey. *International Journal of Telemedicine and Applications*, *1-5*. doi:10.1155/2016/3929741 PMID:27688752

Que, S. K., Fraga-Braghiroli, N., Grant-Kels, J. M., Rabinovitz, H. S., Oliviero, M., & Scope, A. (2015). Through the looking glass: Basics and principles of reflectance confocal microscopy. *Journal of the American Academy of Dermatology*, *73*(2), 276–284. doi:10.1016/j.jaad.2015.04.047 PMID:26051696

Que, S. K., Grant-Kels, J. M., Longo, C., & Pellacani, G. (2016). Basics of confocal microscopy and the complexity of diagnosing skin tumors: New imaging tools in clinical practice, diagnostic workflows, cost-estimate, and new trends. *Dermatologic Clinics*, *34*(4), 367–375. doi:10.1016/j.det.2016.05.001 PMID:27692444

Rahman, T., & Amirfar, V. A. (2016). AliveCor Mobile ECG: A smartphone with heart. *Pharmacy Today*, *22*(3), 56. doi:10.1016/j.ptdy.2016.02.026

Ravindran, R., Kashyap, M., Lilis, L., Vivekanantham, S., & Phoenix, G. (2014). Evaluation of an online medical teaching forum. *The Clinical Teacher*, *11*(4), 274–278. doi:10.1111/tct.12139 PMID:24917096

Reznick, R. K., & MacRae, H. (2006). Teaching surgical skills — changes in the wind. *The New England Journal of Medicine*, *355*(25), 2664–2669. doi:10.1056/NEJMra054785 PMID:17182991

Richardson, W. C., Berwick, D. M., Bristow, L. R., Buck, C. R., Cassel, C. K., Chassin, M. R. … Warden, G.L. (2001). Committee on Quality of Health Care in America. Crossing the Quality Chasm: A New Health System for the 21st Century. Institute of Medicine. Washington, DC: National Academies Press.

Robbins, J. A., Bertakis, K. D., Helms, L. J., Azari, R., Callahan, E. J., & Creten, D. A. (1993). The influence of physician practice behaviors on patient satisfaction. *Family Medicine-Kansas City*, *25*, 17–17. PMID:8454118

Rochester, C. D., & Pradel, F. (2008). Students' perceptions and satisfaction with a web-based human nutrition course. *American Journal of Pharmaceutical Education*, *72*(4), 91. doi:10.5688/aj720491 PMID:19002289

Ronquillo, J. G., & Zuckerman, D. M. (2017). Software-related recalls of health information technology and other medical devices: Implications for FDA regulation of digital health. *The Milbank Quarterly*, *95*(3), 535–553. doi:10.1111/1468-0009.12278 PMID:28895231

Rosen, K. R. (2008). The history of medical simulation. *Journal of Critical Care*, *23*(2), 157–166. doi:10.1016/j.jcrc.2007.12.004 PMID:18538206

Rouf, E., Chumley, H. S., & Dobbie, A. E. (2008). Electronic health records in outpatient clinics: Perspectives of third year medical students. *BMC Medical Education*, *8*(1), 13. doi:10.1186/1472-6920-8-13 PMID:18373880

Roy, S., Pantanowitz, L., Amin, M., Seethala, R. R., Ishtiaque, A., Yousem, S. A., ... Hartman, D. J. (2014). Smartphone adapters for digital photomicrography. *Journal of Pathology Informatics*, *5*(1), 24–28. doi:10.4103/2153-3539.137728 PMID:25191623

Ruiz, J. G., Mintzer, M., & Leipzig, R. (2006). The Impact of E-Learning in Medical Education. Academic Medicine, 81(3).

Russo, A., Morescalchi, F., Costagliola, C., Delcassi, L., & Semeraro, F. (n.d.). Comparison of smartphone ophthalmoscopy with slit-lamp biomicroscopy for grading diabetic retinopathy. *American Journal of Ophtalmology, 159*(2), 360-364.

Ryan, G., Lyon, P., Kuma, K., Bell, J., Barnet, S., & Shaw, T. (2007). Online CME: An effective alternative to face-to-face delivery. *Medical Teacher, 29*(8), e251–e257. doi:10.1080/01421590701551698 PMID:18236269

Saco, A., Bombi, J. A., Garcia, A., Ramírez, J., & Ordi, J. (2016). Current status of whole-slide imaging in education. *Pathobiology, 83*(2-3), 79–88. doi:10.1159/000442391 PMID:27101397

Sanna, T., Diener, H. C., Passman, R. S., Di Lazzaro, V., Bernstein, R. A., Morillo, C. A., ... Brachmann, M. D. (2014). Cryptogenic stroke and underlying atrial fibrillation. *The New England Journal of Medicine, 370*(26), 2478–2486. doi:10.1056/NEJMoa1313600 PMID:24963567

Satava, R. M. (2001). Accomplishments and challenges of surgical simulation: Dawning of the next-generation surgical education. *Surgical Endoscopy, 15*(3), 232–241. doi:10.1007004640000369 PMID:11344421

Schnall, R., & Iribarren, S. J. (2015). Review and analysis of existing mobile phone applications for health care-associated infection prevention. *American Journal of Infection Control, 43*(6), 572–576. doi:10.1016/j.ajic.2015.01.021 PMID:25748924

Scoville, S. A., & Buskirk, T. D. (2007). Traditional and virtual microscopy compared experimentally in a classroom setting. *Clinical Anatomy (New York, N.Y.), 20*(5), 565–570. doi:10.1002/ca.20440 PMID:17109440

Shahriari, N., Grant-Kels, J., & Murphy, M. J. (2017). Dermatopathology education in the era of modern technology. *Journal of Cutaneous Pathology, 44*(9), 763–771. doi:10.1111/cup.12980 PMID:28612388

Sherman, S. E. (1989). The history of the ophthalmoscope. *Documenta Ophtalmologica, 71*(2), 221–228. doi:10.1007/BF00163473 PMID:2663401

Simpson, G., & Nicholls, B. (2013). Use of ultrasound in chronic pain medicine. Part 1: Neuraxial and sympathetic blocks. *Continuing Education in Anaesthesia, Critical Care & Pain, 13*(5), 145–151. doi:10.1093/bjaceaccp/mkt013

Sinsky, C., Colligan, L., Li, L., Prgomet, M., Reynolds, Goeders, L., … Blike, G. (2016). Allocation of Physician Time in Ambulatory Practice: A Time and Motion Study in 4 Specialities. *Annals of Internal Medicine.*

Sogunro, O. A. (2015). Motivating factors for adult learners in higher education. *International Journal of Higher Education*, *4*(1), 22–37.

SonoSim. (n.d.). Retrieved from www.sonosim.com

Sosa, E. (1993). Epistemology, Realism, and Truth: The First Philosophical Perspectives Lecture. In *Philosophical Perspectives* (Vol. 7, pp. 1–16). Ridgeview Publishing.

Stanford25. (n.d.). Retrieved from https://stanfordmedicine25.stanford.edu

Stern, D. T., & Papadakis, M. (2006). The developing physician—becoming a professional. *The New England Journal of Medicine*, *355*(17), 1794–1799. doi:10.1056/NEJMra054783 PMID:17065641

Stokes, B. G. (2005). Videogames have changed: Time to consider Serious Games'? *Development Education Journal*, *11*(3), 12.

Strachan, I. W. (2000). Technology leaps all around propel advances in simulators. *National Defense Magazine*. Accessed November 19, 2007 from http://www.nationaldefensemagazine.org

Stuart, R. K., Shikora, S. A., Akerman, P., Lowell, J. A., Baxter, J. K., Apovian, C., ... Bistrian, B. R. (1990). Incidence of arrhythmia with central venous catheter insertion and exchange. *JPEN. Journal of Parenteral and Enteral Nutrition*, *14*(2), 152–155. doi:10.1177/0148607190014002152 PMID:2112623

Sukalich, S., Elliott, J. O., & Ruffner, G. (2014). Teaching medical error disclosure to residents using patient-centered simulation training. *Acad Med J Assoc Am Med Coll*, *89*(1), 136–144. doi:10.1097/ACM.0000000000000046 PMID:24280843

Summers, J. J., Waigandt, A., & Whittaker, T. A. (2005). A comparison of student achievement and satisfaction in an online versusa traditional face-to-face statistics class. *Innovations in Higher Education.*, *29*(3), 233–250. doi:10.100710755-005-1938-x

Swanson, S., Ku, T., & Chou, C. (2011). Assessment of direct ophthalmoscopy using plastic canisters. *Medical Education*, *45*(5), 520–521. doi:10.1111/j.1365-2923.2011.03987.x PMID:21486343

Swing, S. R. (2007). The ACGME outcome project: Retrospective and prospective. *Medical Teacher*, *29*(7), 648–654. doi:10.1080/01421590701392903 PMID:18236251

Sydow, L., & Cheney, S. (2018). 2017 retrospective: A monumental year for the app economy [Blog post]. Retrieved from https://www.appannie.com/en/insights/market-data/app-annie-2017-retrospective/

Szu, H., Hsu, C., Moon, G., Landa, J., Nakajima, H., & Hata, Y. (2013). Smartphone homecare monitoring of hearts. *Applied Computational Intelligence and Soft Computing*, *2013*, 1–10. doi:10.1155/2013/983515

Taekman, J. M., Segall, N., Hobbs, E., & Wright, M. (2007). 3DiTeams–Healthcare team training in a virtual environment. *Anesthesiology*, *107*(A2145), A2145.

Tegtmeyer, K., Ibsen, L., & Goldstein, B. (2001). Computer-assisted learning in critical care: From ENIAC to HAL. *Critical Care Medicine*, *29*(8Suppl), N177–N182. doi:10.1097/00003246-200108001-00006 PMID:11496040

Teixeira, P. J., Carraça, E. V., Markland, D., Silva, M. N., & Ryan, R. M. (2012). Exercise, physical activity, and self-determination theory: A systematic review. *The International Journal of Behavioral Nutrition and Physical Activity*, *9*(1), 78. doi:10.1186/1479-5868-9-78 PMID:22726453

ten Cate, O., & Billett, S. (2014). Competency-based medical education: Origins, perspectives and potentialities. *Medical Education*, *48*(3), 325–332. doi:10.1111/medu.12355 PMID:24528467

The American Board of Anesthesiology. (2016). *Standardized Oral Examination (SOE) and Objective Structured Clinical Examination (OSCE)*. Raleigh, NC: ABA. Accessed from http://www.theaba.org/TRAINING-PROGRAMS/APPLIED-(Staged-Exam)/About-APPLIED-(Staged-Exam)

The Echo Project. (n.d.). Retrieved from https://echo.unm.edu

Thomas, P. A., Kern, D. E., Hughes, M. T., & Chen, B. Y. (Eds.). (2016). *Curriculum Development for Medical Education: A Six-Step Approach*. Baltimore, MD: John Hopkins University Press.

Thompson, L. R., Leung, C. G., Green, B., Lipps, J., Schaffernocker, T., Ledford, C., ... Kman, N. E. (2017). Development of an assessment for Entrustable Professional Activity (EPA) 10: Emergent patient management. *The Western Journal of Emergency Medicine*, *18*(1), 35–42. doi:10.5811/westjem.2016.10.31479 PMID:28116006

Thorstenson, S., Molin, J., & Lundstrom, C. (2014). Implementation of large-scale routine diagnostics using whole slide imaging in Sweden: Digital pathology experiences 2006-2013. *Journal of Pathology Informatics*, *5*(1), 14. doi:10.4103/2153-3539.129452 PMID:24843825

Torsher, L., & Craigo, P. (2014). Simulation in anesthesiology. In A. I. Levine & ... (Eds.), *The Comprehensive Textbook of Healthcare Simulation* (pp. 257–285). New York: Springer.

Townsend, D. (2009). *Cadaver dissection teams at Kansas State University*. Retrieved from https://www.k-state.edu/ksuhonors/courses/BIOL340-Sp10.htm

Treanor, D., Lim, C. H., Magee, D., Bulpitt, A., & Quirke, P. (2009). Tracking with virtual slides: A tool to study diagnostic error in histopathology. *Histopathology*, *55*(1), 37–45. doi:10.1111/j.1365-2559.2009.03325.x PMID:19614765

Treskes, R. W., Gielen, W., Wermer, M. J., Grauss, R. W., Alem, A. P., Dehnavi, R. A., ... Trines, S. A. (2017). Mobile phones in cryptogenic stroke patients bringing single lead ECGs for atrial fibrillation detection (MOBILE-AF): Study protocol for a randomized controlled trial. *Trials*, *18*(1), 402. doi:10.118613063-017-2131-0 PMID:28851409

Triola, M. M., & Holloway, W. J. (2011). Enhanced virtual microscopy for collaborative education. *BMC Medical Education*, *11*(1), 4–10. doi:10.1186/1472-6920-11-4 PMID:21269474

Tsai, C.-C., Chuang, S.-C., Liang, J.-C., & Tsai, M.-J. (2011). Self-efficacy in Internet-based Learning Environments: A Literature Review. *Journal of Educational Technology & Society*, *14*(4), 222–240.

Tuoriniemi, P., & Schott-Baer, D. (2008). Implementing a high-fidelity simulation program in a community college setting. *Nursing Education Perspectives*, *29*(2), 105–109. doi:10.1097/00024776-200803000-00012 PMID:18459626

U.S. Department of Education, Office of Planning, Evaluation, and Policy Development. (2010). *Evaluation of Evidence-Based Practices in Online Learning: A Meta-Analysis and Review of Online Learning Studies*. Washington, DC: Author.

Ulger, F., Esen, S., Dilek, A., Yanik, K., Gunaydin, M., & Leblebicioglu, H. (2009). Are we aware how contaminated our mobile phones with nosocomial pathogens? *Annals of Clinical Microbiology and Antimicrobials*, *8*(1), 7. doi:10.1186/1476-0711-8-7 PMID:19267892

Umudum, H. (2015). Smart phones and microscopic image capturing: Searching, finding, capturing, talking about, as well as sharing microscopic images of pathologic conditions form another type of learning module. *Archives of Pathology & Laboratory Medicine, 139*(7), 847. doi:10.5858/arpa.2014-0436-LE PMID:26125424

UNSW Sydney iLearn Resources. (n.d.). Retrieved from https://teaching.unsw.edu.au/assessment-blog-wiki-or-forum-which-should-you-use

Ventola, C. L. (2014). Mobile devices and apps for health care professionals: uses and benefits. *Pharmacy and Therapeutics, 39*(5), 356-364. Retrieved from https://www.ncbi.nlm.nih.gov/pmc/articles/PMC4029126/pdf/ptj3905356.pdf

Virtual Heroes 3diteams. (n.d.). Retrieved from http://www.virtualheroes.com/projects/3diteams

Von der Pütten, A., Krämer, N., & Gratch, J. (2010). How our Personality Shapes our Interactions with Virtual Characters-implications for Research and Development. In *Proceedings of the 10th International Conference on Intelligent Virtual Agents* (pp. 208-221). Springer.

Wald, H. S., Dube, C. E., & Anthony, D. C. (2007). Untangling the Web—The impact of Internet use on health care and the physician–patient relationship. *Patient Education and Counseling, 68*(3), 218–224. doi:10.1016/j.pec.2007.05.016 PMID:17920226

Wald, H. S., George, P., Reis, S. P., & Taylor, J. S. (2014). Electronic health record training in undergraduate medical education: Bridging theory to practice with curricula for empowering patient-and relationship-centered care in the computerized setting. *Academic Medicine, 89*(3), 380–386. doi:10.1097/ACM.0000000000000131 PMID:24448045

Walkowski, S., Lundin, M., Szymas, J., & Lundin, J. (2014). Students' performance during practical examination on whole slide images using view path tracking. *Diagnostic Pathology, 9*(1), 208–215. doi:10.118613000-014-0208-6 PMID:25358824

Walrod, B. J., Schroeder, A., Conroy, M. J., Boucher, L. C., Bockbrader, M., Way, D. P., ... Bahner, D. P. (2018). Does Ultrasound-Enhanced Instruction of Musculoskeletal Anatomy Improve Physical Examination Skills of First-Year Medical Students? *Journal of Ultrasound in Medicine, 37*(1), 225–232. doi:10.1002/jum.14322 PMID:28795411

Walsh, J. A. III, Topol, E. J., & Steinhubl, S. R. (2014). Novel wireless devices for cardiac monitoring. *Circulation, 130*(7), 573–581. doi:10.1161/CIRCULATIONAHA.114.009024 PMID:25114186

Weaker, F. J., & Herbert, D. C. (2009). Transition of a dental histology course from light to virtual. *Microscopy, 73*(10), 1213–1221. PMID:19805786

Weinberger, S. E., Pereira, A. G., Iobst, W. F., Mechaber, A. J., & Bronze, M. S. (2010). Competency-based education and training in internal medicine. *Annals of Internal Medicine, 153*(11), 751–756. doi:10.7326/0003-4819-153-11-201012070-00009 PMID:21135298

White, T. (n.d.). *Body image: Computerized table lets students do virtual dissection*. Retrieved January 20, 2018, from Https://med.stanford.edu/news/all-news/2011/05/body-image-computerized-table-lets-students-do-virtual-dissection.html

Wiggins, G. (2007, November 15). What is an essential question? *Big Ideas*. Retrieved from http://www.authenticeducation.org/ae_bigideas/article.lasso?artid=53

Wilson, L. O. (2014). *What are essential questions?* Retrieved from https://thesecondprinciple.com/teaching-essentials/essential-questions/

Wilson, A. B., Taylor, M. A., Klein, B. A., Sugrue, M. K., Whipple, E. C., & Brokaw, J. J. (2016). Meta-analysis and review of learner performance and preference: Virtual versus optical microscopy. *Medical Education, 50*(4), 428–440. doi:10.1111/medu.12944 PMID:26995482

Winkelmann, R. R., Farberg, A. S., Glazer, A. M., Cockerell, C. J., Sober, A. J., Siegel, D. M., ... Rigel, D. S. (2017). Integrating skin cancer-related technologies into clinical Practice. *Dermatologic Clinics, 35*(4), 565–576. doi:10.1016/j.det.2017.06.018 PMID:28886814

World Health Organization (WHO). (2010). *Framework for action on Interprofessional education & collaborative practice*. Geneva: World Health Organization. Retrieved from http:/whqlibdoc.who.int/hq/2010/WHO.HRH.HPN 10.3.eng.pdf

Woyke, E. (2014). *The smartphone: Anatomy of an industry* (1st ed.). New York, NY: The New Press.

Yang, D., Wei, Y. K., Xue, F. S., Deng, X. M., & Zhi, J. (2016). Simulation-based airway management training: Application and looking forward. *Journal of Anesthesia, 30*(2), 284–289. doi:10.100700540-015-2116-7 PMID:26671260

Zhou, C., Yu, Y., Xue, R., & Elston, D. M. (2016). High-quality digital photomicrography utilizing a smartphone without adapter. *Journal of Cutaneous Pathology*, *43*(1), 82–84. doi:10.1111/cup.12561 PMID:26280458

Zion Market Research. (2017). *mHealth market by devices, by stakeholder, by service, by therapeutics, and by applications: Global industry perspective, comprehensive analysis, and forecast, 2014 - 2022*. Retrieved from https://www.zionmarketresearch.com/report/mhealth-market

Ziv, A., Ben-David, S., & Ziv, M. (2005). Simulation[-]based medical education: An opportunity to learn from errors. *Medical Teacher*, *27*(3), 193–199. doi:10.1080/01421590500126718 PMID:16011941

Related References

To continue our tradition of advancing information science and technology research, we have compiled a list of recommended IGI Global readings. These references will provide additional information and guidance to further enrich your knowledge and assist you with your own research and future publications.

Abu Seman, S. A., & Ramayah, T. (2017). Are We Ready to App?: A Study on mHealth Apps, Its Future, and Trends in Malaysia Context. In J. Pelet (Ed.), *Mobile Platforms, Design, and Apps for Social Commerce* (pp. 69–83). Hershey, PA: IGI Global. doi:10.4018/978-1-5225-2469-4.ch005

Aggarwal, S., & Azad, V. (2017). A Hybrid System Based on FMM and MLP to Diagnose Heart Disease. In S. Bhattacharyya, S. De, I. Pan, & P. Dutta (Eds.), *Intelligent Multidimensional Data Clustering and Analysis* (pp. 293–325). Hershey, PA: IGI Global. doi:10.4018/978-1-5225-1776-4.ch011

Akaichi, J., & Mhadhbi, L. (2016). A Clinical Decision Support System: Ontology-Driven Approach for Effective Emergency Management. In J. Moon & M. Galea (Eds.), *Improving Health Management through Clinical Decision Support Systems* (pp. 270–294). Hershey, PA: IGI Global. doi:10.4018/978-1-4666-9432-3.ch013

Akerkar, R. (2016). Towards an Intelligent Integrated Approach for Clinical Decision Support. In A. Aggarwal (Ed.), *Managing Big Data Integration in the Public Sector* (pp. 187–205). Hershey, PA: IGI Global. doi:10.4018/978-1-4666-9649-5.ch011

Al-Busaidi, S. S. (2018). Interdisciplinary Relationships Between Medicine and Social Sciences. In M. Al-Suqri, A. Al-Kindi, S. AlKindi, & N. Saleem (Eds.), *Promoting Interdisciplinarity in Knowledge Generation and Problem Solving* (pp. 124–137). Hershey, PA: IGI Global. doi:10.4018/978-1-5225-3878-3.ch009

Al Kareh, T., & Thoumy, M. (2018). The Impact of Health Information Digitization on the Physiotherapist-Patient Relationship: A Pilot Study of the Lebanese Community. *International Journal of Healthcare Information Systems and Informatics, 13*(2), 29–53. doi:10.4018/IJHISI.2018040103

Alenzuela, R. (2017). Research, Leadership, and Resource-Sharing Initiatives: The Role of Local Library Consortia in Access to Medical Information. In S. Ram (Ed.), *Library and Information Services for Bioinformatics Education and Research* (pp. 199–211). Hershey, PA: IGI Global. doi:10.4018/978-1-5225-1871-6.ch012

Ameri, H., Alizadeh, S., & Noughabi, E. A. (2017). Application of Data Mining Techniques in Clinical Decision Making: A Literature Review and Classification. In E. Noughabi, B. Raahemi, A. Albadvi, & B. Far (Eds.), *Handbook of Research on Data Science for Effective Healthcare Practice and Administration* (pp. 257–295). Hershey, PA: IGI Global. doi:10.4018/978-1-5225-2515-8.ch012

Anand, S. (2017). Medical Image Enhancement Using Edge Information-Based Methods. In B. Singh (Ed.), *Computational Tools and Techniques for Biomedical Signal Processing* (pp. 123–148). Hershey, PA: IGI Global. doi:10.4018/978-1-5225-0660-7.ch006

Angjellari-Dajci, F., Sapienza, C., Lawless, W. F., & Kavanagh, K. (2016). Human Capital Accumulation in Medical Simulated Learning Environments: A Framework for Economic Evaluation. In M. Russ (Ed.), *Quantitative Multidisciplinary Approaches in Human Capital and Asset Management* (pp. 65–88). Hershey, PA: IGI Global. doi:10.4018/978-1-4666-9652-5.ch004

Anil, M., Ayyildiz-Tamis, D., Tasdemir, S., Sendemir-Urkmez, A., & Gulce-Iz, S. (2016). Bioinspired Materials and Biocompatibility. In M. Bououdina (Ed.), *Emerging Research on Bioinspired Materials Engineering* (pp. 294–322). Hershey, PA: IGI Global. doi:10.4018/978-1-4666-9811-6.ch011

Anton, J. L., Soriano, J. V., Martinez, M. I., & Garcia, F. B. (2018). Comprehensive E-Learning Appraisal System. In M. Khosrow-Pour, D.B.A. (Ed.), Encyclopedia of Information Science and Technology, Fourth Edition (pp. 5787-5799). Hershey, PA: IGI Global. doi:10.4018/978-1-5225-2255-3.ch503

Arabi, M. (2016). Redesigning the Organizational Structure to Reach Efficiency: The Case of Ministry of Health and Medical Education of Iran. In R. Gholipour & K. Rouzbehani (Eds.), *Social, Economic, and Political Perspectives on Public Health Policy-Making* (pp. 257–294). Hershey, PA: IGI Global. doi:10.4018/978-1-4666-9944-1.ch012

Assis-Hassid, S., Heart, T., Reychav, I., & Pliskin, J. S. (2016). Modelling Factors Affecting Patient-Doctor-Computer Communication in Primary Care. *International Journal of Reliable and Quality E-Healthcare, 5*(1), 1–17. doi:10.4018/IJRQEH.2016010101

Atzori, B., Hoffman, H. G., Vagnoli, L., Messeri, A., & Grotto, R. L. (2018). Virtual Reality as Distraction Technique for Pain Management in Children and Adolescents. In M. Khosrow-Pour, D.B.A. (Ed.), Encyclopedia of Information Science and Technology, Fourth Edition (pp. 5955-5965). Hershey, PA: IGI Global. doi:10.4018/978-1-5225-2255-3.ch518

Audibert, M., Mathonnat, J., Pélissier, A., & Huang, X. X. (2018). The Impact of the New Rural Cooperative Medical Scheme on Township Hospitals' Utilization and Income Structure in Weifang Prefecture, China. In I. Management Association (Ed.), Health Economics and Healthcare Reform: Breakthroughs in Research and Practice (pp. 109-121). Hershey, PA: IGI Global. doi:10.4018/978-1-5225-3168-5.ch007

Ayyachamy, S. (2016). Analysis and Comparison of Developed 2D Medical Image Database Design using Registration Scheme, Retrieval Scheme, and Bag-of-Visual-Words. In N. Dey & A. Ashour (Eds.), *Classification and Clustering in Biomedical Signal Processing* (pp. 149–168). Hershey, PA: IGI Global. doi:10.4018/978-1-5225-0140-4.ch007

Babalola, A. C. (2016). Literacy and Decision Making on Health Issues among Married Women in Southwest Nigeria. In V. Wang (Ed.), *Handbook of Research on Advancing Health Education through Technology* (pp. 191–212). Hershey, PA: IGI Global. doi:10.4018/978-1-4666-9494-1.ch009

Babu, A., & Ayyappan, S. (2017). A Methodological Evaluation of Crypto-Watermarking System for Medical Images. In C. Bhatt & S. Peddoju (Eds.), *Cloud Computing Systems and Applications in Healthcare* (pp. 189–217). Hershey, PA: IGI Global. doi:10.4018/978-1-5225-1002-4.ch010

Bakke, A. (2017). Ethos in E-Health: From Informational to Interactive Websites. In M. Folk & S. Apostel (Eds.), *Establishing and Evaluating Digital Ethos and Online Credibility* (pp. 85–103). Hershey, PA: IGI Global. doi:10.4018/978-1-5225-1072-7.ch005

Bali, S. (2018). Enhancing the Reach of Health Care Through Telemedicine: Status and New Possibilities in Developing Countries. In U. Pandey & V. Indrakanti (Eds.), *Open and Distance Learning Initiatives for Sustainable Development* (pp. 339–354). Hershey, PA: IGI Global. doi:10.4018/978-1-5225-2621-6.ch019

Barrett, T. E. (2018). Essentials for Education and Training for Tomorrow's Physicians. In C. Smith (Ed.), *Exploring the Pressures of Medical Education From a Mental Health and Wellness Perspective* (pp. 230–252). Hershey, PA: IGI Global. doi:10.4018/978-1-5225-2811-1.ch010

Barrett, T. J. (2016). Knowledge in Action: Fostering Health Education through Technology. In V. Wang (Ed.), *Handbook of Research on Advancing Health Education through Technology* (pp. 39–62). Hershey, PA: IGI Global. doi:10.4018/978-1-4666-9494-1.ch003

Berrahal, S., & Boudriga, N. (2017). The Risks of Wearable Technologies to Individuals and Organizations. In A. Marrington, D. Kerr, & J. Gammack (Eds.), *Managing Security Issues and the Hidden Dangers of Wearable Technologies* (pp. 18–46). Hershey, PA: IGI Global. doi:10.4018/978-1-5225-1016-1.ch002

Bhagat, A. P., & Atique, M. (2016). Medical Image Mining Using Fuzzy Connectedness Image Segmentation: Efficient Retrieval of Patients' Stored Images. In W. Karâa & N. Dey (Eds.), *Biomedical Image Analysis and Mining Techniques for Improved Health Outcomes* (pp. 184–209). Hershey, PA: IGI Global. doi:10.4018/978-1-4666-8811-7.ch009

Bhargava, P. (2018). Blended Learning: An Effective Application to Clinical Teaching. In S. Tang & C. Lim (Eds.), *Preparing the Next Generation of Teachers for 21st Century Education* (pp. 302–320). Hershey, PA: IGI Global. doi:10.4018/978-1-5225-4080-9.ch018

Binh, N. T., & Tuyet, V. T. (2016). The Combination of Adaptive Filters to Improve the Quality of Medical Images in New Wavelet Domain. In N. Dey & A. Ashour (Eds.), *Classification and Clustering in Biomedical Signal Processing* (pp. 46–76). Hershey, PA: IGI Global. doi:10.4018/978-1-5225-0140-4.ch003

Bird, J. L. (2017). Writing Healing Narratives. In V. Bryan & J. Bird (Eds.), *Healthcare Community Synergism between Patients, Practitioners, and Researchers* (pp. 1–28). Hershey, PA: IGI Global. doi:10.4018/978-1-5225-0640-9.ch001

Bottrighi, A., Leonardi, G., Piovesan, L., & Terenziani, P. (2016). Knowledge-Based Support to the Treatment of Exceptions in Computer Interpretable Clinical Guidelines. *International Journal of Knowledge-Based Organizations*, *6*(3), 1–27. doi:10.4018/IJKBO.2016070101

Bougoulias, K., Kouris, I., Prasinos, M., Giokas, K., & Koutsouris, D. (2017). Ob/Gyn EMR Software: A Solution for Obstetricians and Gynecologists. In A. Moumtzoglou (Ed.), *Design, Development, and Integration of Reliable Electronic Healthcare Platforms* (pp. 101–111). Hershey, PA: IGI Global. doi:10.4018/978-1-5225-1724-5.ch006

Bouslimi, R., Ayadi, M. G., & Akaichi, J. (2018). Medical Image Retrieval in Healthcare Social Networks. *International Journal of Healthcare Information Systems and Informatics, 13*(2), 13–28. doi:10.4018/IJHISI.2018040102

Bouzaabia, O., Bouzaabia, R., & Mejri, K. (2017). Role of Internet in the Development of Medical Tourism Service in Tunisia. In A. Capatina & E. Rancati (Eds.), *Key Challenges and Opportunities in Web Entrepreneurship* (pp. 211–241). Hershey, PA: IGI Global. doi:10.4018/978-1-5225-2466-3.ch009

Briz-Ponce, L., Juanes-Méndez, J. A., & García-Peñalvo, F. J. (2016). The Role of Gender in Technology Acceptance for Medical Education. In M. Cruz-Cunha, I. Miranda, R. Martinho, & R. Rijo (Eds.), *Encyclopedia of E-Health and Telemedicine* (pp. 1013–1027). Hershey, PA: IGI Global. doi:10.4018/978-1-4666-9978-6.ch079

Briz-Ponce, L., Juanes-Méndez, J. A., & García-Peñalvo, F. J. (2016). A Research Contribution to the Analysis of Mobile Devices in Higher Education from Medical Students' Point of View. In L. Briz-Ponce, J. Juanes-Méndez, & F. García-Peñalvo (Eds.), *Handbook of Research on Mobile Devices and Applications in Higher Education Settings* (pp. 196–221). Hershey, PA: IGI Global. doi:10.4018/978-1-5225-0256-2.ch009

Brown-Jackson, K. L. (2018). Telemedicine and Telehealth: Academics Engaging the Community in a Call to Action. In S. Burton (Ed.), *Engaged Scholarship and Civic Responsibility in Higher Education* (pp. 166–193). Hershey, PA: IGI Global. doi:10.4018/978-1-5225-3649-9.ch008

Bwalya, K. J. (2017). Next Wave of Tele-Medicine: Virtual Presence of Medical Personnel. In K. Moahi, K. Bwalya, & P. Sebina (Eds.), *Health Information Systems and the Advancement of Medical Practice in Developing Countries* (pp. 168–180). Hershey, PA: IGI Global. doi:10.4018/978-1-5225-2262-1.ch010

Carlton, E. L., Holsinger, J. W. Jr, & Anunobi, N. (2016). Physician Engagement with Health Information Technology: Implications for Practice and Professionalism. *International Journal of Computers in Clinical Practice, 1*(2), 51–73. doi:10.4018/IJCCP.2016070103

Castillo-Page, L., Eliason, J., Conrad, S. S., & Nivet, M. A. (2016). Diversity in Undergraduate Medical Education: An Examination of Organizational Culture and Climate in Medical Schools. In C. Scott & J. Sims (Eds.), *Developing Workforce Diversity Programs, Curriculum, and Degrees in Higher Education* (pp. 304–326). Hershey, PA: IGI Global. doi:10.4018/978-1-5225-0209-8.ch016

Cebeci, H. I., & Hiziroglu, A. (2016). Review of Business Intelligence and Intelligent Systems in Healthcare Domain. In N. Celebi (Ed.), *Intelligent Techniques for Data Analysis in Diverse Settings* (pp. 192–206). Hershey, PA: IGI Global. doi:10.4018/978-1-5225-0075-9.ch009

Celik, G. (2018). Determining Headache Diseases With Genetic Algorithm. In U. Kose, G. Guraksin, & O. Deperlioglu (Eds.), *Nature-Inspired Intelligent Techniques for Solving Biomedical Engineering Problems* (pp. 249–262). Hershey, PA: IGI Global. doi:10.4018/978-1-5225-4769-3.ch012

Chakraborty, C., Gupta, B., & Ghosh, S. K. (2016). Mobile Telemedicine Systems for Remote Patient's Chronic Wound Monitoring. In A. Moumtzoglou (Ed.), *M-Health Innovations for Patient-Centered Care* (pp. 213–239). Hershey, PA: IGI Global. doi:10.4018/978-1-4666-9861-1.ch011

Chakraborty, S., Chatterjee, S., Ashour, A. S., Mali, K., & Dey, N. (2018). Intelligent Computing in Medical Imaging: A Study. In N. Dey (Ed.), *Advancements in Applied Metaheuristic Computing* (pp. 143–163). Hershey, PA: IGI Global. doi:10.4018/978-1-5225-4151-6.ch006

Chavez, A., & Kovarik, C. (2017). Open Source Technology for Medical Practice in Developing Countries. In K. Moahi, K. Bwalya, & P. Sebina (Eds.), *Health Information Systems and the Advancement of Medical Practice in Developing Countries* (pp. 33–59). Hershey, PA: IGI Global. doi:10.4018/978-1-5225-2262-1.ch003

Chen, E. T. (2016). Examining the Influence of Information Technology on Modern Health Care. In P. Manolitzas, E. Grigoroudis, N. Matsatsinis, & D. Yannacopoulos (Eds.), *Effective Methods for Modern Healthcare Service Quality and Evaluation* (pp. 110–136). Hershey, PA: IGI Global. doi:10.4018/978-1-4666-9961-8.ch006

Chin, S. (2016). Surviving Sandy: Recovering Collections after a Natural Disaster. In E. Decker & J. Townes (Eds.), *Handbook of Research on Disaster Management and Contingency Planning in Modern Libraries* (pp. 366–388). Hershey, PA: IGI Global. doi:10.4018/978-1-4666-8624-3.ch016

Chojnacki, M., & Wójcik, A. (2016). Security and the Role of New Technologies and Innovation in Medical Ethics. In A. Rosiek & K. Leksowski (Eds.), *Organizational Culture and Ethics in Modern Medicine* (pp. 52–77). Hershey, PA: IGI Global. doi:10.4018/978-1-4666-9658-7.ch003

Cılız, N., Yıldırım, H., & Temizel, Ş. (2016). Structure Development for Effective Medical Waste and Hazardous Waste Management System. In U. Akkucuk (Ed.), *Handbook of Research on Waste Management Techniques for Sustainability* (pp. 303–327). Hershey, PA: IGI Global. doi:10.4018/978-1-4666-9723-2.ch016

Ciufudean, C. (2018). Innovative Formalism for Biological Data Analysis. In M. Khosrow-Pour, D.B.A. (Ed.), Encyclopedia of Information Science and Technology, Fourth Edition (pp. 1814-1824). Hershey, PA: IGI Global. doi:10.4018/978-1-5225-2255-3.ch158

Ciufudean, C., & Ciufudean, O. (2016). Tele-Monitoring for Medical Diagnosis Availability. In M. Cruz-Cunha, I. Miranda, R. Martinho, & R. Rijo (Eds.), *Encyclopedia of E-Health and Telemedicine* (pp. 401–411). Hershey, PA: IGI Global. doi:10.4018/978-1-4666-9978-6.ch032

Colaguori, R., & Danesi, M. (2017). Medical Semiotics: A Revisitation and an Exhortation. *International Journal of Semiotics and Visual Rhetoric*, *1*(1), 11–18. doi:10.4018/IJSVR.2017010102

Cole, A. W., & Salek, T. A. (2017). Adopting a Parasocial Connection to Overcome Professional Kakoethos in Online Health Information. In M. Folk & S. Apostel (Eds.), *Establishing and Evaluating Digital Ethos and Online Credibility* (pp. 104–120). Hershey, PA: IGI Global. doi:10.4018/978-1-5225-1072-7.ch006

Contreras, E. C., & Puente, G. J. (2016). How to Identify Rheumatic Diseases by General Physicians. In T. Gasmelseid (Ed.), *Advancing Pharmaceutical Processes and Tools for Improved Health Outcomes* (pp. 136–166). Hershey, PA: IGI Global. doi:10.4018/978-1-5225-0248-7.ch006

D'Andrea, A., Ferri, F., & Grifoni, P. (2016). RFID Technologies in Healthcare Setting: Applications and Future Perspectives. *International Journal of Computers in Clinical Practice*, *1*(1), 15–27. doi:10.4018/IJCCP.2016010102

Damianakis, A., Kallonis, P., Loudos, G., Tsatsos, D., & Tsoukalis, A. (2016). Exploiting 3D Medical Equipment Simulations to Support Biomedical Engineering Academic Courses: Design Methodology and Implementation in a Small Scale National Project. In B. Khan (Ed.), *Revolutionizing Modern Education through Meaningful E-Learning Implementation* (pp. 277–295). Hershey, PA: IGI Global. doi:10.4018/978-1-5225-0466-5.ch015

Demiroz, E. (2016). Principles of Instructional Design for E-Learning and Online Learning Practices: Implications for Medical Education. In V. Wang (Ed.), *Handbook of Research on Advancing Health Education through Technology* (pp. 419–451). Hershey, PA: IGI Global. doi:10.4018/978-1-4666-9494-1.ch018

Deperlioglu, O. (2018). Intelligent Techniques Inspired by Nature and Used in Biomedical Engineering. In U. Kose, G. Guraksin, & O. Deperlioglu (Eds.), *Nature-Inspired Intelligent Techniques for Solving Biomedical Engineering Problems* (pp. 51–77). Hershey, PA: IGI Global. doi:10.4018/978-1-5225-4769-3.ch003

Dey, N., & Ashour, A. S. (2018). Meta-Heuristic Algorithms in Medical Image Segmentation: A Review. In N. Dey (Ed.), *Advancements in Applied Metaheuristic Computing* (pp. 185–203). Hershey, PA: IGI Global. doi:10.4018/978-1-5225-4151-6.ch008

Dey, N., Ashour, A. S., & Althoupety, A. S. (2017). Thermal Imaging in Medical Science. In V. Santhi (Ed.), *Recent Advances in Applied Thermal Imaging for Industrial Applications* (pp. 87–117). Hershey, PA: IGI Global. doi:10.4018/978-1-5225-2423-6.ch004

Di Virgilio, F., Camillo, A. A., & Camillo, I. C. (2017). The Impact of Social Network on Italian Users' Behavioural Intention for the Choice of a Medical Tourist Destination. *International Journal of Tourism and Hospitality Management in the Digital Age*, *1*(1), 36–49. doi:10.4018/IJTHMDA.2017010103

Dias, C. M., Ribeiro, A. G., & Furtado, S. F. (2016). An Overview about the Use of Healthcare Applications on Mobile Devices. In M. Cruz-Cunha, I. Miranda, R. Martinho, & R. Rijo (Eds.), *Encyclopedia of E-Health and Telemedicine* (pp. 285–298). Hershey, PA: IGI Global. doi:10.4018/978-1-4666-9978-6.ch024

Dogra, A. K., & Dogra, P. (2017). The Medical Tourism Industry in the BRIC Nations: An Indian Analysis. In M. Dhiman (Ed.), *Opportunities and Challenges for Tourism and Hospitality in the BRIC Nations* (pp. 320–336). Hershey, PA: IGI Global. doi:10.4018/978-1-5225-0708-6.ch020

Drowos, J. L., & Wood, S. K. (2017). Preparing Future Physicians to Adapt to the Changing Health Care System: Promoting Humanism through Curricular Design. In V. Bryan & J. Bird (Eds.), *Healthcare Community Synergism between Patients, Practitioners, and Researchers* (pp. 106–125). Hershey, PA: IGI Global. doi:10.4018/978-1-5225-0640-9.ch006

Dulam, K. (2017). Medical Patents and Impact on Availability and Affordability of Essential Medicines in India. In R. Aggarwal & R. Kaur (Eds.), *Patent Law and Intellectual Property in the Medical Field* (pp. 41–57). Hershey, PA: IGI Global. doi:10.4018/978-1-5225-2414-4.ch003

Dutta, P. (2017). Decision Making in Medical Diagnosis via Distance Measures on Interval Valued Fuzzy Sets. *International Journal of System Dynamics Applications*, *6*(4), 63–83. doi:10.4018/IJSDA.2017100104

Edoh, T. O., Pawar, P. A., Brügge, B., & Teege, G. (2016). A Multidisciplinary Remote Healthcare Delivery System to Increase Health Care Access, Pathology Screening, and Treatment in Developing Countries: The Case of Benin. *International Journal of Healthcare Information Systems and Informatics*, *11*(4), 1–31. doi:10.4018/IJHISI.2016100101

El Guemhioui, K., & Demurjian, S. A. (2017). Semantic Reconciliation of Electronic Health Records Using Semantic Web Technologies. *International Journal of Information Technology and Web Engineering*, *12*(2), 26–48. doi:10.4018/IJITWE.2017040102

Ellouze, N., Rekhis, S., & Boudriga, N. (2016). Forensic Investigation of Digital Crimes in Healthcare Applications. In O. Isafiade & A. Bagula (Eds.), *Data Mining Trends and Applications in Criminal Science and Investigations* (pp. 169–210). Hershey, PA: IGI Global. doi:10.4018/978-1-5225-0463-4.ch007

Eneanya, A. N. (2016). Health Policy Implementation and Its Barriers: The Case Study of US Health System. In R. Gholipour & K. Rouzbehani (Eds.), *Social, Economic, and Political Perspectives on Public Health Policy-Making* (pp. 42–63). Hershey, PA: IGI Global. doi:10.4018/978-1-4666-9944-1.ch003

Entico, G. J. (2016). Knowledge Management and the Medical Health Librarians: A Perception Study. In J. Yap, M. Perez, M. Ayson, & G. Entico (Eds.), *Special Library Administration, Standardization and Technological Integration* (pp. 52–77). Hershey, PA: IGI Global. doi:10.4018/978-1-4666-9542-9.ch003

Ferradji, M. A., & Zidani, A. (2016). Collaborative Environment for Remote Clinical Reasoning Learning. *International Journal of E-Health and Medical Communications*, *7*(4), 62–81. doi:10.4018/IJEHMC.2016100104

Fisher, J. (2018). Sociological Perspectives on Improving Medical Diagnosis Emphasizing CAD. In M. Khosrow-Pour, D.B.A. (Ed.), Encyclopedia of Information Science and Technology, Fourth Edition (pp. 1017-1024). Hershey, PA: IGI Global. doi:10.4018/978-1-5225-2255-3.ch088

Flores, C. D., Respício, A., Coelho, H., Bez, M. R., & Fonseca, J. M. (2016). Simulation for Medical Training. In M. Cruz-Cunha, I. Miranda, R. Martinho, & R. Rijo (Eds.), *Encyclopedia of E-Health and Telemedicine* (pp. 827–842). Hershey, PA: IGI Global. doi:10.4018/978-1-4666-9978-6.ch064

Frank, E. M. (2018). Healthcare Education: Integrating Simulation Technologies. In V. Bryan, A. Musgrove, & J. Powers (Eds.), *Handbook of Research on Human Development in the Digital Age* (pp. 163–182). Hershey, PA: IGI Global. doi:10.4018/978-1-5225-2838-8.ch008

Garner, G. (2018). Foundations for Yoga Practice in Rehabilitation. In S. Telles & N. Singh (Eds.), *Research-Based Perspectives on the Psychophysiology of Yoga* (pp. 263–307). Hershey, PA: IGI Global. doi:10.4018/978-1-5225-2788-6.ch015

Gasmelseid, T. M. (2016). Improving Pharmaceutical Care through the Use of Intelligent Pharmacoinformatics. In T. Gasmelseid (Ed.), *Advancing Pharmaceutical Processes and Tools for Improved Health Outcomes* (pp. 167–188). Hershey, PA: IGI Global. doi:10.4018/978-1-5225-0248-7.ch007

Gavurová, B., Kováč, V., & Šoltés, M. (2018). Medical Equipment and Economic Determinants of Its Structure and Regulation in the Slovak Republic. In M. Khosrow-Pour, D.B.A. (Ed.), Encyclopedia of Information Science and Technology, Fourth Edition (pp. 5841-5852). Hershey, PA: IGI Global. doi:10.4018/978-1-5225-2255-3.ch508

Ge, X., Wang, Q., Huang, K., Law, V., & Thomas, D. C. (2017). Designing Simulated Learning Environments and Facilitating Authentic Learning Experiences in Medical Education. In J. Stefaniak (Ed.), *Advancing Medical Education Through Strategic Instructional Design* (pp. 77–100). Hershey, PA: IGI Global. doi:10.4018/978-1-5225-2098-6.ch004

Gewald, H., & Gewald, C. (2018). Inhibitors of Physicians' Use of Mandatory Hospital Information Systems (HIS). *International Journal of Healthcare Information Systems and Informatics, 13*(1), 29–44. doi:10.4018/IJHISI.2018010103

Ghosh, D., & Dinda, S. (2017). Health Infrastructure and Economic Development in India. In R. Das (Ed.), *Social, Health, and Environmental Infrastructures for Economic Growth* (pp. 99–119). Hershey, PA: IGI Global. doi:10.4018/978-1-5225-2364-2.ch006

Ghosh, K., & Sen, K. C. (2017). The Potential of Crowdsourcing in the Health Care Industry. In N. Wickramasinghe (Ed.), *Handbook of Research on Healthcare Administration and Management* (pp. 418–427). Hershey, PA: IGI Global. doi:10.4018/978-1-5225-0920-2.ch024

Ghrab, S., & Saad, I. (2016). Identifying Crucial Know-How and Knowing-That for Medical Decision Support. *International Journal of Decision Support System Technology*, *8*(4), 14–33. doi:10.4018/IJDSST.2016100102

Giokas, K., Tsirmpas, C., Anastasiou, A., Iliopoulou, D., Costarides, V., & Koutsouris, D. (2016). Contemporary Heart Failure Treatment Based on Improved Knowledge and Personalized Care of Comorbidities. In D. Fotiadis (Ed.), *Handbook of Research on Trends in the Diagnosis and Treatment of Chronic Conditions* (pp. 301–314). Hershey, PA: IGI Global. doi:10.4018/978-1-4666-8828-5.ch014

Gopalan, V., Chan, E., & Ho, D. T. (2018). Deliberate Self-Harm and Suicide Ideology in Medical Students. In C. Smith (Ed.), *Exploring the Pressures of Medical Education From a Mental Health and Wellness Perspective* (pp. 122–143). Hershey, PA: IGI Global. doi:10.4018/978-1-5225-2811-1.ch005

Goswami, S., Dey, U., Roy, P., Ashour, A., & Dey, N. (2017). Medical Video Processing: Concept and Applications. In N. Dey, A. Ashour, & P. Patra (Eds.), *Feature Detectors and Motion Detection in Video Processing* (pp. 1–17). Hershey, PA: IGI Global. doi:10.4018/978-1-5225-1025-3.ch001

Goswami, S., Mahanta, K., Goswami, S., Jigdung, T., & Devi, T. P. (2018). Ageing and Cancer: The Epigenetic Basis, Alternative Treatment, and Care. In B. Prasad & S. Akbar (Eds.), *Handbook of Research on Geriatric Health, Treatment, and Care* (pp. 206–235). Hershey, PA: IGI Global. doi:10.4018/978-1-5225-3480-8.ch012

Gouva, M. I. (2017). The Psychological Impact of Medical Error on Patients, Family Members, and Health Professionals. In M. Riga (Ed.), *Impact of Medical Errors and Malpractice on Health Economics, Quality, and Patient Safety* (pp. 171–196). Hershey, PA: IGI Global. doi:10.4018/978-1-5225-2337-6.ch007

Gürcü, M., & Tengilimoğlu, D. (2017). Health Tourism-Based Destination Marketing. In A. Bayraktar & C. Uslay (Eds.), *Strategic Place Branding Methodologies and Theory for Tourist Attraction* (pp. 308–331). Hershey, PA: IGI Global. doi:10.4018/978-1-5225-0579-2.ch015

Gürsel, G. (2016). Mobility in Healthcare: M-Health. In A. Panagopoulos (Ed.), *Handbook of Research on Next Generation Mobile Communication Systems* (pp. 485–511). Hershey, PA: IGI Global. doi:10.4018/978-1-4666-8732-5.ch019

Gürsel, G. (2017). For Better Healthcare Mining Health Data. In S. Bhattacharyya, S. De, I. Pan, & P. Dutta (Eds.), *Intelligent Multidimensional Data Clustering and Analysis* (pp. 135–158). Hershey, PA: IGI Global. doi:10.4018/978-1-5225-1776-4.ch006

Guzman-Lugo, G., Lopez-Martinez, M., Lopez-Ramirez, B., & Avila-Vazquez, D. (2016). City-Driven Approach to Determine Health Services Based on Current User Location and Collaborative Information. *International Journal of Knowledge Society Research, 7*(1), 53–62. doi:10.4018/IJKSR.2016010104

Gyaase, P. O., Darko-Lartey, R., William, H., & Borkloe, F. (2017). Towards an Integrated Electronic Medical Records System for Quality Healthcare in Ghana: An Exploratory Factor Analysis. *International Journal of Computers in Clinical Practice, 2*(2), 38–55. doi:10.4018/IJCCP.2017070103

Handayani, P. W., Sandhyaduhita, P. I., Hidayanto, A. N., Pinem, A. A., Fajrina, H. R., Junus, K. M., ... Ayuningtyas, D. (2016). Integrated Hospital Information System Architecture Design in Indonesia. In T. Iyamu & A. Tatnall (Eds.), *Maximizing Healthcare Delivery and Management through Technology Integration* (pp. 207–236). Hershey, PA: IGI Global. doi:10.4018/978-1-4666-9446-0.ch013

Hanel, P. (2017). Is China Catching Up?: Health-Related Applications of Biotechnology. In T. Bas & J. Zhao (Eds.), *Comparative Approaches to Biotechnology Development and Use in Developed and Emerging Nations* (pp. 465–520). Hershey, PA: IGI Global. doi:10.4018/978-1-5225-1040-6.ch016

Harmsen, C. A., & Royle, R. N. (2016). St. Stephen's Hospital Hervey Bay: Study of Developing a Digital Hospital. In J. Moon & M. Galea (Eds.), *Improving Health Management through Clinical Decision Support Systems* (pp. 127–153). Hershey, PA: IGI Global. doi:10.4018/978-1-4666-9432-3.ch006

Harp, D., Shim, R. S., Johnson, J., Harp, J. A., Wilcox, W. C., & Wilcox, J. K. (2016). Race and Gender Inequalities in Medicine and Biomedical Research. In U. Thomas & J. Drake (Eds.), *Critical Research on Sexism and Racism in STEM Fields* (pp. 115–134). Hershey, PA: IGI Global. doi:10.4018/978-1-5225-0174-9.ch006

Hartman, A., & Brown, S. (2017). Synergism through Therapeutic Visual Arts. In V. Bryan & J. Bird (Eds.), *Healthcare Community Synergism between Patients, Practitioners, and Researchers* (pp. 29–48). Hershey, PA: IGI Global. doi:10.4018/978-1-5225-0640-9.ch002

Hazra, J., Chowdhury, A. R., & Dutta, P. (2016). Cluster Based Medical Image Registration Using Optimized Neural Network. In S. Bhattacharyya, P. Banerjee, D. Majumdar, & P. Dutta (Eds.), *Handbook of Research on Advanced Hybrid Intelligent Techniques and Applications* (pp. 551–581). Hershey, PA: IGI Global. doi:10.4018/978-1-4666-9474-3.ch018

Hung, S., Huang, W., Yen, D. C., Chang, S., & Lu, C. (2016). Effect of Information Service Competence and Contextual Factors on the Effectiveness of Strategic Information Systems Planning in Hospitals. *Journal of Global Information Management, 24*(1), 14–36. doi:10.4018/JGIM.2016010102

Iltchev, P., Śliwczyński, A., Szynkiewicz, P., & Marczak, M. (2016). Mobile Health Applications Assisting Patients with Chronic Diseases: Examples from Asthma Care. In A. Moumtzoglou (Ed.), *M-Health Innovations for Patient-Centered Care* (pp. 170–196). Hershey, PA: IGI Global. doi:10.4018/978-1-4666-9861-1.ch009

Iqbal, S., Ahmad, S., & Willis, I. (2017). Influencing Factors for Adopting Technology Enhanced Learning in the Medical Schools of Punjab, Pakistan. *International Journal of Information and Communication Technology Education, 13*(3), 27–39. doi:10.4018/IJICTE.2017070103

Jagan, J., Dalkiliç, Y., & Samui, P. (2016). Utilization of SVM, LSSVM and GP for Predicting the Medical Waste Generation. In G. Hua (Ed.), *Smart Cities as a Solution for Reducing Urban Waste and Pollution* (pp. 224–251). Hershey, PA: IGI Global. doi:10.4018/978-1-5225-0302-6.ch008

Jagiello, K., Sosnowska, A., Mikolajczyk, A., & Puzyn, T. (2017). Nanomaterials in Medical Devices: Regulations' Review and Future Perspectives. *Journal of Nanotoxicology and Nanomedicine, 2*(2), 1–11. doi:10.4018/JNN.2017070101

Jena, T. K. (2018). Skill Training Process in Medicine Through Distance Mode. In U. Pandey & V. Indrakanti (Eds.), *Optimizing Open and Distance Learning in Higher Education Institutions* (pp. 228–243). Hershey, PA: IGI Global. doi:10.4018/978-1-5225-2624-7.ch010

Jesus, Â., & Gomes, M. J. (2016). Web 2.0 Tools in Biomedical and Pharmaceutical Education: Updated Review and Commentary. In T. Gasmelseid (Ed.), *Advancing Pharmaceutical Processes and Tools for Improved Health Outcomes* (pp. 52–78). Hershey, PA: IGI Global. doi:10.4018/978-1-5225-0248-7.ch003

Joseph, V., & Miller, J. M. (2018). Medical Students' Perceived Stigma in Seeking Care: A Cultural Perspective. In C. Smith (Ed.), *Exploring the Pressures of Medical Education From a Mental Health and Wellness Perspective* (pp. 44–67). Hershey, PA: IGI Global. doi:10.4018/978-1-5225-2811-1.ch002

Joyce, B. L., & Swanberg, S. M. (2017). Using Backward Design for Competency-Based Undergraduate Medical Education. In J. Stefaniak (Ed.), *Advancing Medical Education Through Strategic Instructional Design* (pp. 53–76). Hershey, PA: IGI Global. doi:10.4018/978-1-5225-2098-6.ch003

Kaljo, K., & Jacques, L. (2018). Flipping the Medical School Classroom. In M. Khosrow-Pour, D.B.A. (Ed.), Encyclopedia of Information Science and Technology, Fourth Edition (pp. 5800-5809). Hershey, PA: IGI Global. doi:10.4018/978-1-5225-2255-3.ch504

Karon, R. (2016). Utilisation of Health Information Systems for Service Delivery in the Namibian Environment. In T. Iyamu & A. Tatnall (Eds.), *Maximizing Healthcare Delivery and Management through Technology Integration* (pp. 169–183). Hershey, PA: IGI Global. doi:10.4018/978-1-4666-9446-0.ch011

Kasina, H., Bahubalendruni, M. V., & Botcha, R. (2017). Robots in Medicine: Past, Present and Future. *International Journal of Manufacturing, Materials, and Mechanical Engineering*, *7*(4), 44–64. doi:10.4018/IJMMME.2017100104

Katehakis, D. G. (2018). Electronic Medical Record Implementation Challenges for the National Health System in Greece. *International Journal of Reliable and Quality E-Healthcare*, *7*(1), 16–30. doi:10.4018/IJRQEH.2018010102

Katz, A., & Shtub, A. (2016). Design and Build a Wizard of Oz (WOZ) Telemedicine Simulator Platform. In M. Cruz-Cunha, I. Miranda, R. Martinho, & R. Rijo (Eds.), *Encyclopedia of E-Health and Telemedicine* (pp. 128–141). Hershey, PA: IGI Global. doi:10.4018/978-1-4666-9978-6.ch011

Kaur, P. D., & Sharma, P. (2017). Success Dimensions of ICTs in Healthcare. In B. Singh (Ed.), *Computational Tools and Techniques for Biomedical Signal Processing* (pp. 149–173). Hershey, PA: IGI Global. doi:10.4018/978-1-5225-0660-7.ch007

Kaushik, P. (2018). Comorbidity of Medical and Psychiatric Disorders in Geriatric Population: Treatment and Care. In B. Prasad & S. Akbar (Eds.), *Handbook of Research on Geriatric Health, Treatment, and Care* (pp. 448–474). Hershey, PA: IGI Global. doi:10.4018/978-1-5225-3480-8.ch025

Khachane, M. Y. (2017). Organ-Based Medical Image Classification Using Support Vector Machine. *International Journal of Synthetic Emotions*, *8*(1), 18–30. doi:10.4018/IJSE.2017010102

Kirci, P. (2018). Intelligent Techniques for Analysis of Big Data About Healthcare and Medical Records. In N. Shah & M. Mittal (Eds.), *Handbook of Research on Promoting Business Process Improvement Through Inventory Control Techniques* (pp. 559–582). Hershey, PA: IGI Global. doi:10.4018/978-1-5225-3232-3.ch029

Kldiashvili, E. (2016). Cloud Computing as the Useful Resource for Application of the Medical Information System for Quality Assurance Purposes. *International Journal of Computers in Clinical Practice*, *1*(2), 1–23. doi:10.4018/IJCCP.2016070101

Kldiashvili, E. (2018). Cloud Approach for the Medical Information System: MIS on Cloud. In M. Khosrow-Pour (Ed.), *Incorporating Nature-Inspired Paradigms in Computational Applications* (pp. 238–261). Hershey, PA: IGI Global. doi:10.4018/978-1-5225-5020-4.ch008

Kldiashvili, E., Burduli, A., Ghortlishvili, G., & Sheklashvili, I. (2016). Georgian Experience in Telecytology. In M. Cruz-Cunha, I. Miranda, R. Martinho, & R. Rijo (Eds.), *Encyclopedia of E-Health and Telemedicine* (pp. 62–71). Hershey, PA: IGI Global. doi:10.4018/978-1-4666-9978-6.ch006

Ko, H., Mesicek, L., Choi, J., Choi, J., & Hwang, S. (2018). A Study on Secure Contents Strategies for Applications With DRM on Cloud Computing. *International Journal of Cloud Applications and Computing*, *8*(1), 143–153. doi:10.4018/IJCAC.2018010107

Komendziński, T., Dreszer-Drogorób, J., Mikołajewska, E., Mikołajewski, D., & Bałaj, B. (2016). Interdisciplinary Education for Research and Everyday Clinical Practice: Lessons Learned from InteRDoCTor Project. In A. Rosiek & K. Leksowski (Eds.), *Organizational Culture and Ethics in Modern Medicine* (pp. 78–110). Hershey, PA: IGI Global. doi:10.4018/978-1-4666-9658-7.ch004

Komendziński, T., Mikołajewska, E., & Mikołajewski, D. (2018). Cross-Cultural Decision-Making in Healthcare: Theory and Practical Application in Real Clinical Conditions. In A. Rosiek-Kryszewska & K. Leksowski (Eds.), *Healthcare Administration for Patient Safety and Engagement* (pp. 276–298). Hershey, PA: IGI Global. doi:10.4018/978-1-5225-3946-9.ch015

Konecny, L. T. (2018). Medical School Wellness Initiatives. In C. Smith (Ed.), *Exploring the Pressures of Medical Education From a Mental Health and Wellness Perspective* (pp. 209–228). Hershey, PA: IGI Global. doi:10.4018/978-1-5225-2811-1.ch009

Konieczna, A., & Słomkowski, P. (2016). Confrontation of Human Rights in Daily Clinical Situations. In A. Rosiek & K. Leksowski (Eds.), *Organizational Culture and Ethics in Modern Medicine* (pp. 255–281). Hershey, PA: IGI Global. doi:10.4018/978-1-4666-9658-7.ch011

Kromrei, H., Solomonson, W. L., & Juzych, M. S. (2017). Teaching Residents How to Teach. In J. Stefaniak (Ed.), *Advancing Medical Education Through Strategic Instructional Design* (pp. 164–185). Hershey, PA: IGI Global. doi:10.4018/978-1-5225-2098-6.ch008

Kulkarni, S., Savyanavar, A., Kulkarni, P., Stranieri, A., & Ghorpade, V. (2018). Framework for Integration of Medical Image and Text-Based Report Retrieval to Support Radiological Diagnosis. In M. Kolekar & V. Kumar (Eds.), *Biomedical Signal and Image Processing in Patient Care* (pp. 86–122). Hershey, PA: IGI Global. doi:10.4018/978-1-5225-2829-6.ch006

Kumar, A., & Sarkar, B. K. (2018). Performance Analysis of Nature-Inspired Algorithms-Based Bayesian Prediction Models for Medical Data Sets. In U. Singh, A. Tiwari, & R. Singh (Eds.), *Soft-Computing-Based Nonlinear Control Systems Design* (pp. 134–155). Hershey, PA: IGI Global. doi:10.4018/978-1-5225-3531-7.ch007

Kurtz, R. S. (2016). Fortitude: A Study of African Americans in Surgery in New York City. In U. Thomas & J. Drake (Eds.), *Critical Research on Sexism and Racism in STEM Fields* (pp. 153–169). Hershey, PA: IGI Global. doi:10.4018/978-1-5225-0174-9.ch009

Labbadi, W., & Akaichi, J. (2017). Efficient Algorithm for Answering Fuzzy Medical Requests in Pervasive Healthcare Information Systems. *International Journal of Healthcare Information Systems and Informatics, 12*(2), 46–64. doi:10.4018/IJHISI.2017040103

Lagumdzija, A., & Swing, V. K. (2017). Health, Digitalization, and Individual Empowerment. In F. Topor (Ed.), *Handbook of Research on Individualism and Identity in the Globalized Digital Age* (pp. 380–402). Hershey, PA: IGI Global. doi:10.4018/978-1-5225-0522-8.ch017

Lamey, T. W., & Davidson-Shivers, G. V. (2017). Instructional Strategies and Sequencing. In J. Stefaniak (Ed.), *Advancing Medical Education Through Strategic Instructional Design* (pp. 30–52). Hershey, PA: IGI Global. doi:10.4018/978-1-5225-2098-6.ch002

Leon, G. (2017). The Role of Forensic Medicine in Medical Errors. In M. Riga (Ed.), *Impact of Medical Errors and Malpractice on Health Economics, Quality, and Patient Safety* (pp. 144–170). Hershey, PA: IGI Global. doi:10.4018/978-1-5225-2337-6.ch006

Lidia, B., Federica, G., & Maria, V. E. (2016). The Patient-Centered Medicine as the Theoretical Framework for Patient Engagement. In G. Graffigna (Ed.), *Promoting Patient Engagement and Participation for Effective Healthcare Reform* (pp. 25–39). Hershey, PA: IGI Global. doi:10.4018/978-1-4666-9992-2.ch002

Love, L., & McDowelle, D. (2018). Developing a Comprehensive Wellness Program for Medical Students. In C. Smith (Ed.), *Exploring the Pressures of Medical Education From a Mental Health and Wellness Perspective* (pp. 190–208). Hershey, PA: IGI Global. doi:10.4018/978-1-5225-2811-1.ch008

Lovell, K. L. (2017). Development and Evaluation of Neuroscience Computer-Based Modules for Medical Students: Instructional Design Principles and Effectiveness. In J. Stefaniak (Ed.), *Advancing Medical Education Through Strategic Instructional Design* (pp. 262–276). Hershey, PA: IGI Global. doi:10.4018/978-1-5225-2098-6.ch013

Lubin, R., & Hamlin, M. D. (2018). Medical Student Burnout: A Social Cognitive Learning Perspective on Medical Student Mental Health and Wellness. In C. Smith (Ed.), *Exploring the Pressures of Medical Education From a Mental Health and Wellness Perspective* (pp. 92–121). Hershey, PA: IGI Global. doi:10.4018/978-1-5225-2811-1.ch004

Luk, C. Y. (2018). Moving Towards Universal Health Coverage: Challenges for the Present and Future in China. In B. Fong, A. Ng, & P. Yuen (Eds.), *Sustainable Health and Long-Term Care Solutions for an Aging Population* (pp. 19–45). Hershey, PA: IGI Global. doi:10.4018/978-1-5225-2633-9.ch002

Mahat, M., & Pettigrew, A. (2017). The Regulatory Environment of Non-Profit Higher Education and Research Institutions and Its Implications for Managerial Strategy: The Case of Medical Education and Research. In L. West & A. Worthington (Eds.), *Handbook of Research on Emerging Business Models and Managerial Strategies in the Nonprofit Sector* (pp. 336–351). Hershey, PA: IGI Global. doi:10.4018/978-1-5225-2537-0.ch017

Maitra, I. K., & Bandhyopadhyaay, S. K. (2017). Adaptive Edge Detection Method towards Features Extraction from Diverse Medical Imaging Technologies. In S. Bhattacharyya, S. De, I. Pan, & P. Dutta (Eds.), *Intelligent Multidimensional Data Clustering and Analysis* (pp. 159–192). Hershey, PA: IGI Global. doi:10.4018/978-1-5225-1776-4.ch007

Mangu, V. P. (2017). Mobile Health Care: A Technology View. In C. Bhatt & S. Peddoju (Eds.), *Cloud Computing Systems and Applications in Healthcare* (pp. 1–18). Hershey, PA: IGI Global. doi:10.4018/978-1-5225-1002-4.ch001

Manirabona, A., Fourati, L. C., & Boudjit, S. (2017). Investigation on Healthcare Monitoring Systems: Innovative Services and Applications. *International Journal of E-Health and Medical Communications*, *8*(1), 1–18. doi:10.4018/IJEHMC.2017010101

Mannai, M. M., & Karâa, W. B. (2016). Biomedical Image Processing Overview. In W. Karâa & N. Dey (Eds.), *Biomedical Image Analysis and Mining Techniques for Improved Health Outcomes* (pp. 1–12). Hershey, PA: IGI Global. doi:10.4018/978-1-4666-8811-7.ch001

Manzoor, A. (2016). RFID in Health Care-Building Smart Hospitals for Quality Healthcare. *International Journal of User-Driven Healthcare*, *6*(2), 21–45. doi:10.4018/IJUDH.2016070102

Marwan, M., Kartit, A., & Ouahmane, H. (2018). A Framework to Secure Medical Image Storage in Cloud Computing Environment. *Journal of Electronic Commerce in Organizations*, *16*(1), 1–16. doi:10.4018/JECO.2018010101

Masoud, M. P., Nejad, M. K., Darebaghi, H., Chavoshi, M., & Farahani, M. (2018). The Decision Support System and Conventional Method of Telephone Triage by Nurses in Emergency Medical Services: A Comparative Investigation. *International Journal of E-Business Research*, *14*(1), 77–88. doi:10.4018/IJEBR.2018010105

McDonald, W. G., Martin, M., & Salzberg, L. D. (2018). From Medical Student to Medical Resident: Graduate Medical Education and Mental Health in the United States. In C. Smith (Ed.), *Exploring the Pressures of Medical Education From a Mental Health and Wellness Perspective* (pp. 145–169). Hershey, PA: IGI Global. doi:10.4018/978-1-5225-2811-1.ch006

Medhekar, A. (2017). The Role of Social Media for Knowledge Dissemination in Medical Tourism: A Case of India. In R. Chugh (Ed.), *Harnessing Social Media as a Knowledge Management Tool* (pp. 25–54). Hershey, PA: IGI Global. doi:10.4018/978-1-5225-0495-5.ch002

Medhekar, A., & Haq, F. (2018). Urbanization and New Jobs Creation in Healthcare Services in India: Challenges and Opportunities. In U. Benna & I. Benna (Eds.), *Urbanization and Its Impact on Socio-Economic Growth in Developing Regions* (pp. 198–218). Hershey, PA: IGI Global. doi:10.4018/978-1-5225-2659-9.ch010

Mehta, G., Dutta, M. K., & Kim, P. S. (2016). An Efficient and Lossless Cryptosystem for Security in Tele-Ophthalmology Applications Using Chaotic Theory. *International Journal of E-Health and Medical Communications*, *7*(4), 28–47. doi:10.4018/IJEHMC.2016100102

Mehta, P. (2017). Framework of Indian Healthcare System and its Challenges: An Insight. In V. Bryan & J. Bird (Eds.), *Healthcare Community Synergism between Patients, Practitioners, and Researchers* (pp. 247–271). Hershey, PA: IGI Global. doi:10.4018/978-1-5225-0640-9.ch011

Metelmann, B., & Metelmann, C. (2016). M-Health in Prehospital Emergency Medicine: Experiences from the EU funded Project LiveCity. In A. Moumtzoglou (Ed.), *M-Health Innovations for Patient-Centered Care* (pp. 197–212). Hershey, PA: IGI Global. doi:10.4018/978-1-4666-9861-1.ch010

Mi, M. (2017). Informal Learning in Medical Education. In J. Stefaniak (Ed.), *Advancing Medical Education Through Strategic Instructional Design* (pp. 225–244). Hershey, PA: IGI Global. doi:10.4018/978-1-5225-2098-6.ch011

Miglioretti, M., Mariani, F., & Vecchio, L. (2016). Could Patient Engagement Promote a Health System Free From Malpractice Litigation Risk? In G. Graffigna (Ed.), *Promoting Patient Engagement and Participation for Effective Healthcare Reform* (pp. 240–264). Hershey, PA: IGI Global. doi:10.4018/978-1-4666-9992-2.ch012

Misra, S. C., & Bisui, S. (2016). Feasibility of Large Scale Implementation of Personalized Medicine in the Current Scenario. *International Journal of E-Health and Medical Communications*, *7*(2), 30–49. doi:10.4018/IJEHMC.2016040103

Misra, S. C., Bisui, S., & Fantazy, K. (2016). Identifying Critical Changes in Adoption of Personalized Medicine (PM) in Healthcare Management. *International Journal of E-Health and Medical Communications*, *7*(3), 1–15. doi:10.4018/IJEHMC.2016070101

Mohammadian, M., Hatzinakos, D., Spachos, P., & Jentzsh, R. (2016). An Intelligent and Secure Framework for Wireless Information Technology in Healthcare for User and Data Classification in Hospitals. In V. Wang (Ed.), *Handbook of Research on Advancing Health Education through Technology* (pp. 452–479). Hershey, PA: IGI Global. doi:10.4018/978-1-4666-9494-1.ch019

Mokeddem, S., & Atmani, B. (2016). Assessment of Clinical Decision Support Systems for Predicting Coronary Heart Disease. *International Journal of Operations Research and Information Systems*, *7*(3), 57–73. doi:10.4018/IJORIS.2016070104

Mokrzycka, A., & Kowalska-Bobko, I. (2016). Public Health Legislation and Patient's Rights: Health2020 Strategy, European Perspective. In A. Rosiek & K. Leksowski (Eds.), *Organizational Culture and Ethics in Modern Medicine* (pp. 298–322). Hershey, PA: IGI Global. doi:10.4018/978-1-4666-9658-7.ch013

Moon, J. D., & Galea, M. P. (2016). Overview of Clinical Decision Support Systems in Healthcare. In J. Moon & M. Galea (Eds.), *Improving Health Management through Clinical Decision Support Systems* (pp. 1–27). Hershey, PA: IGI Global. doi:10.4018/978-1-4666-9432-3.ch001

Mosadeghrad, A. M., & Woldemichael, A. (2017). Application of Quality Management in Promoting Patient Safety and Preventing Medical Errors. In M. Riga (Ed.), *Impact of Medical Errors and Malpractice on Health Economics, Quality, and Patient Safety* (pp. 91–112). Hershey, PA: IGI Global. doi:10.4018/978-1-5225-2337-6.ch004

Moumtzoglou, A. (2017). Digital Medicine: The Quality Standpoint. In A. Moumtzoglou (Ed.), *Design, Development, and Integration of Reliable Electronic Healthcare Platforms* (pp. 179–195). Hershey, PA: IGI Global. doi:10.4018/978-1-5225-1724-5.ch011

Moumtzoglou, A., & Pouliakis, A. (2018). Population Health Management and the Science of Individuality. *International Journal of Reliable and Quality E-Healthcare, 7*(2), 1–26. doi:10.4018/IJRQEH.2018040101

Mpofu, C. (2016). International Medical Experiences Outbound New Zealand: An Economic and Medical Workforce Strategy. In D. Velliaris & D. Coleman-George (Eds.), *Handbook of Research on Study Abroad Programs and Outbound Mobility* (pp. 446–469). Hershey, PA: IGI Global. doi:10.4018/978-1-5225-0169-5.ch018

Mukhtar, W. F., & Abuelyaman, E. S. (2017). Opportunities and Challenges of Big Data in Healthcare. In N. Wickramasinghe (Ed.), *Handbook of Research on Healthcare Administration and Management* (pp. 47–58). Hershey, PA: IGI Global. doi:10.4018/978-1-5225-0920-2.ch004

Munugala, S., Brar, G. K., Syed, A., Mohammad, A., & Halgamuge, M. N. (2018). The Much Needed Security and Data Reforms of Cloud Computing in Medical Data Storage. In M. Lytras & P. Papadopoulou (Eds.), *Applying Big Data Analytics in Bioinformatics and Medicine* (pp. 99–113). Hershey, PA: IGI Global. doi:10.4018/978-1-5225-2607-0.ch005

Narasimhamurthy, A. (2016). An Overview of Machine Learning in Medical Image Analysis: Trends in Health Informatics. In N. Dey & A. Ashour (Eds.), *Classification and Clustering in Biomedical Signal Processing* (pp. 23–45). Hershey, PA: IGI Global. doi:10.4018/978-1-5225-0140-4.ch002

Ngara, R. (2017). Multiple Voices, Multiple Paths: Towards Dialogue between Western and Indigenous Medical Knowledge Systems. In P. Ngulube (Ed.), *Handbook of Research on Theoretical Perspectives on Indigenous Knowledge Systems in Developing Countries* (pp. 332–358). Hershey, PA: IGI Global. doi:10.4018/978-1-5225-0833-5.ch015

O'Connor, Y., & Heavin, C. (2018). Defining and Characterising the Landscape of eHealth. In M. Khosrow-Pour, D.B.A. (Ed.), Encyclopedia of Information Science and Technology, Fourth Edition (pp. 5864-5875). Hershey, PA: IGI Global. doi:10.4018/978-1-5225-2255-3.ch510

Ochonogor, W. C., & Okite-Amughoro, F. A. (2018). Building an Effective Digital Library in a University Teaching Hospital (UTH) in Nigeria. In A. Tella & T. Kwanya (Eds.), *Handbook of Research on Managing Intellectual Property in Digital Libraries* (pp. 184–204). Hershey, PA: IGI Global. doi:10.4018/978-1-5225-3093-0.ch010

Olaniran, B. A. (2016). ICTs, E-health, and Multidisciplinary Healthcare Teams: Promises and Challenges. *International Journal of Privacy and Health Information Management, 4*(2), 62–75. doi:10.4018/IJPHIM.2016070105

Olaniran, B. A. (2016). ICT Use and Multidisciplinary Healthcare Teams in the Age of e-Health. *International Journal of Reliable and Quality E-Healthcare, 5*(1), 18–31. doi:10.4018/IJRQEH.2016010102

Olivares, S. L., Cruz, A. G., Cabrera, M. V., Regalado, A. I., & García, J. E. (2017). An Assessment Study of Quality Model for Medical Schools in Mexico. In S. Mukerji & P. Tripathi (Eds.), *Handbook of Research on Administration, Policy, and Leadership in Higher Education* (pp. 404–439). Hershey, PA: IGI Global. doi:10.4018/978-1-5225-0672-0.ch016

Omidoyin, E. O., Opeke, R. O., & Osagbemi, G. K. (2016). Utilization Pattern and Privacy Issues in the use of Health Records for Research Practice by Doctors: Selected Nigerian Teaching Hospitals as Case Study. *International Journal of Privacy and Health Information Management, 4*(1), 1–11. doi:10.4018/IJPHIM.2016010101

Omoruyi, E. A., & Omidele, F. (2018). Resident Physician and Medical Academic Faculty Burnout: A Review of Current Literature. In C. Smith (Ed.), *Exploring the Pressures of Medical Education From a Mental Health and Wellness Perspective* (pp. 171–189). Hershey, PA: IGI Global. doi:10.4018/978-1-5225-2811-1.ch007

Osop, H., & Sahama, T. (2016). Data-Driven and Practice-Based Evidence: Design and Development of Efficient and Effective Clinical Decision Support System. In J. Moon & M. Galea (Eds.), *Improving Health Management through Clinical Decision Support Systems* (pp. 295–328). Hershey, PA: IGI Global. doi:10.4018/978-1-4666-9432-3.ch014

Ossowski, R., & Izdebski, P. (2016). Ethical Aspects of Talking to a Patient. In A. Rosiek & K. Leksowski (Eds.), *Organizational Culture and Ethics in Modern Medicine* (pp. 203–235). Hershey, PA: IGI Global. doi:10.4018/978-1-4666-9658-7.ch009

Pandian, P. S. (2016). An Overview of Telemedicine Technologies for Healthcare Applications. *International Journal of Biomedical and Clinical Engineering, 5*(2), 29–52. doi:10.4018/IJBCE.2016070103

Papadopoulou, P., Lytras, M., & Marouli, C. (2018). Bioinformatics as Applied to Medicine: Challenges Faced Moving from Big Data to Smart Data to Wise Data. In M. Lytras & P. Papadopoulou (Eds.), *Applying Big Data Analytics in Bioinformatics and Medicine* (pp. 1–25). Hershey, PA: IGI Global. doi:10.4018/978-1-5225-2607-0.ch001

Paraskou, A., & George, B. P. (2018). An Overview of Reproductive Tourism. In *Legal and Economic Considerations Surrounding Reproductive Tourism: Emerging Research and Opportunities* (pp. 1–17). Hershey, PA: IGI Global. doi:10.4018/978-1-5225-2694-0.ch001

Park, S., & Moon, J. (2016). Strategic Approach towards Clinical Information Security. In J. Moon & M. Galea (Eds.), *Improving Health Management through Clinical Decision Support Systems* (pp. 329–359). Hershey, PA: IGI Global. doi:10.4018/978-1-4666-9432-3.ch015

Pereira, D., Castro, A., Gomes, P., Areias, J. C., Reis, Z. S., Coimbra, M. T., & Cruz-Correia, R. (2016). Digital Auscultation: Challenges and Perspectives. In M. Cruz-Cunha, I. Miranda, R. Martinho, & R. Rijo (Eds.), *Encyclopedia of E-Health and Telemedicine* (pp. 910–927). Hershey, PA: IGI Global. doi:10.4018/978-1-4666-9978-6.ch070

Peters, R. A., & Cruz, M. (2016). The States as Generators of Incremental Change in American Health Care Policy: 1935 to 1965. In R. Gholipour & K. Rouzbehani (Eds.), *Social, Economic, and Political Perspectives on Public Health Policy-Making* (pp. 86–114). Hershey, PA: IGI Global. doi:10.4018/978-1-4666-9944-1.ch005

Phuritsabam, B., & Devi, A. B. (2017). Information Seeking Behavior of Medical Scientists at Jawaharlal Nehru Institute of Medical Science: A Study. In S. Ram (Ed.), *Library and Information Services for Bioinformatics Education and Research* (pp. 177–187). Hershey, PA: IGI Global. doi:10.4018/978-1-5225-1871-6.ch010

Pieczka, B. (2018). Management of Risk and Adverse Events in Medical Entities. In A. Rosiek-Kryszewska & K. Leksowski (Eds.), *Healthcare Administration for Patient Safety and Engagement* (pp. 31–46). Hershey, PA: IGI Global. doi:10.4018/978-1-5225-3946-9.ch003

Poduval, J. (2016). Curriculum Development. In *Optimizing Medicine Residency Training Programs* (pp. 45–102). Hershey, PA: IGI Global. doi:10.4018/978-1-4666-9527-6.ch003

Poduval, J. (2016). Ethics and Professionalism. In *Optimizing Medicine Residency Training Programs* (pp. 103–133). Hershey, PA: IGI Global. doi:10.4018/978-1-4666-9527-6.ch004

Poduval, J. (2016). Management Skills and Leadership. In *Optimizing Medicine Residency Training Programs* (pp. 182–205). Hershey, PA: IGI Global. doi:10.4018/978-1-4666-9527-6.ch008

Poduval, J. (2016). Medicine Residency Training. In *Optimizing Medicine Residency Training Programs* (pp. 1–27). Hershey, PA: IGI Global. doi:10.4018/978-1-4666-9527-6.ch001

Poduval, J. (2016). Personal Issues. In *Optimizing Medicine Residency Training Programs* (pp. 206–221). Hershey, PA: IGI Global. doi:10.4018/978-1-4666-9527-6.ch009

Poduval, J. (2017). Medical Errors: Impact on Health Care Quality. In M. Riga (Ed.), *Impact of Medical Errors and Malpractice on Health Economics, Quality, and Patient Safety* (pp. 33–60). Hershey, PA: IGI Global. doi:10.4018/978-1-5225-2337-6.ch002

Politis, D., Stagiopoulos, P., Aidona, S., Kyriafinis, G., & Constantinidis, I. (2018). Autonomous Learning and Skill Accreditation: A Paradigm for Medical Studies. In A. Kumar (Ed.), *Optimizing Student Engagement in Online Learning Environments* (pp. 266–296). Hershey, PA: IGI Global. doi:10.4018/978-1-5225-3634-5.ch012

Pomares-Quimbaya, A., Gonzalez, R. A., Quintero, S., Muñoz, O. M., Bohórquez, W. R., García, O. M., & Londoño, D. (2016). A Review of Existing Applications and Techniques for Narrative Text Analysis in Electronic Medical Records. In M. Cruz-Cunha, I. Miranda, R. Martinho, & R. Rijo (Eds.), *Encyclopedia of E-Health and Telemedicine* (pp. 796–811). Hershey, PA: IGI Global. doi:10.4018/978-1-4666-9978-6.ch062

Pomares-Quimbaya, A., González, R. A., Sierra, A., Daza, J. C., Muñoz, O., García, A., ... Bohórquez, W. R. (2017). ICT for Enabling the Quality Evaluation of Health Care Services: A Case Study in a General Hospital. In A. Moumtzoglou (Ed.), *Design, Development, and Integration of Reliable Electronic Healthcare Platforms* (pp. 196–210). Hershey, PA: IGI Global. doi:10.4018/978-1-5225-1724-5.ch012

Pouliakis, A., Margari, N., Karakitsou, E., Archondakis, S., & Karakitsos, P. (2018). Emerging Technologies Serving Cytopathology: Big Data, the Cloud, and Mobile Computing. In I. El Naqa (Ed.), *Emerging Developments and Practices in Oncology* (pp. 114–152). Hershey, PA: IGI Global. doi:10.4018/978-1-5225-3085-5.ch005

Queirós, A., Silva, A. G., Ferreira, A., Caravau, H., Cerqueira, M., & Rocha, N. P. (2016). Assessing Mobile Applications Considered Medical Devices. In M. Cruz-Cunha, I. Miranda, R. Martinho, & R. Rijo (Eds.), *Encyclopedia of E-Health and Telemedicine* (pp. 111–127). Hershey, PA: IGI Global. doi:10.4018/978-1-4666-9978-6.ch010

Raffaeli, L., Spinsante, S., & Gambi, E. (2016). Integrated Smart TV-Based Personal e-Health System. *International Journal of E-Health and Medical Communications, 7*(1), 48–64. doi:10.4018/IJEHMC.2016010103

Rai, A., Kothari, R., & Singh, D. P. (2017). Assessment of Available Technologies for Hospital Waste Management: A Need for Society. In R. Singh, A. Singh, & V. Srivastava (Eds.), *Environmental Issues Surrounding Human Overpopulation* (pp. 172–188). Hershey, PA: IGI Global. doi:10.4018/978-1-5225-1683-5.ch010

Ramamoorthy, S., & Sivasubramaniam, R. (2018). Image Processing Including Medical Liver Imaging: Medical Image Processing from Big Data Perspective, Ultrasound Liver Images, Challenges. In M. Lytras & P. Papadopoulou (Eds.), *Applying Big Data Analytics in Bioinformatics and Medicine* (pp. 380–392). Hershey, PA: IGI Global. doi:10.4018/978-1-5225-2607-0.ch016

Rathor, G. P., & Gupta, S. K. (2017). Improving Multimodality Image Fusion through Integrate AFL and Wavelet Transform. In V. Tiwari, B. Tiwari, R. Thakur, & S. Gupta (Eds.), *Pattern and Data Analysis in Healthcare Settings* (pp. 143–157). Hershey, PA: IGI Global. doi:10.4018/978-1-5225-0536-5.ch008

Rawat, D. B., & Bhattacharya, S. (2016). Wireless Body Area Network for Healthcare Applications. In N. Meghanathan (Ed.), *Advanced Methods for Complex Network Analysis* (pp. 343–358). Hershey, PA: IGI Global. doi:10.4018/978-1-4666-9964-9.ch014

Rea, P. M. (2016). Advances in Anatomical and Medical Visualisation. In M. Pinheiro & D. Simões (Eds.), *Handbook of Research on Engaging Digital Natives in Higher Education Settings* (pp. 244–264). Hershey, PA: IGI Global. doi:10.4018/978-1-5225-0039-1.ch011

Rexhepi, H., & Persson, A. (2017). Challenges to Implementing IT Support for Evidence Based Practice Among Nurses and Assistant Nurses: A Qualitative Study. *Journal of Electronic Commerce in Organizations, 15*(2), 61–76. doi:10.4018/JECO.2017040105

Reychav, I., & Azuri, J. (2016). Including Elderly Patients in Decision Making via Electronic Health Literacy. In M. Cruz-Cunha, I. Miranda, R. Martinho, & R. Rijo (Eds.), *Encyclopedia of E-Health and Telemedicine* (pp. 241–249). Hershey, PA: IGI Global. doi:10.4018/978-1-4666-9978-6.ch020

Richards, D., & Caldwell, P. H. (2016). Gamification to Improve Adherence to Clinical Treatment Advice: Improving Adherence to Clinical Treatment. In D. Novák, B. Tulu, & H. Brendryen (Eds.), *Handbook of Research on Holistic Perspectives in Gamification for Clinical Practice* (pp. 47–77). Hershey, PA: IGI Global. doi:10.4018/978-1-4666-9522-1.ch004

Rissman, B. (2016). Medical Conditions Associated with NLD. In B. Rissman (Ed.), *Medical and Educational Perspectives on Nonverbal Learning Disability in Children and Young Adults* (pp. 27–66). Hershey, PA: IGI Global. doi:10.4018/978-1-4666-9539-9.ch002

Rosiek, A. (2018). The Assessment of Actions of the Environment and the Impact of Preventive Medicine for Public Health in Poland. In A. Rosiek-Kryszewska & K. Leksowski (Eds.), *Healthcare Administration for Patient Safety and Engagement* (pp. 106–119). Hershey, PA: IGI Global. doi:10.4018/978-1-5225-3946-9.ch006

Rosiek, A., Leksowski, K., Goch, A., Rosiek-Kryszewska, A., & Leksowski, Ł. (2016). Medical Treatment and Difficult Ethical Decisions in Interdisciplinary Hospital Teams. In A. Rosiek & K. Leksowski (Eds.), *Organizational Culture and Ethics in Modern Medicine* (pp. 121–153). Hershey, PA: IGI Global. doi:10.4018/978-1-4666-9658-7.ch006

Rosiek, A., & Rosiek-Kryszewska, A. (2018). Managed Healthcare: Doctor Life Satisfaction and Its Impact on the Process of Communicating With the Patient. In A. Rosiek-Kryszewska & K. Leksowski (Eds.), *Healthcare Administration for Patient Safety and Engagement* (pp. 244–261). Hershey, PA: IGI Global. doi:10.4018/978-1-5225-3946-9.ch013

Rosiek-Kryszewska, A., Leksowski, Ł., Rosiek, A., Leksowski, K., & Goch, A. (2016). Clinical Communication in the Aspect of Development of New Technologies and E-Health in the Doctor-Patient Relationship. In A. Rosiek & K. Leksowski (Eds.), *Organizational Culture and Ethics in Modern Medicine* (pp. 18–51). Hershey, PA: IGI Global. doi:10.4018/978-1-4666-9658-7.ch002

Rosiek-Kryszewska, A., & Rosiek, A. (2018). The Involvement of the Patient and his Perspective Evaluation of the Quality of Healthcare. In A. Rosiek-Kryszewska & K. Leksowski (Eds.), *Healthcare Administration for Patient Safety and Engagement* (pp. 121–144). Hershey, PA: IGI Global. doi:10.4018/978-1-5225-3946-9.ch007

Rosiek-Kryszewska, A., & Rosiek, A. (2018). The Impact of Management and Leadership Roles in Building Competitive Healthcare Units. In A. Rosiek-Kryszewska & K. Leksowski (Eds.), *Healthcare Administration for Patient Safety and Engagement* (pp. 13–30). Hershey, PA: IGI Global. doi:10.4018/978-1-5225-3946-9.ch002

Roşu, S. M., Păvăloiu, I. B., Dragoi, G., Apostol, C. G., & Munteanu, D. (2016). Telemedicine Based on LMDS in the Urban/Metropolitan Area: A Romanian Case Study. In M. Cruz-Cunha, I. Miranda, R. Martinho, & R. Rijo (Eds.), *Encyclopedia of E-Health and Telemedicine* (pp. 96–109). Hershey, PA: IGI Global. doi:10.4018/978-1-4666-9978-6.ch009

Rouzbehani, K. (2017). Health Policy Implementation: Moving Beyond Its Barriers in United States. In N. Wickramasinghe (Ed.), *Handbook of Research on Healthcare Administration and Management* (pp. 541–552). Hershey, PA: IGI Global. doi:10.4018/978-1-5225-0920-2.ch032

Ruiz, I. M., Cohen, D. S., & Marco, Á. M. (2016). ISO/IEEE11073 Family of Standards: Trends and Applications on E-Health Monitoring. In M. Cruz-Cunha, I. Miranda, R. Martinho, & R. Rijo (Eds.), *Encyclopedia of E-Health and Telemedicine* (pp. 646–660). Hershey, PA: IGI Global. doi:10.4018/978-1-4666-9978-6.ch050

Sam, S. (2017). Mobile Phones and Expanding Human Capabilities in Plural Health Systems. In K. Moahi, K. Bwalya, & P. Sebina (Eds.), *Health Information Systems and the Advancement of Medical Practice in Developing Countries* (pp. 93–114). Hershey, PA: IGI Global. doi:10.4018/978-1-5225-2262-1.ch006

Sankaranarayanan, S., & Ganesan, S. (2016). Applications of Intelligent Agents in Health Sector-A Review. *International Journal of E-Health and Medical Communications*, *7*(1), 1–30. doi:10.4018/IJEHMC.2016010101

Santos-Trigo, M., Suaste, E., & Figuerola, P. (2018). Technology Design and Routes for Tool Appropriation in Medical Practices. In M. Khosrow-Pour, D.B.A. (Ed.), Encyclopedia of Information Science and Technology, Fourth Edition (pp. 3794-3804). Hershey, PA: IGI Global. doi:10.4018/978-1-5225-2255-3.ch329

Sarivougioukas, J., Vagelatos, A., Parsopoulos, K. E., & Lagaris, I. E. (2018). Home UbiHealth. In M. Khosrow-Pour, D.B.A. (Ed.), Encyclopedia of Information Science and Technology, Fourth Edition (pp. 7765-7774). Hershey, PA: IGI Global. doi:10.4018/978-1-5225-2255-3.ch675

Sarkar, B. K. (2017). Big Data and Healthcare Data: A Survey. *International Journal of Knowledge-Based Organizations*, *7*(4), 50–77. doi:10.4018/IJKBO.2017100104

Saxena, K., & Banodha, U. (2017). An Essence of the SOA on Healthcare. In R. Bhadoria, N. Chaudhari, G. Tomar, & S. Singh (Eds.), *Exploring Enterprise Service Bus in the Service-Oriented Architecture Paradigm* (pp. 283–304). Hershey, PA: IGI Global. doi:10.4018/978-1-5225-2157-0.ch018

Schmeida, M., & McNeal, R. (2016). Consulting Online Healthcare Information: E-Caregivers as Knowledgeable Decision Makers. *International Journal of Computers in Clinical Practice*, *1*(1), 42–52. doi:10.4018/IJCCP.2016010104

Sen, K., & Ghosh, K. (2018). Incorporating Global Medical Knowledge to Solve Healthcare Problems: A Framework for a Crowdsourcing System. *International Journal of Healthcare Information Systems and Informatics*, *13*(1), 1–14. doi:10.4018/IJHISI.2018010101

Shakdher, A., & Pandey, K. (2017). REDAlert+: Medical/Fire Emergency and Warning System using Android Devices. *International Journal of E-Health and Medical Communications*, *8*(1), 37–51. doi:10.4018/IJEHMC.2017010103

Shekarian, E., Abdul-Rashid, S. H., & Olugu, E. U. (2017). An Integrated Fuzzy VIKOR Method for Performance Management in Healthcare. In M. Tavana, K. Szabat, & K. Puranam (Eds.), *Organizational Productivity and Performance Measurements Using Predictive Modeling and Analytics* (pp. 40–61). Hershey, PA: IGI Global. doi:10.4018/978-1-5225-0654-6.ch003

Shi, J., Erdem, E., & Liu, H. (2016). Expanding Role of Telephone Systems in Healthcare: Developments and Opportunities. In A. Dwivedi (Ed.), *Reshaping Medical Practice and Care with Health Information Systems* (pp. 87–131). Hershey, PA: IGI Global. doi:10.4018/978-1-4666-9870-3.ch004

Shijina, V., & John, S. J. (2017). Multiple Relations and its Application in Medical Diagnosis. *International Journal of Fuzzy System Applications*, *6*(4), 47–62. doi:10.4018/IJFSA.2017100104

Shipley, N., & Chakraborty, J. (2018). Big Data and mHealth: Increasing the Usability of Healthcare Through the Customization of Pinterest – Literary Perspective. In J. Machado, A. Abelha, M. Santos, & F. Portela (Eds.), *Next-Generation Mobile and Pervasive Healthcare Solutions* (pp. 46–66). Hershey, PA: IGI Global. doi:10.4018/978-1-5225-2851-7.ch004

Singh, A., & Dutta, M. K. (2017). A Reversible Data Hiding Scheme for Efficient Management of Tele-Ophthalmological Data. *International Journal of E-Health and Medical Communications, 8*(3), 38–54. doi:10.4018/IJEHMC.2017070103

Sivaji, A., Radjo, H. K., Amin, M., & Abu Hashim, M. A. (2016). Design of a Hospital Interactive Wayfinding System: Designing for Malaysian Users. In N. Mohamed, T. Mantoro, M. Ayu, & M. Mahmud (Eds.), *Critical Socio-Technical Issues Surrounding Mobile Computing* (pp. 88–123). Hershey, PA: IGI Global. doi:10.4018/978-1-4666-9438-5.ch005

Skourti, P. K., & Pavlakis, A. (2017). The Second Victim Phenomenon: The Way Out. In M. Riga (Ed.), *Impact of Medical Errors and Malpractice on Health Economics, Quality, and Patient Safety* (pp. 197–222). Hershey, PA: IGI Global. doi:10.4018/978-1-5225-2337-6.ch008

Smith, C. R. (2018). Medical Students' Quest Towards the Long White Coat: Impact on Mental Health and Well-Being. In C. Smith (Ed.), *Exploring the Pressures of Medical Education From a Mental Health and Wellness Perspective* (pp. 1–42). Hershey, PA: IGI Global. doi:10.4018/978-1-5225-2811-1.ch001

Smith, S. I., & Dandignac, M. (2018). Perfectionism: Addressing Lofty Expectations in Medical School. In C. Smith (Ed.), *Exploring the Pressures of Medical Education From a Mental Health and Wellness Perspective* (pp. 68–91). Hershey, PA: IGI Global. doi:10.4018/978-1-5225-2811-1.ch003

Sobrinho, Á. A., Dias da Silva, L., Perkusich, A., Cunha, P., Pinheiro, M. E., & Melo de Medeiros, L. (2016). Towards Medical Systems to Aid the Detection and Treatment of Chronic Diseases. In D. Fotiadis (Ed.), *Handbook of Research on Trends in the Diagnosis and Treatment of Chronic Conditions* (pp. 50–69). Hershey, PA: IGI Global. doi:10.4018/978-1-4666-8828-5.ch003

Soczywko, J., & Rutkowska, D. (2018). The Patient/Provider Relationship in Emergency Medicine: Organization, Communication, and Understanding. In A. Rosiek-Kryszewska & K. Leksowski (Eds.), *Healthcare Administration for Patient Safety and Engagement* (pp. 74–105). Hershey, PA: IGI Global. doi:10.4018/978-1-5225-3946-9.ch005

Sołtysik-Piorunkiewicz, A., Furmankiewicz, M., & Ziuziański, P. (2016). Web Healthcare Applications in Poland: Trends, Standards, Barriers and Possibilities of Implementation and Usage of E-Health Systems. In I. Deliyannis, P. Kostagiolas, & C. Banou (Eds.), *Experimental Multimedia Systems for Interactivity and Strategic Innovation* (pp. 258–283). Hershey, PA: IGI Global. doi:10.4018/978-1-4666-8659-5.ch013

Soni, P. (2018). Implications of HIPAA and Subsequent Regulations on Information Technology. In M. Gupta, R. Sharman, J. Walp, & P. Mulgund (Eds.), *Information Technology Risk Management and Compliance in Modern Organizations* (pp. 71–98). Hershey, PA: IGI Global. doi:10.4018/978-1-5225-2604-9.ch004

Spinelli, R., & Benevolo, C. (2016). From Healthcare Services to E-Health Applications: A Delivery System-Based Taxonomy. In A. Dwivedi (Ed.), *Reshaping Medical Practice and Care with Health Information Systems* (pp. 205–245). Hershey, PA: IGI Global. doi:10.4018/978-1-4666-9870-3.ch007

Srivastava, A., & Aggarwal, A. K. (2018). Medical Image Fusion in Spatial and Transform Domain: A Comparative Analysis. In M. Anwar, A. Khosla, & R. Kapoor (Eds.), *Handbook of Research on Advanced Concepts in Real-Time Image and Video Processing* (pp. 281–300). Hershey, PA: IGI Global. doi:10.4018/978-1-5225-2848-7.ch011

Srivastava, S. K., & Roy, S. N. (2018). Recommendation System: A Potential Tool for Achieving Pervasive Health Care. In J. Machado, A. Abelha, M. Santos, & F. Portela (Eds.), *Next-Generation Mobile and Pervasive Healthcare Solutions* (pp. 111–127). Hershey, PA: IGI Global. doi:10.4018/978-1-5225-2851-7.ch008

Stancu, A. (2016). Correlations and Patterns of Food and Health Consumer Expenditure. In A. Jean-Vasile (Ed.), *Food Science, Production, and Engineering in Contemporary Economies* (pp. 44–101). Hershey, PA: IGI Global. doi:10.4018/978-1-5225-0341-5.ch003

Stanimirovic, D. (2017). Digitalization of Death Certification Model: Transformation Issues and Implementation Concerns. In S. Saeed, Y. Bamarouf, T. Ramayah, & S. Iqbal (Eds.), *Design Solutions for User-Centric Information Systems* (pp. 22–43). Hershey, PA: IGI Global. doi:10.4018/978-1-5225-1944-7.ch002

Stavros, A., Vavoulidis, E., & Nasioutziki, M. (2016). The Use of Mobile Health Applications for Quality Control and Accreditational Purposes in a Cytopathology Laboratory. In A. Moumtzoglou (Ed.), *M-Health Innovations for Patient-Centered Care* (pp. 262–283). Hershey, PA: IGI Global. doi:10.4018/978-1-4666-9861-1.ch013

Sukkird, V., & Shirahada, K. (2018). E-Health Service Model for Asian Developing Countries: A Case of Emergency Medical Service for Elderly People in Thailand. In M. Khosrow-Pour (Ed.), *Optimizing Current Practices in E-Services and Mobile Applications* (pp. 214–232). Hershey, PA: IGI Global. doi:10.4018/978-1-5225-5026-6.ch011

Sygit, B., & Wąsik, D. (2016). Patients' Rights and Medical Personnel Duties in the Field of Hospital Care. In A. Rosiek & K. Leksowski (Eds.), *Organizational Culture and Ethics in Modern Medicine* (pp. 282–297). Hershey, PA: IGI Global. doi:10.4018/978-1-4666-9658-7.ch012

Sygit, B., & Wąsik, D. (2016). The Idea of Human Rights in Conditions of Hospital Treatment. In A. Rosiek & K. Leksowski (Eds.), *Organizational Culture and Ethics in Modern Medicine* (pp. 236–254). Hershey, PA: IGI Global. doi:10.4018/978-1-4666-9658-7.ch010

Talbot, T. B. (2017). Making Lifelike Medical Games in the Age of Virtual Reality: An Update on "Playing Games with Biology" from 2013. In B. Dubbels (Ed.), *Transforming Gaming and Computer Simulation Technologies across Industries* (pp. 103–119). Hershey, PA: IGI Global. doi:10.4018/978-1-5225-1817-4.ch006

Tamposis, I., Pouliakis, A., Fezoulidis, I., & Karakitsos, P. (2016). Mobile Platforms Supporting Health Professionals: Need, Technical Requirements, and Applications. In A. Moumtzoglou (Ed.), *M-Health Innovations for Patient-Centered Care* (pp. 91–114). Hershey, PA: IGI Global. doi:10.4018/978-1-4666-9861-1.ch005

Tiago, M. T., Tiago, F., Amaral, F. E., & Silva, S. (2016). Healthy 3.0: Healthcare Digital Dimensions. In A. Dwivedi (Ed.), *Reshaping Medical Practice and Care with Health Information Systems* (pp. 287–322). Hershey, PA: IGI Global. doi:10.4018/978-1-4666-9870-3.ch010

Tripathy, B. (2016). Application of Rough Set Based Models in Medical Diagnosis. In S. Dash & B. Subudhi (Eds.), *Handbook of Research on Computational Intelligence Applications in Bioinformatics* (pp. 144–168). Hershey, PA: IGI Global. doi:10.4018/978-1-5225-0427-6.ch008

Turcu, C. E., & Turcu, C. O. (2017). Social Internet of Things in Healthcare: From Things to Social Things in Internet of Things. In C. Reis & M. Maximiano (Eds.), *Internet of Things and Advanced Application in Healthcare* (pp. 266–295). Hershey, PA: IGI Global. doi:10.4018/978-1-5225-1820-4.ch010

Unwin, D. W., Sanzogni, L., & Sandhu, K. (2017). Developing and Measuring the Business Case for Health Information Technology. In K. Moahi, K. Bwalya, & P. Sebina (Eds.), *Health Information Systems and the Advancement of Medical Practice in Developing Countries* (pp. 262–290). Hershey, PA: IGI Global. doi:10.4018/978-1-5225-2262-1.ch015

Urooj, S., & Singh, S. P. (2016). Wavelet Transform-Based Soft Computational Techniques and Applications in Medical Imaging. In P. Saxena, D. Singh, & M. Pant (Eds.), *Problem Solving and Uncertainty Modeling through Optimization and Soft Computing Applications* (pp. 339–363). Hershey, PA: IGI Global. doi:10.4018/978-1-4666-9885-7.ch016

Vasant, P. (2018). A General Medical Diagnosis System Formed by Artificial Neural Networks and Swarm Intelligence Techniques. In U. Kose, G. Guraksin, & O. Deperlioglu (Eds.), *Nature-Inspired Intelligent Techniques for Solving Biomedical Engineering Problems* (pp. 130–145). Hershey, PA: IGI Global. doi:10.4018/978-1-5225-4769-3.ch006

Waegemann, C. P. (2016). mHealth: History, Analysis, and Implementation. In A. Moumtzoglou (Ed.), M-Health Innovations for Patient-Centered Care (pp. 1-19). Hershey, PA: IGI Global. doi:10.4018/978-1-4666-9861-1.ch001

Watfa, M. K., Majeed, H., & Salahuddin, T. (2016). Computer Based E-Healthcare Clinical Systems: A Comprehensive Survey. *International Journal of Privacy and Health Information Management*, *4*(1), 50–69. doi:10.4018/IJPHIM.2016010104

Wietholter, J. P., Coetzee, R., Nardella, B., Kincaid, S. E., & Slain, D. (2016). International Healthcare Experiences: Caring While Learning and Learning While Caring. In D. Velliaris & D. Coleman-George (Eds.), *Handbook of Research on Study Abroad Programs and Outbound Mobility* (pp. 470–496). Hershey, PA: IGI Global. doi:10.4018/978-1-5225-0169-5.ch019

Witzke, K., & Specht, O. (2017). M-Health Telemedicine and Telepresence in Oral and Maxillofacial Surgery: An Innovative Prehospital Healthcare Concept in Structurally Weak Areas. *International Journal of Reliable and Quality E-Healthcare*, *6*(4), 37–48. doi:10.4018/IJRQEH.2017100105

Wójcik, A., & Chojnacki, M. (2016). Behavior and Ethical Problems in the Functioning of the Operating Theater (Case Study). In A. Rosiek & K. Leksowski (Eds.), *Organizational Culture and Ethics in Modern Medicine* (pp. 154–179). Hershey, PA: IGI Global. doi:10.4018/978-1-4666-9658-7.ch007

Wolk, K., & Marasek, K. P. (2016). Translation of Medical Texts using Neural Networks. *International Journal of Reliable and Quality E-Healthcare*, *5*(4), 51–66. doi:10.4018/IJRQEH.2016100104

Wong, A. K., & Lo, M. F. (2018). Using Pervasive Computing for Sustainable Healthcare in an Aging Population. In B. Fong, A. Ng, & P. Yuen (Eds.), *Sustainable Health and Long-Term Care Solutions for an Aging Population* (pp. 187–202). Hershey, PA: IGI Global. doi:10.4018/978-1-5225-2633-9.ch010

Wu, W., Martin, B. C., & Ni, C. (2017). A Systematic Review of Competency-Based Education Effort in the Health Professions: Seeking Order Out of Chaos. In K. Rasmussen, P. Northrup, & R. Colson (Eds.), *Handbook of Research on Competency-Based Education in University Settings* (pp. 352–378). Hershey, PA: IGI Global. doi:10.4018/978-1-5225-0932-5.ch018

Yadav, N., Aliasgari, M., & Poellabauer, C. (2016). Mobile Healthcare in an Increasingly Connected Developing World. *International Journal of Privacy and Health Information Management, 4*(2), 76–97. doi:10.4018/IJPHIM.2016070106

Yadav, S., Ekbal, A., Saha, S., Pathak, P. S., & Bhattacharyya, P. (2017). Patient Data De-Identification: A Conditional Random-Field-Based Supervised Approach. In S. Saha, A. Mandal, A. Narasimhamurthy, S. V, & S. Sangam (Eds.), Handbook of Research on Applied Cybernetics and Systems Science (pp. 234-253). Hershey, PA: IGI Global. doi:10.4018/978-1-5225-2498-4.ch011

Yu, B., Wijesekera, D., & Costa, P. C. (2017). Informed Consent in Healthcare: A Study Case of Genetic Services. In A. Moumtzoglou (Ed.), *Design, Development, and Integration of Reliable Electronic Healthcare Platforms* (pp. 211–242). Hershey, PA: IGI Global. doi:10.4018/978-1-5225-1724-5.ch013

Yu, B., Wijesekera, D., & Costa, P. C. (2017). Informed Consent in Electronic Medical Record Systems. In I. Management Association (Ed.), Healthcare Ethics and Training: Concepts, Methodologies, Tools, and Applications (pp. 1029-1049). Hershey, PA: IGI Global. doi:10.4018/978-1-5225-2237-9.ch049

Yu, M., Li, J., & Wang, W. (2017). Creative Life Experience among Students in Medical Education. In C. Zhou (Ed.), *Handbook of Research on Creative Problem-Solving Skill Development in Higher Education* (pp. 158–184). Hershey, PA: IGI Global. doi:10.4018/978-1-5225-0643-0.ch008

Zarour, K. (2017). Towards a Telehomecare in Algeria: Case of Diabetes Measurement and Remote Monitoring. *International Journal of E-Health and Medical Communications, 8*(4), 61–80. doi:10.4018/IJEHMC.2017100104

Zavyalova, Y. V., Korzun, D. G., Meigal, A. Y., & Borodin, A. V. (2017). Towards the Development of Smart Spaces-Based Socio-Cyber-Medicine Systems. *International Journal of Embedded and Real-Time Communication Systems*, *8*(1), 45–63. doi:10.4018/IJERTCS.2017010104

Zeinali, A. A. (2018). Word Formation Study in Developing Naming Guidelines in the Translation of English Medical Terms Into Persian. In M. Khosrow-Pour, D.B.A. (Ed.), Encyclopedia of Information Science and Technology, Fourth Edition (pp. 5136-5147). Hershey, PA: IGI Global. doi:10.4018/978-1-5225-2255-3.ch446

Ziminski, T. B., Demurjian, S. A., Sanzi, E., & Agresta, T. (2016). Toward Integrating Healthcare Data and Systems: A Study of Architectural Alternatives. In T. Iyamu & A. Tatnall (Eds.), *Maximizing Healthcare Delivery and Management through Technology Integration* (pp. 270–304). Hershey, PA: IGI Global. doi:10.4018/978-1-4666-9446-0.ch016

Ziminski, T. B., Demurjian, S. A., Sanzi, E., Baihan, M., & Agresta, T. (2016). An Architectural Solution for Health Information Exchange. *International Journal of User-Driven Healthcare*, *6*(1), 65–103. doi:10.4018/IJUDH.2016010104

Zineldin, M., & Vasicheva, V. (2018). Reducing Medical Errors and Increasing Patient Safety: TRM and 5 Q's Approaches for Better Quality of Life. In *Technological Tools for Value-Based Sustainable Relationships in Health: Emerging Research and Opportunities* (pp. 87–115). Hershey, PA: IGI Global. doi:10.4018/978-1-5225-4091-5.ch005

About the Contributors

Erdem Demiroz is faculty at Trakya University, School of Education, Department of Computer Education and Learning Technologies. He has a bachelor's degree in Computer Education and Instructional and Learning Technologies (CEIT); MA with an emphasis on General Curriculum and Instructional Leadership (CIL) and Instructional and Learning Technologies (ILTs); and PhD with emphasis on Teacher Education and Curriculum Studies (formerly Curriculum and Instructional Leadership) and Mathematics and Statistics. He is a dedicated teacher and a scholar. As an active technology user, who have extensive background in ILTs, his general research interests focus on ILTs in general, best practices of using ILTs not only in K-12 education but also in higher education and its effects on learning processes and on student learning outcomes. His research interests include but are not limited to course redesign and flipped learning with heavy use of ILTs, virtual learning environments, online teaching practices and design, learning theories in virtual learning, artificial intelligence, gaming and educational game design educational practices, human-computer interaction, kinesthetic learning in virtual settings, etc. Finally, he is the Erasmus +, Farabi and Mevlana Programs coordinator of the CEIT department, and Vice Provost of the Trakya University Continuing Education Center.

Steven D. Waldman, M.D., J.D., serves as Associate Dean and Chair of the Department Medical Humanities and Bioethics at the University of Missouri-Kansas City School of Medicine. He holds joint academic appointments as Clinical Professor of Anesthesiology and Professor of Medical Humanities and Bioethics. The author of 35 textbooks and numerous academic articles on the specialty of interventional pain management, ultrasound, and medical education, Dr. Waldman also continues his clinical work as an interventional pain management physician as well as an active member of the medical staff at Truman Medical Center.

* * *

Cheryll Albold, PhD, is an Assistant Professor of Medical Education and she currently serves as the Designated Institutional Administrator for the Mayo Clinic School of Graduate Medical Education, one of five accredited schools in the Mayo Clinic College of Medicine and Science. In this role, she is partnered with the Dean and Designated Institutional Official (DIO) to provide administrative oversight for Sponsoring Institution and program accreditation activities governing 290 plus graduate medical education programs, enrolling physicians in training, located in Minnesota, Florida, and Arizona.

Joyce (Joy) Balls-Berry, Ph.D., is an Assistant Professor of Epidemiology and the Co-Director for the Mayo Clinic Center for Clinical and Translational Science Community Engagement Program. Her work as a scientist centers on increasing awareness of the importance of collaborative research in diverse communities. Dr. Balls-Berry is the principal investigator of a number of health disparities research studies and recently received a PCORI award. The focus of the PCORI award is to expand the efforts of the Minority Women in Research Network, which she established in 2011. The network's mission is to promote community and patient engagement in research conducted by minority women scientists and their stakeholders interested in research collaborations, academic scholarship, innovation, and dissemination. As an educator, Dr. Balls-Berry received the Mayo Clinic Teacher of Year and CCaTS Educator of the Year awards.

Raveena Basra, MD, is a first-year Internal Medicine resident at Olive View-UCLA Medical Center in Sylmar, California. She graduated from the UMKC School of Medicine in 2018.

Jordann Dhuse is a second year medical student at the University of Missouri Kansas City School of Medicine. She is a Curriculum Ambassador for the UMKC School of Medicine Council on Curriculum, an Admission Ambassador, a Color Officer, and a tutor. She is also an officer of the Emergency Medicine Interest Group and is interested in simulation education.

Charles Donohoe, M.D., is an Associate Professor and Chair in the Department of Neurology and Cognitive Neuroscience at the University of Missouri-Kansas City School of Medicine. He was born in New York City, attended medical school at the Albert Einstein College of Medicine in Bronx, New York graduating in 1972. He completed his internal medicine internship at Albert Einstein College of Medicine, and neurology residency at the Mount Sinai Hospital School of Medicine in New York City. He has practiced clinical neurology in Kansas City since 1977. He is board certified in Neurology by the American Board of Psychiatry and Neurology, in Neurorehabilitation by the American Society of Neurorehabilitation, and in Neuroimaging by the United Council for Neurologic Subspecialties. He holds professional memberships in the American Academy of Neurology, American Academy of Clinical Neurophysiology and the American Society of Neuroimaging. His interests include multiple sclerosis, neurorehabilitation, magnetic resonance imaging/ultrasound, pain management, and telemedicine. He has published numerous journal articles, book chapters and given many oral presentations at medical conferences. He is an associate clinical professor of medical education at the UMKC School of Medicine and has been an active member of the board of the Sirridge Office of Medical Humanities since its inception.

Stefanie R. Ellison, M.D. FACEP, is the Associate Dean for Learning Initiatives at the UMKC School of Medicine and a Professor of Emergency Medicine at Truman Medical Center. She graduated from TMC/UMKC Emergency Medicine residency program in June 2000 and joined the faculty at Truman Medical Center. She is board certified in Emergency Medicine and is a core faculty for the Emergency Medicine residency at Truman Medical Center. She served as the Associate Dean and Chair for the Council on Curriculum at the UMKC School of Medicine from 2000-2017 and was a member of the UMKC SOM Council on Curriculum for over ten years. She served as the Emergency Medicine Clerkship director from 2004-2015. She is an active member of the UMKC Interprofessional Education (IPE) Steering Committee and the Co-convener of the UMKC IPE Curriculum and Assessment Working Group since 2011. Her research interests include curriculum development, simulation in medical education, medical communication and interpersonal skills, and the sexual assault patient. She is currently focusing on Interprofessional Education and acute care recognition and management curriculum development in undergraduate medical education. She is also working to integrate competency-based teaching and assessment in undergraduate medical education, specifically in the areas of communication and interpersonal skills and professionalism. She has presented and published in IPE curriculum as well as for the EM clerkship and residency in the area of communication and interpersonal skills. She is also active in developing and implementing a curriculum in Interprofessional Education across the UMKC Health Science Programs and simulation in the EM clerkship curriculum.

James L. Fishback, MD, is a Chancellor's Club Distinguished Teaching Professor Emeritus of Pathology and Laboratory Medicine at the University of Kansas, School of Medicine, Kansas City, KS. He was instrumental in the implementation of KU's (former) technology-intensive, integrated undergraduate medical curriculum, which began in August of 2006. The curriculum utilizes the tablet PC and Microsoft OneNote® as the primary integrating platform, with Aperio® (now Leitz®)

microscope simulator for histopathology labs, video podcasts, and computerized testing facilities. The KU basic science program expanded to 3 geographically separate campuses in the summer of 2011, with high definition televideo lectures simultaneously transmitted to Wichita and Salina, KS. Dr. Fishback also served as Chief Flight Surgeon and Commander, 442nd Medical Squadron, with the rank of Colonel, in the United States Air Force Reserve, 442nd Fighter Wing, Whiteman AFB, MO. He was previously a flight surgeon with the 303rd Fighter Squadron, and is an Operation Iraqi Freedom veteran. He retired effective 7 Sept 2008, with more than 23 years of service. Specialties: Curriculum development, educational technology, infectious disease pathology, bioterrorism, clinical microbiology, autopsy pathology, graduate medical education, and continuing education.

Morgan E. Gonder, M.D., received her bachelor's of science from Sewanee: The University of the South and her medical degree from The University of Missouri- Kansas City. She is currently an anesthesiology resident at the University of Kansas. She looks forward to a future career as an anesthesia educator and provider.

Jane M. Grant-Kels is the Vice Chair of the Department of Dermatology, Director of the Cutaneous Oncology Center and Melanoma Programs, and Professor of Dermatology, Pathology, and Pediatrics at UConn Health. She was founding chair of the Department of Dermatology, founding director emeritus of the dermatology residency program, and founding director emeritus of the dermatopathology laboratory. Dr. Grant-Kels received her BA from Smith College and her medical degree from Cornell University Medical College. She trained in pediatrics and dermatology at the New York Hospital of Cornell Medical Center and completed a dermatopathology fellowship at NYU. Dr. Grant-Kels has a particular interest in melanoma, reflectance confocal microscopy, and the education of medical students, residents, and fellows.

Sean Gratton is an Assistant Professor of Neurology and Ophthalmology at the University of Missouri--Kansas City. He practices as a neurologist at Truman Medical Center, and as a Neuro-ophthalmologist at Sabates Eye Centers in Kansas City. He is the Neurology Residency Program Director at UMKC.

Lauren Haar, Ph.D., is a Research Associate in the Department of Pharmacology & Molecular Therapeutics at Loyola University Chicago. She has contributed to the development of medical education programming for communities underrepresented in health science professions and is currently serving as a Responsible Conduct of Research Program fellow at the Neiswanger Institute for Bioethics.

David John received both his B.A. and M.D. from the University of Missouri-Kansas City in 1977. After an internal medicine residency at the University of Hawaii and a rheumatology fellowship at the Rackham Arthritis Research Unit, University of Michigan, he was an Associate Clinical Professor at the University of Hawaii John A. Burns School of Medicine and he maintained a full private practice in Honolulu. Dr. John served at various times on the Boards of Waikiki Health Center, the Life Foundation (Chair, 2010-2011), Hawaii Medical Association Physicians' Health Committee (Pu'ulu Lapa'au), the latter as Chair from 2010 to 2017. Since April, 2017, Dr. John has been an Assistant Professor of Medicine at the University of Missouri-Kansas City School of Medicine. Dr. John has been involved in multiple organizations supportive of the arts and of youth at risk. One focus at this time is that of preserving humanism and the art of medicine in medical education and practice.

Deborah Kaercher received her B.A. in Philosophy and Political Science from the University of Missouri, Kansas City. Dr. Kaercher received her Doctorate of Philosophy from Edith Cowan University, Perth, AU. Her professional background is in public health and technology based start-ups. She was founding Vice-President and Executive Director of the Women and Family Health Information Network, establishing operations in 1997 with a coalition of over thirty community and non-profit members in the south Texas area. This Network was later adopted by the University of Texas Health Sciences Center in San Antonio in 2004. Her most recent publication was included in Feminist Popular Education in Transnational Debates: Building Pedagogies of Possibility. She has authored numerous articles on end-of-life for the Rivard Report in 2016 and 2017 and other media outlets. She is the playwright of Flannery's Stone, Leviathan, and co-writer of The Face of Time. She is currently working on a book of poetry and a work of fiction. The Acts Project is and arts, humanities and theatre based organization that supports programming around end of life. Her non-profit is dedicated to humanizing the end of life experience through the arts, humanities, theatre, education and resource development. Dr. Kaercher oversees a new initiative the non-profit launched in January, 2018; this endeavor is the capstone project for a team of five seniors at the McCombs School of Business at the University of Texas, Austin. The project team is building the technology infrastructure for a new national portal for The Final Acts Project: TAD-Resources (Transitions and Decisions: Resources for End of Life and Advance Care Planning. Dr. Kaercher also serves on the Patient Institute and The Women's Health Initiative at the UTHSCSA.

Simon Kaja, Ph.D., serves as the Dr. John P. and Therese E. Mulcahy Endowed Professor in Ophthalmology at Loyola University Chicago. Trained in Molecular Biology, Medicine and Neuroscience, Dr. Kaja's research interest lies in the pathophysiology of ophthalmic and neurodegenerative disorders. Dr. Kaja is an experienced medical educator and actively contributes to the creation of novel online learning environments and online curricula in the medical and graduate curriculum. In addition, he actively contributes to advancing the use of telemedicine in ophthalmology.

Robert M. Klein, PhD, is Vice Chancellor for Academic and Student Affairs and Chancellor's Club Professor of Anatomy & Cell Biology at the University of Kansas Medical Center (KUMC). He earned his Ph.D. from New York University and completed postdoctoral work at Marquette University. Dr. Klein has been a faculty member at KUMC since 1975 and earned the rank of professor in 1987. During Dr. Klein's academic career, he has been honored with an American Council on Education Fellowship and was Associate Dean for Professional Development and Faculty Affairs in the School of Medicine for 11 years. Dr. Klein has earned numerous teaching awards, including the Chancellor's Distinguished Teaching Award, the Bohan Teaching Professorship, The International Association of Medical Science Educators' Master Teacher Award, The Alpha Omega Alpha Robert J. Glaser AAMC Teaching Award, and was twice honored with the Kemper Teaching Excellence Award. He is an honorary member of the Alpha Omega Alpha Honor Medical Society, a Fellow of the American Association of Anatomists, and the 2010 Honorary KU Medical Alumnus. Dr. Klein was named a 2018 Icon of Education by Ingram's Magazine. His research career spans more than 30 years at KUMC where he has dedicated much of his career to mentoring of graduate and medical students, as well as junior faculty.

Michael J. Murphy is a professor of dermatology and dermatopathology, attending dermatopathologist, and director of the Immunopathology Laboratory within the Department of Dermatology at the UConn Health Center. He graduated from the medical school at University College Dublin, Ireland. Dr. Murphy completed his residency and chief residency in anatomic pathology at the Beth Israel Deaconess Medical Center, Harvard Medical School in Boston, MA, and his fellowship in dermatopathology at Albany Medical College, Albany, NY. Dr. Murphy has a particular interest in the role of molecular technologies in the diagnosis and management of skin disorders, and the education of medical students, residents, and fellows on this subject.

Imran Nizamuddin, BA, is a medical student at the University of Missouri-Kansas City in Kansas City, MO. He anticipates graduating in May 2019 and will go on to a residency program in Internal Medicine. He has an interest in community health and the use of medical applications on mobile devices to benefit patient care.

Nurry Pirani, MD, FACP, is the Associate Dean and Chair for the Council on Curriculum and an Assistant Professor of Internal Medicine at the University of Missouri - Kansas City School of Medicine. She graduated from the UMKC Internal Medicine residency program in 2011. She served as the Associate Program Director for the Internal Medicine residency from 2013-2017. She practices Internal Medicine at Truman Medical Center and serves as a Docent/Mentor at the UMKC School of Medicine.

Kristin M. Torre received her BS in Biology from Boston College in 2013. Currently, she is a third year medical student at the University of Connecticut and is pursuing dermatology. She worked at a dermatology practice in Boston before entering medical school and recently was a research fellow in the dermatology clinical trials department at UConn during her second year. She writes and presents on topics related to medical education, molecular technologies, and clinical dermatology.

Vivek Vallurupalli is a medical student at the University of Missouri-Kansas City in Kansas City, MO. He anticipates graduating in May 2019 and will go on to a residency program in Anesthesiology. He has an interest in utilization of medical applications and technological advances to facilitate patient care.

Sai Vanam, MD, is a first-year Internal Medicine resident at the University of California-San Diego. He graduated from the UMKC School of Medicine in 2018.

Index

www.ingramcontent.com/pod-product-compliance
Lightning Source LLC
LaVergne TN
LVHW061540290926
849162LV00004B/864